# Materials
# Management for
# Health Services

# Materials Management for Health Services

**Arnold Reisman**
Case Western Reserve
University

**LexingtonBooks**
D.C. Heath and Company
Lexington, Massachusetts
Toronto

**Library of Congress Cataloging in Publication Data**

Reisman, Arnold, 1934 (Aug. 2)-
    Materials management for health services.

    Includes bibliographical references and index.
    1. Health facilities—Materials management.
I. Title. [DNLM: 1. Equipment and supplies, Hospital. 2. Delivery of health
care—Organization and administration—United States. 3. Health services—
Organization and administration—United States.WX 147 R377m]
RA971.33.R44            362.1′068′7            79-3524
ISBN 0-669-03458-4

Published simultaneously in Canada

Printed in the United States of America

International Standard Book Number: 0-669-03458-4

Library of Congress Catalog Card Number: 79-3524

*To Maya, grandchild number one.*
*May she and her generation learn*
*to live at peace with the world.*
*May their world be peaceful.*

# Contents

| List of Figures | xi |
|---|---|
| List of Tables | xvii |
| Preface | xix |
| Acknowledgments | xxi |

**Chapter 1**     **Overview**                            1

| The Health-Services Materials-Management Environment | 1 |
|---|---|
| Importance of Materials Management in the Health Services | 5 |
| Materials Management and Other Institutional Functions | 6 |
| Basic Materials-Management-System Components | 8 |
| Importance of a Good Materials-Management System at the Institutional Level | 11 |
| Example of Documentation of an Existing Standard-Stock MMS in a Multifacility Health Center | 14 |
| Example of a Physical-Inventory Count and Analysis of Findings | 16 |
| Appendix 1A: Checklist for an Effective Materials-Management Department | 21 |

**Chapter 2**     **Managerial Infrastructure**          25

| Organizational Structures for Materials Management | 25 |
|---|---|
| Organizational Structures | 33 |
| Materials-Distribution Structures | 37 |
| Examples of MMS Alternatives for a Multifacility HMO | 42 |
| Management by Objectives | 47 |
| MMS Control Indexes | 52 |
| Systems and Procedures | 53 |
| Purchasing | 61 |

Purchasing-Department Ethics                                    81
Receiving and Central-Stores Activities                        83
Materials Storage                                               86
Charging and Billing                                            89
Appendix 2A: Checklist for an Effective Supply-
    Cart-Exchange System                                        93
Appendix 2B: Checklist for Evaluating a
    Materials-Management Infrastructure                         95
Appendix 2C: Checklist for Determining if an
    MBO Program Exists                                         103
Appendix 2D: Checklist for MMS Audits and
    Evaluations                                                109
Appendix 2E: Checklist and Audit Procedures
    for Vendor Competition                                     111
Appendix 2F: Checklist and Audit Procedures
    for Purchasing                                             117
Appendix 2G: Checklist and Audit Procedures
    for Receiving                                              145
Appendix 2H: Checklist and Audit Procedures
    for Distribution                                           149

Chapter 3    **Materials-Management Information Systems**      153

Information and Data                                           153
Planning an MMIS Project                                      154
Information Requested for Materials-
    Management Reports                                         158
MMIS Characteristics                                           163
Computers and MMIS                                            166
Computer-Selection Considerations                             178
Documentation of Systems and Procedures                      181
Appendix 3A: Checklists and Audit Procedures
    for Materials-Management Information
    Systems                                                   193

Chapter 4    **Decision Rules**                                209

Materials-Inventory Control: An Analogy                       209
Materials-Inventory Decision Guidelines                       212
Economic-Lot-Size-Equation Modifications and
    Aids to Computation                                       228
Worksheets for Various Economic-Lot-Size
    Equations                                                 230

# Contents

An Interactive Computer Program for Various
Economic-Lot-Size Equations                    236
The History of Inventory-Control Theory        238
Classification of Characteristics of Inventory-
Control Problems                               240
Measures of Materials Service Performance      242
Break-Even Analysis                            263
ABC Analysis                                   269
Make or Buy                                    271
Calculation of Inventory-Related Unit Costs    272
Setup or Ordering Costs                        273
Inventory Carrying Costs                       277
Shortage Costs                                 278
Substitutability, Urgency, and Costs           295
Standardization                                296
Reusables                                      297
Materials Distribution                         302
Appendix 4A: Checklists and Audit Procedures
for Decision Rules                             309
Appendix 4B: Checklists and Audit Procedures
for Standardization                            315
Appendix 4C: Checklists and Audit Procedures
for Processing, Handling, and Value
Analysis                                       319

**Chapter 5**    **Techniques for MMS Improvement and
Control Studies**                              327

Graphic Techniques for MMS Improvement and
Control Studies                                327
Simulation                                     360
Appendix 5A: Checklist for Evaluating MMS
Systems and Procedures                         365

**Chapter 6**    **Data Collection**                          367

Types of Data                                  367
Means for Data Acquisition                     368

**Selected
References**    **Purchasing and Materials Management**       381

**Appendix A**    **Glossary of Terms**                         389

**Appendix B**    **Recommended Materials-Processing Procedures
and Equipment**                                          469

**Index**                                                479

**About the Author**                                     489

# List of Figures

| 1-1 | Distribution of Hospital Expenses | 2 |
|---|---|---|
| 1-2 | Payroll as a Percentage of Total Hospital Costs | 3 |
| 1-3 | Major Functions of a Materiel-Management System | 7 |
| 1-4 | Material Flow | 9 |
| 1-5 | Components of a Materials-Management System | 10 |
| 1-6 | Materials and Information Flow of Standard-Stock Items | 16 |
| 2-1 | A Representative Materials-Management Organizational Chart | 27 |
| 2-2 | A Purchasing-Department Organization Chart | 28 |
| 2-3 | Areas of Responsibility—Supply and Distribution | 29 |
| 2-4 | Areas of Responsibility—Processing | 30 |
| 2-5 | Director of Purchasing: Job Description | 32 |
| 2-6 | Purchasing Buyer: Job Description | 33 |
| 2-7 | Hierarchical Organization | 34 |
| 2-8 | Matrix-Type Organization Structures | 35 |
| 2-9 | Distribution Alternatives | 38 |
| 2-10 | A General View of an Exchange-Cart System in Operation | 40 |
| 2-11 | Physical Components of an Exchange-Cart System | 41 |
| 2-12 | Data Collection and Use | 48 |
| 2-13 | Materials-Management Procedures | 49 |
| 2-14 | Charging System | 50 |
| 2-15 | Interaction of Purchasing with Other Organizational Units | 62 |
| 2-16 | Office-Supplies Requisition Form | 80 |
| 2-17 | Storage by Coordinate Index | 87 |
| 3-1 | Inventory-Control Setup/Change Form, A | 167 |

3-2     Inventory-Control Setup/Change Form, B                        169

3-3     Input Audit Register                                          170

3-4     Input Register                                                171

3-5     Purchase-Price-Variance Report, A                             173

3-6     Purchase-Price-Variance Report, B                             174

3-7     Inventory-Control Setup/Change Form, C                        176

3-8     Procedure Flow Chart for Ordering Office Equipment            177

3-9     Materials-Management System: Information Available
        and Desired                                                   182

3-10    A Multiechelon Materials-Management System                    183

3-11    Example of Procurement Procedures for Nonstandard-
        Stock Items                                                   184

3-12    Files of Nonstandard Stock                                    187

4-1     Inventory Concepts                                            209

4-2     Graphical Inventory Concepts                                  211

4-3     Effect of Extreme Inventory Policies on Inventory
        Level under Constant-Demand and Constant-Lead-
        Time Conditions                                               212

4-4     Cost of Review                                                213

4-5     Example of Materials-Management-System Lead
        Times                                                         215

4-6     Idealized Structure of Inventory Levels in Relation
        to Time                                                       217

4-7     The Relationship between Costs and Lot Sizes                  221

4-8     Graduated Quantity Discounts, Total Cost of Q Units           223

4-9     Cash Discounts, Total Cost of Q Units                         225

4-10    Graduated Quantity Discounts, Stocking Cost                   226

4-11    Cash Discounts, Stocking Cost                                 227

4-12    Computation Process for Finding Minimum EOQ in a
        Volume-Discount Environment                                   229

4-13    Basic EOQ Concept                                             230

| 4-14 | Worksheet for Case I: Calculation of Basic Economic Lot Size | 231 |
|---|---|---|
| 4-15 | EOQ with Shortages Permitted | 232 |
| 4-16 | Worksheet for Case II: Calculation of Economic Lot Size with Shortages Allowed | 233 |
| 4-17 | EOQ with Deliveries over a Period of Time | 234 |
| 4-18 | Worksheet for Case III: Calculation of Economic Lot Size with Production Spread over Time | 235 |
| 4-19 | EOQ with Shortages Permitted and Deliveries over a Period of Time | 236 |
| 4-20 | Worksheet for Case IV: Calculation of Economic Lot Size with Production Spread over Time and Shortages Allowed | 237 |
| 4-21 | Worksheet for Case V: Calculation of Lot Size and Number of Cycles | 239 |
| 4-22 | Worksheet for Case VI: Multiple Items with Space Constraint | 244 |
| 4-23 | Worksheet for Case VII: Multiple Items with Budgetary Constraint | 250 |
| 4-24 | Plot of Square Roots of $X$, 100-100,000 | 255 |
| 4-25 | Plot of Square Roots of $X$, 1,000,000-1,000,000,000 | 256 |
| 4-26 | Inventory Models | 258 |
| 4-27 | Sample Computer Solutions of the Various EOQ Cases | 260 |
| 4-28 | Break-Even Analysis | 264 |
| 4-29 | Break-Even Chart for Linear Systems | 265 |
| 4-30 | Net-Revenue Curves for Linear Systems | 266 |
| 4-31 | Graphical Solution of a Break-Even Problem | 267 |
| 4-32 | ABC Analysis | 270 |
| 4-33 | Worksheet for Ordering- and/or Setup-Cost Calculations | 274 |
| 4-34 | Worksheets for Inventory-Holding-Cost Parameter Calculations | 280 |

4-35    Worksheets for Holding-Cost Calculations                        286

4-36    Worksheet for Shortage-Cost Calculation                         288

4-37    An Example of Central-Processing-Department
        Material Flow                                                   300

4-38    Material Flow                                                   303

4-39    Materials-Distribution Subsystem                               304

4-40    Space Relationship-Material Support Services                   305

4-41    Transportation-Distribution Issues                             306

5-1     MMS Activities Involving People, Information, and/
        or Materials                                                   328

5-2     Operator Chart: Tasks Performed by a Hospital-
        Cafeteria Worker                                               331

5-3     Micromotion Analysis or Simo Chart for Opening a
        Corrugated Case                                                332

5-4     Man-Flow Process Chart for Pharmacy Clerk's Role
        in an Outpatient Clinic—Function: To Receive, Fill,
        and Deliver Prescriptions                                      334

5-5     Blood-Sample-Collection Flow-Process Chart                     335

5-6     Product-Flow Process Diagram for Hemostat Sterili-
        zation in Two Dimensions                                       336

5-7     Product-Flow Process Diagram for Hemostat Sterili-
        zation and Utilization in Three Dimensions                     338

5-8     Procedure Flow Chart for Ordering Office Equipment             339

5-9     Operation Process Chart of Intravenous-Solution
        Prescription                                                   340

5-10    Assembly Chart of a Medical Record after Patient
        Discharge                                                      341

5-11    Summary of Flow-Chart Symbols                                  342

5-12    Example of a Tight and an Open Layout of a System
        Chart for the Same System                                      345

5-13    Task Delegation                                                346

5-14    Computer-Service Selection-Decision Table                      347

| 5-15 | Incidence Matrix | 348 |
|---|---|---|
| 5-16 | Precedence Diagram | 349 |
| 5-17 | Precedence Matrix | 350 |
| 5-18 | Bill of Materials for IV Solutions | 351 |
| 5-19 | Explosion Chart | 352 |
| 5-20 | Input-Output Matrix | 353 |
| 5-21 | Gantt Milestone Chart | 355 |
| 5-22 | Gantt Chart with Rectangles Removed and Replaced with Arrows | 356 |
| 5-23 | Gantt Chart Partially Transferred to a PERT Network | 356 |
| 5-24 | Complete Transformation of Gantt Chart to a PERT Network | 357 |
| 5-25 | PERT Network: Earliest Expected and Latest Allowable Times, $T_E$ and $T_L$, Respectively | 358 |
| 5-26 | Operations-Function-Flow Schematic | 359 |
| 6-1 | ABC Usage-Analysis Curve | 374 |

# List of Tables

**1-1**   Total Estimated Expenditures for Hospital Supplies, 1970-1978   4

**1-2**   Distribution of Total Annual Regional Purchase Value and Number of Line Items, by Family   15

**1-3**   Distribution of the Regional On-Hand Inventory of Standard-Stock Sutures   17

**1-4**   Distribution of the Regional On-Hand Inventory of Standard-Stock Syringes   18

**1-5**   Total Dollar Value of Nonstandard Sutures on Hand in Each Facility   19

**2-1**   Advantages and Disadvantages of Centralization   43

**2-2**   Advantages and Disadvantages of Decentralization   44

**2-3**   Suggested Base-Statistic Parameters for Clinical Departments   54

**2-4**   Study by a Task Force of Hospital Financial Management Association on Shur Statistics   55

**3-1**   Issue-Unit Designation   178

**4-1**   A Taxonomic Scheme for Classification of Inventory-Control Systems   243

**4-2**   Example of a Break-Even Numerical Solution   268

**4-3**   Sampling Strata and Numbers of Line Items   271

**4-4**   Item Substitution   292

**5-1**   Classification, Information Displayed, and Use of Tools for Systems Description and Analysis   329

**5-2**   Standard Definitions for Terms Used in Charting Information Processes   343

**6-1**   Distribution of the Detailed Sampling-Plan Purchase Values of Items   375

# Preface

Health-care-delivery services make up the third largest sector of the U.S. economy. This sector is fast approaching 10 percent of the gross national product; translated into dollars, this means an "industry" with over $200 billion in annual expenditures. Although 50 to 60 percent of these expenditures are personnel-related, materials-related expenditures are nevertheless significant and are steadily rising in percentage terms.

Purchasers of health services, such as employers, labor unions, the government, and the public, are increasingly calling for the containment of health-care-related costs. Effective management of materials is one area where costs can be contained without sacrificing the quality or the accessibility of health care.

Effective management of materials addresses the apparently conflicting objectives of minimizing materials-related costs while simultaneously reducing the incidence of stockouts. Indeed, it is possible to make intelligent tradeoffs between materials-related costs and the desired levels of materials accessibility. Moreover, not all materials in any one institution require the same degree of accessibility. It is wasteful and not necessarily desirable to take the position that stockouts must *never* occur for *all* items at *all* stocking locations.

A materials-management system must be capable of addressing, speedily and economically, the informational issues of who *has* what, where, and when. Moreover, such a system must provide prescriptions for who *ought* to have what, where, and when. Finally, the system should be kept in *control*. This requires a management infrastructure with clear-cut lines of responsibility and authority for maintaining the proper stocks in the proper locations at the proper time.

This book provides an integrated approach to the many issues of concern in the proper management of materials. An extensive glossary of terms used by materials managers, buyers, producers, sellers, shippers, data processors, and so on is provided as an aid in this integrative process. Each major chapter is followed by appendixes in the form of checklists, with questions relevant to the issues discussed; these, in turn, are often followed by detailed audit procedures that might be invoked or at least considered in maintaining a well-functioning materials-management system. The various economic-lot-size, cost-parameter evaluations, and other decision rules usually expressed in mathematical equations have been reduced to easy-to-follow worksheets requiring no more than the simplest arithmetic operations of addition, substraction, multiplication, and division.

Current and prospective workers in the health-care services who are concerned with proper purchasing, storing, distribution, stocking, and replenishing of consumables, reusables, and disposables should find this a basic and readable text.

# Acknowledgments

I am indebted to a number of individuals who were instrumental in bringing this book from the idea stage to manuscript completion. Thanks are due to Allen H. Aardsma, Director of the Materials Management Resource Center, American Hospital Association; Don G. Soth, Director, Corporate Communications, American Sterilizer Company; Paul Widman, Director of Operations, and Thomas Tisdale, Director of Inventory Control, the Cleveland Clinic Foundation; Paul Buchsbaum, Associate Vice President, Operations, Cleveland Metropolitan General Hospital; Carl Apfelbach, Marketing Project Manager, Scientific Products, American Hospital Supply Company, for their suggestions and generosity in sharing invaluable resource materials. The manuscript was greatly enhanced through the editorial suggestions made by Richard Buxbaum, Vice President, Institutional Services, Greater Cleveland Hospital Association; Philip Salmonowitz, Director, Materials Management, Marymount Hospital of Cleveland; and Richard Osborne, Director of the Center for Management Development, Case Western Reserve University. All of the MBA students in the fall 1979 operations management course at CWRU have contributed to the glossary of terms and to the checklist and detailed-audit-procedures sections. Of these, Jim Moy, Joel C. Sluga, and Janice M. Caster deserve special mention for a job well done. Thanks also go to Mr. Shravan Kotha and Dr. Shahriar Javad for contributing to the chapter on decision rules and to Emanuel Escueta for helping to proofread the manuscript. Jane Cerny and Linda Hossner deserve thanks for diligently typing the various manuscript drafts.

The development of this book was partially funded by a grant from the Cleveland Foundation; for this I am most grateful.

# 1 Overview

## The Health-Services Materials-Management Environment

Health providers—physicians, nurses, physical therapists, laboratory technicians, and so on—are *consumers* of materials. They consume what might be termed *consumables*, *reusables*, and *disposables*. They are generally quite *intolerent* of shortages or stockouts, but normally they are not fully *sensitive* to costs. Health-service *administrators*, on the other hand, are called on to satisfy both the *needs* of the providers and the pressures for *cost containment*.

It would be easy to minimize stockouts or shortages simply by overstocking all materials at *user* locations, as well as at all *backup* locations. But to maintain an optimum balance between the competing objectives of minimizing costs and maximizing *service levels* (nonstockout transactions) is not a trivial problem. It requires knowledge of historical and current usage rates, as well as projections of future rates. Moreover, it requires knowledge of unit purchasing (including price breaks), inventory stocking or holding, and reordering costs, as well as of the costs of shortages in cases where a more costly item is substituted for a stocked-out one; when its resupply is expedited; where a sale is lost; and, worst of all, where a service is deferred or not provided. Finally, it requires current knowledge and projections of replenishment lead times.

Clearly, the desired or demanded service levels must be established. Optimizing between costs and service levels requires a knowledge of certain analytical techniques in order to develop decision rules for replenishment policies. In addition, it requires an appreciation of simulation techniques to validate and/or pretest such decision rules. Finally, a management infrastructure to maintain and keep all systems in control is essential.

According to [1] and as shown in figure 1-1, 27 percent of a typical hospital annual budget was spent on materiel purchases, including materials such as consumables, reusables and disposables, as well as some of the more durable equipment and instrumentation. W.K. Henning [2], in a recent survey, claims that 42 cents of every budget dollar was spent on the *materials* component of *materiel* management. Moreover, out of the 60 percent of the budget in the "labor" category, 19 percent can be allocated to materials-management functions by both service-function administrators and patient-care staffs. Thus 46 cents of every dollar spent by a typical

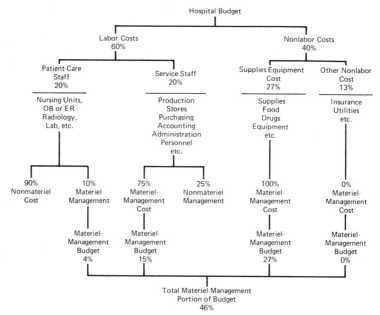

Source: AMSCO Fact Summary, SC-2533, March 1977, Exhibit 3. p. 2, © AMSCO Systems. Reprinted with permission.

**Figure 1-1.** Distribution of Hospital Expenses

hospital in 1977 was attributable to materiel procurement and management functions [2]. If one adds the costs of monies *tied up* in materials inventories, this figure may rise even higher. According to the 1978 edition of *Hospital Statistics*, published by the American Hospital Association, the combined budgets of hospitals reported on during the same year, 1977, exceeded $63 billion. Using these figures, the expenditure for materiel-related activities in the hospital industry during that year was in the neighborhood of $30 billion. Since 1977 hospital expenditures have risen at a higher rate than any other economic indicator. Moreover, since 1960 nonpayroll expenditures have been increasing in percentage terms vis-à-vis payroll expenditures [3, 4, 5]. See figure 1-2.

Focusing on materials-related expenditures exclusive of durables, table 1-1 shows that during 1978 American hospitals spent $16.5 billion on the following item categories: drugs and pharmacy supplies, equipment (noncapital), food and dietary supplies, housekeeping supplies and linen, laboratory supplies, maintenance supplies, medical and surgical supplies, office supplies and stationery, radiology supplies, and sterile supplies.

These figures indicate that expenditures for hospital supplies increased steadily throughout the 1970s, with a temporary lull in 1974. The rate of increase rose significantly through the early 1970s, until the price controls of the Economic Stabilization Program (ESP) had their full effect in 1974. Ac-

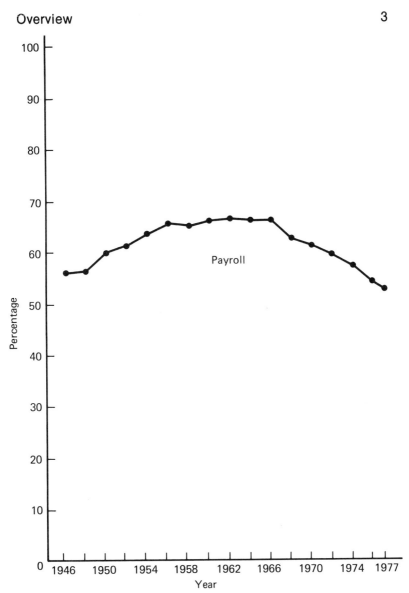

The author is indebted to Dr. S. Javad for the use of this diagram.

**Figure 1-2.** Payroll as a Percentage of Total Hospital Costs

cording to Allen H. Aardsma, director of the Materials Management Resource Center of the American Hospital Association (Personal Communication), prior to the mid-1970s price increases accounted for roughly one-third of the increase in supplies expenditures, with increased demand and utilization accounting for the remaining two-thirds. Following ESP, prices jumped considerably. However, after 1975 the rate of increase for supplies expenditures actually declined significantly. Effective purchasing

**Table 1-1**
**Total Estimated Expenditures for Hospital Supplies, 1970-1978**

| Year | Billions of Dollars | Percentage Increase over Preceding Year | Percentage of Total Hospital Expenditures |
|------|---------------------|-----------------------------------------|-------------------------------------------|
| 1970 | 4.8 | — | 18.8 |
| 1971 | 5.5 | 14.6 | 19.1 |
| 1972 | 6.8 | 23.6 | 20.8 |
| 1973 | 8.6 | 26.5 | 23.7 |
| 1974 | 8.8 | 2.3 | 21.2 |
| 1975 | 10.8 | 22.7 | 22.2 |
| 1976 | 12.7 | 17.6 | 22.7 |
| 1977 | 14.8 | 16.5 | 23.3 |
| 1978 | 16.5 | 11.5 | 23.3 |

Source: Allen H. Aardsma, personal communication.

practices and cost-containment methods have controlled the increase in demand and utilization. In fact, according to Aardsma, since 1975 price increases—and therefore inflation—have accounted for somewhat more than half the increases in supplies expenditures.

As previously indicated, total supplies expenditures expressed as a percentage of total hospital expenditures demonstrated steady increases in the early 1970s. Following significant movement in 1973 and 1974 as a result of ESP, supplies expenditures continued to account for a larger percentage of total hospital expenditures, apparently reaching a plateau in 1977.

Returning to the figures of table 1-1, if annual hospital purchases of supplies are indeed $16.5 billion dollars, and if it is conservatively assumed that on the average hospital inventories turn over ten times a year, then the *maximum* dollar value of supplies inventory was $1.65 billion, and the average inventory on hand was conservatively half of that or $0.825 billion during 1978. If the cost of borrowed money during 1978 is taken as 10 percent then American hospitals spent 82.5 million on monies tied up in supplies inventory. However, the cost of capital is not the only cost associated with managing (as opposed to owning) inventory. Allen Aardsma suggests that *obsolescence* amounts to 7 to 9 percent storage costs account for 5 to 6 percent; *paperwork* and/or administrative costs account for 3 percent; and *pilferage and loss* add another 2 to 3 percent—for an additional total of 17-18 percent of the value of the average inventory. These factors, therefore, add another $140.25 million to the costs of inventory management, for a conservative total of 222.75 million. Enlightened materials-management practices could have easily reduced the average inventories held in hospitals by at least 10 to 20 percent, thus saving the patients and/or third-party payers $22.27 million to $44.55 million without adversely affecting the quality or accessibility of health care. This is a conservative estimate for 1978.

## Importance of Materials Management in the Health Services

Financial sections of newspapers often carry references to the status of inventories in the industrial and retailing sectors. The following types of commentaries abound: "A cleanup of the heavy carryover of this year's inventory of cars, and brisk early sales of next year's models, would lead to a high automobile production and would stimulate a comfortable rise in the output of steel, copper, glass, tires, textiles, and other material."

The values of inventories in industry are watched carefully by investors and are regarded as bellwethers of industry. Raw-material-inventory buildups indicate optimism regarding future sales of a product. Permitting inventories to become depleted indicates pessimism within a particular industry.

Inventory is of such great consequence to the industrial manufacturer and the retailer that it shows up in the most important financial reports, the balance sheet and the profit-and-loss statements. Yet many hospital and clinical administrators do not know and, with the systems and procedures in place in their institutions, have no way of finding out the dollar value of total inventories carried at any one time. Even more disconcerting in these days of cost-containment pressures is the fact that some top-level hospital administrators do not know their annual expenditures on materials.

Because materials are stocked in both *formal* and *informal* stocking locations, the physical inventory at the central stores or central supply rooms is often merely the tip of an iceberg. The *informal* or unknown inventory may often *exceed* the inventory of the central stores or central supply rooms by a factor of three or more.

In at least two otherwise well-managed institutions, a physical count of certain consumables such as sutures or syringes uncovered a stockpile throughout the institution equivalent to three or more *years' supply*. Such inventory *noncontrol* is difficult to rationalize in relation to a typical delivery lead time of a week or two for such items.

The American Hospital Association on 27-28 September 1978 recognized the importance of materials management systems in hospitals by having it's council on management approve the following set of principles.

Hospitals are encouraged to develop a systematic, cost-effective approach to managing and controlling both supplies and equipment by utilizing a materials-management system of coordinating materials acquisition, storage, processing, and distribution.

Since hospitals are facing a changing environment that includes greater external-agency involvement and public accountability as well as increasing requirements to operate with limited resources, each functional unit within the hospital must be managed in the most effective and efficient manner possible.

This is especially important for those functions related to supplies and equipment: materials acquisition, storage, processing, and distribution. External regulatory agencies are setting standards that are affecting materials-related functions, which in turn may affect a hospital's reimbursement or accreditation. The hospital administration needs to be assured that each of these functions is within compliance limits.

Expenditures for supplies and equipment account for an increasingly larger portion of each hospital operating dollar; this fact, combined with inflationary pressures and the need to operate with limited resources, requires that every materials-related function operate with increased efficiency and improved productivity, consistent with quality patient care.

Since these materials-related functions are interdependent, decisions made regarding one function may have a significant effect on the other functions. Therefore, these functions must be coordinated to complement each other and to more effectively contribute to the hospital's overall goals and objectives.

If the hospital utilizes a materials-management system of coordinating materials acquisition, storage, processing, and distribution, the hospital's administration can systematically assign the responsibility and accountability for the management and control of supplies and equipment from their inception of need through their ultimate disposal.

These principles were approved by the Board of Directors of the American Society for Hospital Purchasing and Materials Management on 21 February 1971.

## Materials Management and Other Institutional Functions

E.S. Buffa [6] likens the information system of an organization to the nervous system of the human body. He builds on that analogy by saying that "perhaps the inventory represents the lifeblood." Although his book is intended primarily for the manufacturing or industrial sector, both analogies pertain to the health-care-institutional setting. Without the proper materials at the right time, in the right quantities, and at the right place, few procedures can be performed at effective levels.

Figure 1-3 depicts the interrelationship between the *traditional* materials-management functions—warehousing, storing, distribution, inventory control, purchasing, and receiving and inspection—the health-provider and/or health-service operation; the inventory data base; and the financial-policy functions within an institution. The interrelationships are graphically depicted through the information-flow, materials-flow, order-flow, and cash-flow channels. It can be seen that materials flow from vendors through the receiving and inspection activities, into the warehousing,

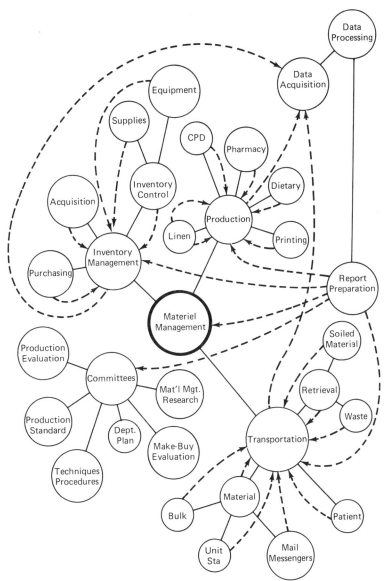

**Figure 1-3.** Major Functions of a Materiel-Management System

storing, and distribution functions within the institution, to the provider and service operation. On the other hand, replenishment orders originate somewhere in the provider and service operations and are transmitted through inventory control to purchasing, resulting in orders being placed with vendors. All the functions within an institution interact with one another through information-flow channels. Thus, the purchasing department transmits relevant information on availability, lead time, quality, and so on, from vendors to inventory control. Inventory control obtains information regarding stock status either directly from the warehousing and storing functions or through the inventory data base. Similarly, it obtains usage information directly from the provider and service operations or through the inventory data base. Inventory control also obtains information regarding the institutional financial policies current at the time, specifically regarding its cost of capital. It then combines all this information in its requisitioning or replenishment orders, which are placed with vendors through purchasing.

Following the lead of American industry, health-provider institutions are increasingly recognizing the need for an integrated approach to the management of materials. The International Material Management Society defines hospital-materials management as "an organizational concept that provides a centralized supply system from procurement through movement and distribution, to point-of-use, and to the reprocessing or final breakdown into the environment, resulting in maximum patient care and cost containment" [7].

Figure 1-4 shows the physical flow of materials (solid lines) in a typical health-care institution, after they have reached the institution. The information-flow channels are indicated by dashed lines. Each of the functional units, such as receiving, stores, and consumer departments, transmits timely transactions data to the data-processing department (this does not necessarily imply the use of electronic data processing). In turn, they receive timely and relevant reports on status, usage, and so on. These reports are used for maintaining and controlling stocks at proper levels in each of the various stocking locations. This is accomplished by preestablished replenishment policies, such as the min-max, the reorder-point economic ordering quantity, and other decision-making guidelines or *decision rules*. Clearly, the parameters of any given decision rule must be constantly reviewed and updated if necessary. Among these reviewables are the various inventory-related unit costs, such as unit carrying, reorder, and set-up costs; delivery lead times; and forecasts of usage. A good materials-management information system, regardless of its degree of computerization, is indispensible to a well-run materials-management system.

**Basic Materials-Management-System Components**

As indicated in figure 1-5, a total materials-management system (MMS) integrates three basic ideas: a *management infrastructure*, a materials-management *information system* (MMIS), and a set of *decision rules* for all

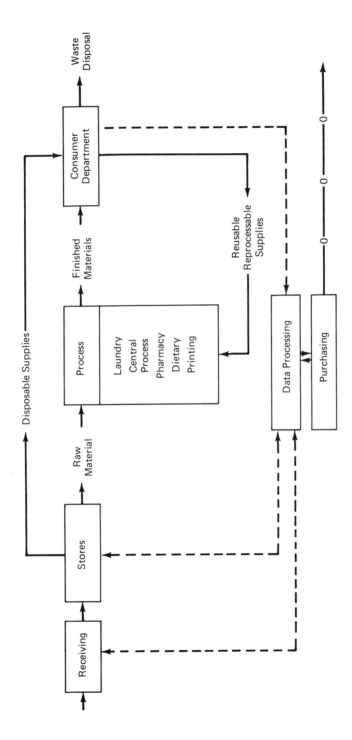

The author is indebted to Don Soth of the American Sterilizer Company for the use of this diagram.

**Figure 1-4. Material Flow**

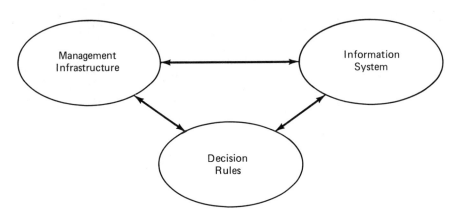

**Figure 1-5.** Components of a Materials-Management System

repetitive decisions (for example, replenishment of stocks). These three components of a materials-management system clearly must permeate the organization both vertically and horizontally. Specifically, it is not sufficient to have a well-managed and well-informed purchasing or central-storeroom operation. Materials management must reach into each and every stocking location throughout the institution. For example, in a multifacility regional health center, the materials-management system must be operative at the regional, the facility, the departmental, and in some cases the module or doctor's office levels.

More specifically, a good materials-management system requires:

> *Management infrastructure*: An infrastructure that maintains and enforces the materials management system including clear-cut
>> Authority for ordering items
>> Responsibility for ordering items
>> Knowledge of decision rules
>> Accountability for ordering items
>
> *Information System*: A system that provides concise, timely, and current information:
>> On materials status
>>> Who has
>>>> What
>>>> When
>>>> Where
>>>> How much

On materials-related transactions
   Who ordered
      What
      When
      Where
      In what quantities
   Who received
      What
      When
      Where
      In what quantities
   What has been the usage
      In units
      In dollars
*Decision rules*: Rules governing the optimal management (replenishment) of materials:
   Who *ought* to have
      What
      Where
      When
      How much

As will be shown in chapter 4, the decision rules should strike an optimum balance between the various inventory-related costs for any given rate of stockouts deemed permissible by management. Clearly, some items must never be out of stock in some locations.

## Importance of a Good Materials-Management System at the Institutional Level

Before expanding on the subject of inventories, we should emphasize the importance of good control over the materials used in a health-care institution. This will be done from three different perspectives or points of view.

### The Ultimate User's Perspective

The health provider:

   Desires to have the proper materials in the proper hygienic condition, at the proper place, at the proper time.

Desires to minimize delays in obtaining the right materials as and when needed.

Desires to minimize travel time and distance in obtaining materials when needed.

Desires to minimize or reduce to zero the time and effort spent in replenishing materials, keeping records, and filling out forms.

The patient:

Desires to have his or her needs satisfied with speed and economy and at a satisfactory level of quality. Often issues of economy are of more concern to the third-party payers than to the patient.

Depends on the reliability of the materials being used in his or her behalf.

*The Facility Administrator's Perspective*

The administrator endeavors to:

Maximize the availability and accessibility of materials.

Minimize costs of:
    Holding inventory.
    Reordering.
    Handling.
    Distribution.
    Setup/manufacture.
    Deterioration, spoilage, shrinkage, theft.

Minimize space usage
    In central processing departments and/or supply rooms.
    In provider departments.
    In provider modules.

Minimize incidence of materials-related crisis intervention:
    Stockouts of critical items.
    Wrong materials
        Function.
        Quality.
        Size.
        Shape.

Maximize goodwill of the health providers—the ultimate users:
>   Doctors.
>   Nurses.
>   Therapists.

Maximize goodwill of the patients.


*The Senior Manager's Perspective*

Top administration:

>   Desires to maximize accessibility and availability of materials to all legitimate users.

>   Desires to minimize total material-related costs.
>>   Material:
>>>   Cost of capital tied up in materials.
>>>   Cost of spoilage and/or shrinkage.
>>>   Cost of improper usage, such as substitution of costlier items.
>>>   Cost of storage space.
>>>   Cost of material shipping.
>>>   Cost of insurance and/or taxes.
>>   Personnel:
>>>   Wages and benefits to personnel handling materials and/or materials-related information on a full- or part-time basis.
>>   Information:
>>>   Cost of data:
>>>>   Collection.
>>>>   Transmission.
>>>>   Porcessing.
>>>>   Storage.
>>>   Cost of reports:
>>>>   Generation.
>>>>   Distribution.


   In summary, this book is concerned with the management of materials, namely, the *management of disposables, consumables, and reusables* in order to satisfy the needs of the ultimate materials user as well as the needs and constraints at the various levels of administration. Examples of actual materials-management problems encountered in health-care institutions are used throughout this book for illustrative purposes. Two such examples are described in the following paragraphs.

**Example of Documentation of an Existing Standard-Stock MMS
in a Multifacility Health Center**

Prior to launching a redesign of an MMS, it is often a good idea to document what exists. This is called a *system description* and is analogous to a physician's workup of a new patient prior to prescribing a treatment for patient-perceived symptoms. Such a description was in fact done by the author in one regional health center for its standard-stock items. The results are discussed in this section.

The study identified eighteen general groups of standard-stock items comprising approximately 1,700 line items and constituting $1 million in annual purchases. The number of line items in a family ranged from 22 (bulbs) to 292 (forms). The dollar value of annual regional purchases ranged from $1,527.61 (parts) to $164,575.35 (drugs and pharmaceuticals).

Table 1-2 exhibits the eighteen general groups of standard-stock items with their annual regional purchase amounts, number of line items, and other relevant information. Comparison of the third and fifth columns of the table reveals two family types: (1) expensive families—those with a much higher percentage of total annual purchases than the percentage of total number of items in the inventory, for examples, disposable linen and operating-room packs, housekeeping and maintenance, intravenous (IV) supplies, laboratory and radiology supplies; (2) nonstandardized or inexpensive families—those with a much higher percentage of total number of items in the inventory than the percentage of total annual regional purchases, for example, forms and office supplies. These latter families are prime candidates for any standardization program.

Figure 1-6 displays the materials and information flow of the standard-stock items. Some of the use locations requisition their needed items from the central stock room (CSR); others request them from the warehouse; and still others place their orders to the vendors directly. The warehouse-distribution staff uses three trucks, the main function of which is to carry mail and medical charts and to distribute materials from the central warehouse to facilities. Warehouse-purchase quantities were generated using an inventory computer package, but computer decisions were overridden 25 to 30 percent of the time by the chief purchasing agent and three of his associates in consideration of projected increases in item costs, freight charges, or lack of space at the central warehouse. Transshipment of items among the facility CSRs did occur occasionally, on a lending basis, mainly during off-hours or weekends. The receiving of items at facilities with a CSR was accomplished by a receiving clerk, whereas at the facilities without a CSR the item was simply left in a hallway. This caused an interruption in the flow of information, among many other significant control problems. At the department and/or module levels, nursing personnel performed the

**Table 1-2**
**Distribution of Total Annual Regional Purchase Value and Number of Line Items by Family**

| Family | Annual Regional Purchase | Percentage of Total Annual Regional Purchase Value | Number of Items | Percentage of Total Number of Items in Inventory |
|---|---|---|---|---|
| Anesthesia and hypodermic supplies | $ 31,557.55 | 2.95 | 54 | 3.27 |
| Bulb | 6,110.19 | .57 | 22 | 1.33 |
| Catheters | 17,670.03 | 1.65 | 25 | 1.52 |
| Dietary | 39,907.60 | 3.73 | 40 | 2.42 |
| Disposable linen and operating-room packs | 133,018.24 | 12.42 | 48 | 2.91 |
| Drugs and pharmaceuticals | 164,575.35 | 15.37 | 243 | 14.73 |
| Pharmaceutical supplies | 10,754.35 | 1.00 | 21 | 1.27 |
| Forms | 62,263.73 | 5.81 | 292 | 17.70 |
| Housekeeping and maintenance | 39,537.41 | 3.69 | 28 | 1.70 |
| IV supplies | 61,478.51 | 5.74 | 52 | 3.15 |
| Laboratory supplies | 109,717.38 | 10.24 | 92 | 5.58 |
| Medical/surgical | 118,868.51 | 11.10 | 142 | 8.61 |
| Office supplies | 33,480.86 | 3.13 | 217 | 13.15 |
| Parts | 1,527.61 | .14 | 88 | 5.33 |
| Patient care | 7,127.14 | .67 | 15 | .91 |
| Radiology | 120,258.15 | 11.23 | 41 | 2.48 |
| Surgical dressing and material | 86,917.93 | 8.12 | 163 | 9.88 |
| Sutures | 26,202.27 | 2.44 | 67 | 4.06 |
| Total in the region | $1,070,972.81 | | 1,650 | |

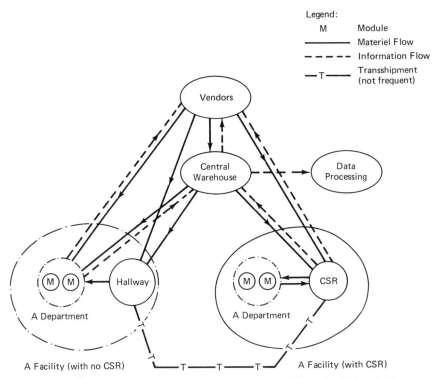

**Figure 1-6.** Materials and Information Flow of Standard-Stock Items

functions of ordering, receiving, and storing of materials. The original shipping slip was taken back to the warehouse by the truck driver, who was also the delivery clerk, and was then sent to data processing. Clearly, the procedures for dealing with emergent situations were radically different from those described here and even less suited for accountability.

This kind of documentation is necessary in order to identify and define problem areas. It is the first phase of problem solving.

**Example of a Physical-Inventory Count and Analysis of Findings**

A physical count of two categories of materials was made in order to establish the potential payoff of system redesign during the course of a materials-management study in a health center providing primary and acute care. The two categories of materials involved sutures and syringes, including insulin but excluding "bulb catheter tip" types.

In the standard-stock-syringe category there were 15 line items. Standard-stock sutures numbered 64 line items. The line-item count of nonstandard-stock sutures was 242. Most of these were in operating rooms and in labor and delivery rooms. There were no nonstandard-stock syringes. The pysical-inventory count was performed at all use locations, at the pharmacies, and at the central warehouse. It was executed in a short time span—half of one day—so as to avoid any double-counting of materials in transit from one facility to another or from the central warehouse to facilities.

The data of the physical-inventory count were analyzed using a computer program that sorted the items into syringe and suture categories, as well as by total on-hand dollar value and total number of units on hand. It reported the on-hand dollar values and on-hand number of units for each item by department, by facility, in the central warehouse, and in the whole region.

Table 1-3 summarizes the result of the physical-inventory count of standard-stock sutures on hand in the region. The calculations are based on the number of item units. It can be seen that approximately 90 percent of

**Table 1-3**
**Distribution of the Regional On-Hand Inventory of Standard-Stock Sutures**

| Number of Lead Times of Regional On-Hand Inventory | Number of Line Items | Relative Frequency | Cumulative Relative Frequency |
|---|---|---|---|
| 1-<3 | 6 | 10.53 | 10.53 |
| 3-<5 | 5 | 8.77 | 19.30 |
| 5-<7 | 7 | 12.29 | 31.59 |
| 7-<9 | 10 | 17.55 | 49.14 |
| 9-<11 | 9 | 15.80 | 64.94 |
| 11-<13 | 5 | 8.77 | 73.71 |
| 13-<15 | 3 | 5.26 | 78.97 |
| 15-<17 | 3 | 5.26 | 84.23 |
| 17-<19 | 1 | 1.75 | 85.98 |
| 19-<21 | 0 | 0.00 | 85.98 |
| 21-<23 | 3 | 5.26 | 91.24 |
| 23-<25 | 1 | 1.75 | 92.98 |
| 25-<27 | 2 | 3.51 | 96.50 |
| 27-<29 | 1 | 1.75 | 98.25 |
| 29-<32 | 1 | 1.75 | 100.00 |
| Total | 57 | 100.00 | |

Notes: (1) Vendor lead time for all the line items of the suture category is less than five weeks. (2) Only the sutures, for which the annual regional units purchased have been available, are reported here.

the line items had more than three lead times' supply on hand and in inventory in the region. It was disconcerting to find that for more than 50 percent of the items there were on-hand inventories of more than nine lead times' usage (forty-five weeks). No special needs could be identified to justify such oversupply. Finally, line items with on-hand inventories of more than two years' supply in the region were not uncommon.

Table 1-4 shows the outcome of the physical-inventory count for standard-stock syringes. Note that data in this part are even more interesting. All the line items have on-hand inventories in the region of more than two lead times. Twenty percent of the line items have on-hand inventories exceeding thirty-five lead times (105 weeks); one item has more than three and one-half years of annual regional usage on hand.

It should be added that most of these on-hand inventories were spread across departments in each facility rather than in the CSR or the central warehouse, supposedly the logistic support systems for all use locations. These excessive inventories occupy expensive storage areas within the use locations, departments, CSRs, and central warehouse, thus limiting the availability of stocking areas for other times. Even though this much on-hand inventory existed at the various locations in the institution, *stockouts* at use locations did occur. Hence, high inventory levels do not necessarily eliminate stockout problems.

For the *nonstandard* sutures only the total dollar value of on-hand inventory in each facility was reported (see table 1-5). Note that in the calculations for the region, the on-hand inventory at facility I ($78.07) is not

**Table 1-4**
**Distribution of the Regional On-Hand Inventory of Standard-Stock Syringes**

| Number of Lead Times of Regional On-Hand Inventory | Number of Line Items | Relative Frequency | Cumulative Relative Frequency |
|---|---|---|---|
| 2-<4 | 2 | 13.33 | 13.33 |
| 4-<6 | 5 | 33.34 | 46.67 |
| 6-<8 | 2 | 13.33 | 60.00 |
| 8-<10 | 3 | 20.00 | 80.00 |
| 10-<35 | 0 | 00.00 | 80.00 |
| 35-<42 | 2 | 13.33 | 93.33 |
| 42-<60 | 0 | 00.00 | 93.33 |
| 60-<62 | 1 | 6.67 | 100.00 |
| Total | 15 | 100.00 | |

Note: Vendor lead time for all the syringes is less than three weeks.

**Table 1-5**
**Total Dollar Value of Nonstandard Sutures on Hand in Each Facility**

| | Total for Nonstandard Sutures | | |
| Facility | Total On-Hand Inventory (1) | Total Annual Purchases (2) | Months of Supply On-Hand [(1)/(2)] × 12 |
|---|---|---|---|
| I | $    78.07 | — | — |
| II | 834.67 | $ 1,464.88 | 6.84 |
| III | 22,641.24 | 11,720.07 | 23.18 |
| IV | 9,493.87 | 16,599.79 | 6.86 |
| Total for the region | $32,969.78 | $29,784.74 | 13.28 |

added to those of the others because the annual purchases of the facility were not available. The region has more than thirteen months' annual regional supply of nonstandard-stock sutures on hand. Facility III leads the way by stocking close to two years' supply.

Based on the results of the physical-inventory count, some of the sutures that were one to four years old were returned to vendors for a total credit of approximately $14,000—a one-shot 23 percent expenditure reduction based on the total regional on-hand inventory of sutures, or a one-shot 20-percent reduction based on the annual regional purchases of sutures. However, this is a conservative figure, since the returned items are the ones not used anymore. Other sutures were found that have not been used for the past two or three years; however, their future use was possible. These sutures were kept for insurance purposes. Also, the 20-percent figure addresses the inactive and not the overstocked items. Since the annual regional purchases of nonstandard stock over all the items was not available, no projection of the total possible one-shot savings could be made. This rather disturbing picture of a materials-management system that has gone out of control is fortunately not typical, though not uncommon. However, in at least one other center, otherwise well managed, a physical count of sutures revealed an inventory corresponding to over three years' supply. Clearly, reduction of unnecessary overstocking of materials frees up funds for other purposes and reduces the costs associated with money that is tied up. These considerations become ever more consequential as interest rates increase or stay at their current double-digit levels.

Appendix 1A provides a list of questions in the form of a *checklist* that can be used by administrators or in-house consultants for evaluating materials-management infrastructures in health-care institutions. The checklist is intended to complement and to expand the materials covered in the chapter.

**References**

1. *AMSCO Fact Summary*, SC-2533. Erie, Pa.: AMSCO Systems, 1977.
2. Henning, William K. "The Financial Impact of Materials Management." *Hospital Financial Management* (February 1980).
3. *Hospitals*, JAHA 34, pt. 2, August 1, 1960.
4. American Hospital Association (AHA). *Hospital Statistics*. Chicago, Ill.: AHA, 1972, 1975, 1978 eds.
5. Javad, Shahriar. "Multi-Echelon Inventory Systems in Health Care Delivery Organizations." Unpublished Ph.D. thesis, Case Western Reserve University, 1980.
6. Buffa, Elwood S., and Miller, Jeffrey G. *Production-Inventory Systems: Planning and Control*, Homewood, Ill.: Richard D. Irwin, 1979.
7. Lucia, S.R. "Material Logistics Operations Determine Material Transport Systems." Unpublished papers in *International Materials Management Society Hospital Material Management Papers*. Monroeville, Pa.

# Appendix 1A: Checklist for an Effective Materials-Management Department

|  | *Comments (Provide data on "yes" answers. Explain "no" answers.)* | |
| --- | --- | --- |
|  | *Yes* | *No* |

Does the department:

1. Supervise, assign, and direct the activities of all personnel performing materials functions? \_\_\_\_\_ \_\_\_\_\_

2. Evaluate the performance, at least annually, of the key supervisory personnel of the Department of Materials Management, that is, purchasing agent, chief pharmacist, CSR supervisor, central-stores supervision, and so on? \_\_\_\_\_ \_\_\_\_\_

3. Negotiate prime-supplier contracts with major suppliers and distributors? \_\_\_\_\_ \_\_\_\_\_

4. Set the appropriate and necessary fiduciary, ethical, and professional tone for the materials-management effort both intra- and interdepartmentally? \_\_\_\_\_ \_\_\_\_\_

5. Establish and maintain a good professional rapport with the medical staff, administration, nursing service, patient-care areas, and all other hospital departments? \_\_\_\_\_ \_\_\_\_\_

6. Confer regularly on at least a monthly basis with all personnel of the department in a group session to discuss plans, objectives, problems, and so on, and record minutes of such meetings, a copy of which is forwarded to administration? \_\_\_\_\_ \_\_\_\_\_

21

*Comments*
*(Provide data*
*on "yes" answers.*
*Explain "no"*
*answers.)*

*Yes          No*

7. Establish review, and appropriately update departmental policies and procedures
in accordance with the institution's
policies?                                                          _____          _____

8. Review and make the appropriate recommendations in reference to all new supplies and instruments for the department
and the entire institution?                                _____          _____

9. Update on a regular basis all departmental managerial tools such as organization charts, policies, procedures, job
descriptions, departmental orientation
plans, and so on?                                           _____          _____

10. Prepare the annual departmental budget
and assure adherence on a monthly basis
to this budget?                                               _____          _____

11. Confer at least bimonthly on a regular
basis with the administration for the purpose of coordinating the materials-
management efforts with the objectives
and plans of top management?                        _____          _____

12. In conjunction with administration,
establish realistic, attainable goals for the
department on an annual basis?                      _____          _____

13. Relate directly and through the proper
committees with the medical staff concerning all aspects of materials manage-
ment?                                                            _____          _____

14. Develop, schedule, conduct, and document in-service and continuing-education
programs for the personnel of the depart-
ment?                                                            _____          _____

*Comments*
*(Provide data*
*on "yes" answers.*
*Explain "no"*
*answers.)*
*Yes          No*

15. Take responsibility for the controlling, counting, and reporting of all hospital-supply inventories, both "official" and "unofficial," on a regular basis?             \_\_\_\_\_       \_\_\_\_\_

16. Establish and maintain the proper and appropriate professional and ethical relationships with all sales representatives?             \_\_\_\_\_       \_\_\_\_\_

17. Conduct the business affairs of the department according to the principles and guidelines of the "prudent-buyer" philosophy?             \_\_\_\_\_       \_\_\_\_\_

18. Meet or exceed standards of compliance for all the accreditation and regulatory bodies, commissions, and so on, in reference to supply management?             \_\_\_\_\_       \_\_\_\_\_

19. Support and participate in bona fide efforts of group purchasing and shared services with other hospitals and related health facilities?             \_\_\_\_\_       \_\_\_\_\_

20. Submit monthly reports to top management concerning the functional and administrative phases of the department?             \_\_\_\_\_       \_\_\_\_\_

21. Initiate and participate in all legitimate supply price comparison studies?             \_\_\_\_\_       \_\_\_\_\_

22. Perform the appropriate committee functions as assigned?             \_\_\_\_\_       \_\_\_\_\_

# 2 Managerial Infrastructure

## Organizational Structures for Materials Management

### Degree of MMS Centralization

The organizational structure of a health-care institution must seriously address issues of rational and cost-effective management of materials. Organizational structures could take a range of forms, including at one extreme the fully *decentralized* form, where each subunit of an organization does its own replenishment, buying, stocking, and so on. Under this approach radiology may maintain its own stocks of supplies both of film and of everything else, as will internal medicine, the pharmacy, the dietary unit, and so forth. At the other extreme is a *highly centralized* structure with all replenishments at all levels of the organization being the sole responsibility of the central materials-management department. Under this schema, central personnel not only purchase and stock the warehouse but are, in fact, responsible for maintaining stocks in every unit and subunit of the institution. An example of a workable centralized system is the *cart system*, whereby the materials needs of every subunit of the institution are brought into each module or department on a portable cart on a periodic, at times even a daily, basis by central materials personnel. In this system, the cart serves as the working storage shelving for materials needed by the unit.

In between these *extremes* there is clearly a whole range of materials-systems configurations. In one configuration, a department using a unique high-dollar-volume material might be allowed to replenish, indeed even purchase, that particular material while using the central supply system for all its other needs. An example of this might be the radiology department being responsible for stocking and perhaps even buying its own X-ray film, while relying on central stores for its paper cups, paper gowns, and paper slippers. A variant of this might be a case where all storage of X-ray film takes place in the radiology department; however, the actual purchasing is performed by a central purchasing department on request from radiology either directly from a vendor or through some regional group-purchasing arrangement, such as those offered in several localities by regional hospital associations.

Clearly, arguments can be advanced in favor of materials-management system (MMS) configurations at any point between and including the two extremes. Arguments in favor of the *decentralized* format recognize that the

25

channels of communication in the requisitioning process are thus kept to a minimum, as is the replenishment or the distribution pipeline. Furthermore, this approach at its extreme does not require central or intermediate warehousing points and thus cuts down on space, personnel, and total on-hand inventory requirements. Furthermore, it can be said that this organizational form is much more responsive to the needs of the ultimate user, who normally is a health-care provider and is intolerant of materials shortages. A corollary to this argument might be the fact that generally health providers' time and equipment costs are relatively high compared with the costs of the materials consumed in providing services. Therefore, "the tail must not wag the dog," and the materials should be there waiting for the user, rather than vice versa.

Arguments in favor of a *centralized* system point to the professionalism that can be brought to managing materials throughout the requisitioning cycle. Specifically, professional buyers can obtain better deals for a given material or group of materials, especially when armed with the purchasing power of the entire institution. The alternative is to have this function performed by people whose professional orientation is quite different from that of the purchasing function, for example, people whose professional orientation is toward providing health-care services. Similar arguments could be made for the development of rational stocking procedures throughout the institution based on accurate and timely knowledge of usage and of *who* has *what*, and *when*. This approach allows for intrainstitutional transfers on a by-exception basis and hence for a potential reduction of total inventory carried throughout the institution.

These arguments also address issues of movement toward *standardization* of stocked items throughout the institution. As discussed in a subsequent section on *value analysis*, creative substitutions could often be made that would result in a reduction of unit as well as total costs, without any reduction in function of the material in question. Thus, the argument goes, a centralized materials-management system can significantly reduce an institution's materials-related costs without jeopardizing the availability, accessibility, and usability of materials. Moreover, the argument can be made that health providers under this system are freed to do what they are best trained and suited for. Figures 2-1 and 2-2 indicate an organizational structure in which materials management is centralized. In such settings, the director of materials management typically reports to either the director or the vice president for operations, who in turn has equal standing with other division chiefs, such as those of medicine, surgery, laboratory, and so on.

From figure 2-1 it is seen that materials management encompasses purchasing, distribution, and processing. Figures 2-2, 2-3, and 2-4, respectively, delineate the various positions that make up the purchasing, distribution, and processing departments. It should also be noted from figure 2-2

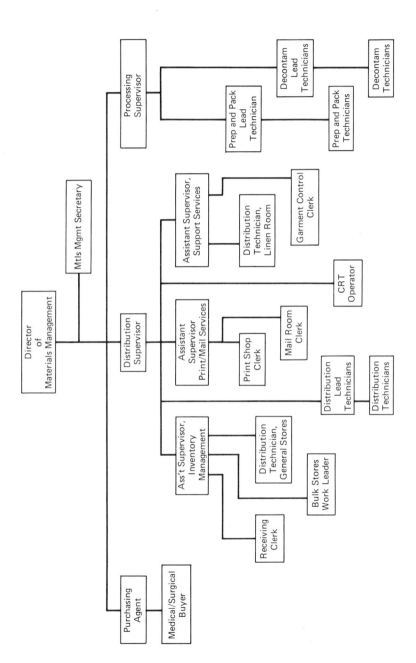

Reproduced with permission from Dr. A. A. Aardsma, director, Materials Management Resource Center, American Hospital Association.

**Figure 2-1.** A Representative Materials-Management Organizational Chart

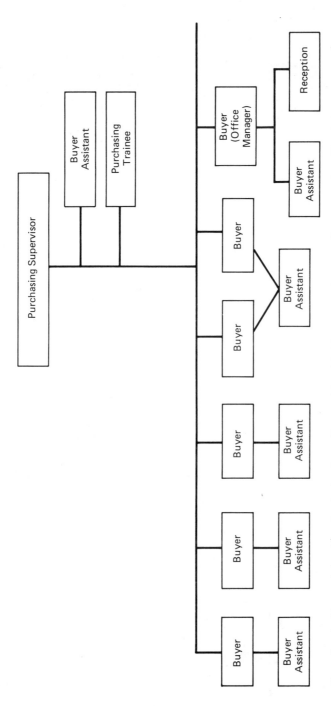

Reproduced with permission from Dr. A. Aardsma, director, Materials Management Resource Center, American Hospital Association.

**Figure 2-2.** A Purchasing-Department Organization Chart

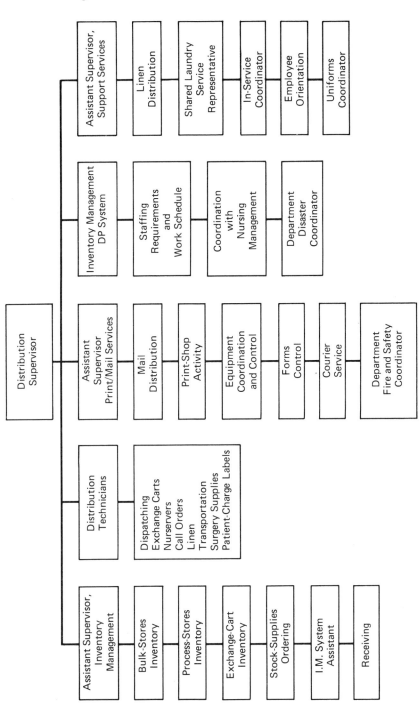

Reproduced with permission from Dr. A. Aardsma, director, Materials Management Resource Center, American Hospital Association.

**Figure 2-3. Areas of Responsibility—Supply and Distribution**

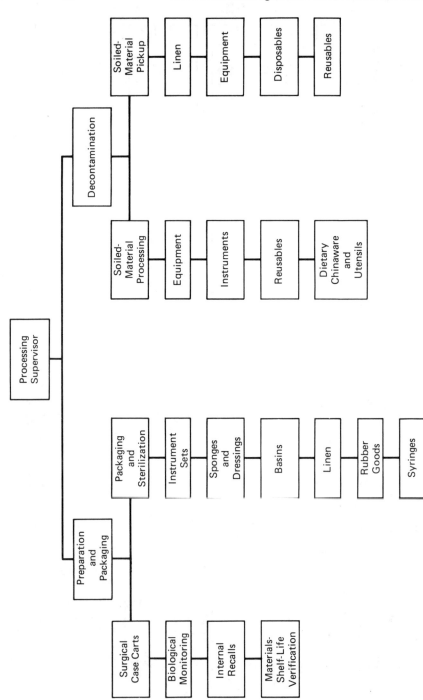

Reproduced with permission from Dr. A. Aardsma, director, Materials Management Resource Center, American Hospital Association.

**Figure 2-4.** Areas of Responsibility—Processing

that each buyer is responsible for some subset of the clinical and/or administrative departments in an institution. Thus, buyer X is concerned with administration, animals, human dialysis, lab stock supplies, laboratory medicine, and so forth; buyer Y is concerned with anesthesia, diabetic recheck, medical records and statistics, and so forth. Figures 2-5 and 2-6 show job descriptions for key positions in the purchasing department.

*Example of a Mixed MMS Organization (Centralized and Decentralized)*

One large health-maintenance organization (HMO) has five geographically dispersed facilities within a metropolitan area. Each facility has a number of departments ranging from thirty-four to fifty-four per facility. Three of the facilities have a central supply room (CSR). The CSRs were originally designed to prepare, process, and sterilize reusable materials. In reality, however, they are used for materials receipt, storage, and intrafacility distribution as well. Each department has a number of use locations, referred to as modules. In addition to facilities, CSRs, departments, and modules—which are *physical* configurations—the HMO has two entities that are basically used for *accounting* and *financial* purposes and that fundamentally represent *logical* detachments. Usually each department belongs to one entity, but there are instances of a department belonging to both entities.

The whole system has a central warehouse, which interacts between the CSRs and modules and the vendors. It works as a logistical support system for the five facilities, the three CSRs, and the use locations. Finally, several vendors function as the supply system for departments, CSRs, and the central warehouse.

This HMO separates materiel into two categories:

1.  *capital materiel*—equipment and supplies that are durable that have a life span of five years or more or a unit cost of $100 or more.
2.  *expensed materials*—all items not covered in the first category.

The expensed materials—perishable, reusable, disposable, and consumable—in turn can be subdivided into two major categories:

1.  *Standard-stock items*—the items inventoried in the warehouse on a regular basis, as well as the most-frequently used items and those with long lead times (say, ten weeks or more). These are managed by a computer. Their total number hovers around 1,700, and their annual regional purchase value is a bit over $1 million.

The position of Director of Purchasing is a staff function exercising line responsibility within the Department of Purchasing. This position is responsible to the designated Administrative Director.

The Director of Purchasing administers and directs the program to purchase materials, supplies and equipment for Foundation use, and coordinates the activities of workers within his area of responsibility.

The Director of Purchasing is responsible for reviewing requests for medical equipment, furnishings, supplies, building materials, and other items to assure that requisitions meet with purchasing policies. He is responsible for providing consultation to department heads to resolve discrepancies or to assist them in preparing requisitions, when necessary. He is responsible for establishing programs which provide ongoing analysis of market conditions and statistical data. He is involved in interviewing vendors and reviewing catalogues and other source material to obtain information on items for purchase. He is responsible for comparing prices, establishing specifications, and determining delivery dates and directs the preparation and mailing of purchase orders to merchandising firms or their representative. He is responsible for the preparation of bid instructions on orders or equipment. He may, when appropriate, submit purchase orders on acceptable bids to administrative personnel or the Equipment Committee for approval.

The Director of Purchasing will examine purchase records to ascertain that his staff has complied with all procurement procedures.

The Director of Purchasing reviews advertising literature, trade journals, magazines, and other publications to keep abreast of market conditions, cost prices and new products. He is responsible for determining, with the consultation of department heads, the quality, effectiveness and durability of products which are purchased. He is responsible for arranging with vendors for replacement of defective items which have been purchased.

The Director of Purchasing is responsible for establishing procedures and for assigning duties to personnel in his area of responsibility. He is responsible for the organization and staffing of his department in such a manner that it allows for the vigorous pursuit of its objectives as described in the policy statement for the Purchasing Department. He is responsible for interviewing and hiring of new employees in his area of responsibility. He will conduct periodic staff meetings to inform members of his department of changes in policies and procedures and he is responsible for the compilation and preparation of periodic reports relating to his area of responsibility.

The Director of Purchasing maintains fiscal responsibility for the activities carried on within his department. Accordingly, he will prepare an annual budget for personnel and equipment required in his department. He is also responsible for assisting all other departments in the Foundation with the preparation of their capital budgets.

The Director of Purchasing acts as the agent of the Cleveland Clinic Foundation. The Foundation is obligated by his decisions when they are within the scope of his defined authority, responsibility and in the best interest of the Foundation. The agent/principle relationship applies and the Director of Purchasing assumes no personal responsibility when he acts within the defined scope of his job responsibility.

The Director of Purchasing may be required to perform other duties and assume additional responsibilities as directed by the appropriate administrative director responsible for the Purchasing Department.

Reproduced with permission of Mr. Paul Widman, vice president, Operations, Cleveland Clinic Foundation.

**Figure 2-5.** Director of Purchasing: Job Description

The Purchasing Buyer reports to the Assistant Director of Purchasing, and is responsible for coordinating the entire purchasing support to the department(s) he may be assigned. This includes interviews with company representatives, review of departmental requests, vendor selection in accordance with the guidelines established by the Foundation Purchasing Policy. Additionally, he is responsible for assigning the activities of his individual Purchasing Assistant in accordance with those general departmental policies.

The Buyer is responsible for seeking out new and/or alternate products that can improve the operation of the departments they serve or improve the cost picture. He keeps the Assistant Director of Purchasing informed of various activities, problems and projects. May be assigned certain duties that are designed to improve the overall effectiveness of the Purchasing Department.

*Personal Qualifications*

A minimum of two years of college preparation, a high degree of responsibility and integrity, an ability to work well with people and an inquisitive attitude are considered essential.

Reproduced with permission of Mr. Paul Widman, vice president, Operations, Cleveland Clinic Foundation.

**Figure 2-6.** Purchasing Buyer: Job Description

2. *Nonstandard-stock items*—the items that are not inventoried at the central warehouse. Their use is usually limited to a single department, the demand for them is very sporadic. Often, each department places the order directly with the vendor. These are highly specialized items and their number, for all practical purposes, is infinite. They are not managed by a computer and, although no exact cost figures are available, their annual regional purchases are approximated at around two to three times that of standard-stock items (over $2 to $3 million). Moreover, in this institution some of the big-user departments—x-ray, laboratory, emergency room, and operating room—place their orders directly with vendors, bypassing central purchasing, receiving, and warehouse—the places where some professionalism in materials management exists and where control is exerted.

## Organizational Structures

### Hierarchical Organization

The materials-management organizational tables shown in figures 2-1 and 2-2 are specific examples of the traditional chain of command of *hierarchical* forms of organization, depicted in figure 2-7. The attributes of this form of highly centralized organization are:

1. Each person has one boss.

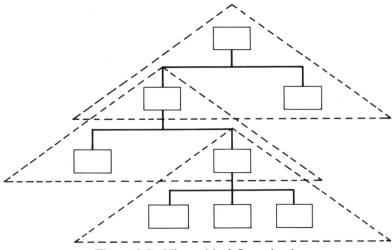

**Figure 2-7.** Hierarchical Organization

2. Each group knows who reports to whom.
3. There is no overlap.
4. There is generally a clear-cut delineation of authority and commensurate responsibility.
5. Structure has a clear vertical hierarchical line.
6. Span of control issues—for example, no person should have more than seven others reporting to him or her—are easily visible.
7. There is vertical control.
8. Even in this type of structure, there is a considerable amount of horizontal flow of work tasks across the organization (frequently known as the informal organization structure).
9. Various methods are used to show the informal structure or horizontal flow. Often the dotted-line concept is resorted to.
10. The structure tends to imply that people do not have two or more bosses, yet this tendency does exist in many organizations.

*Matrix-Type Organization*

Figure 2-8 depicts a *matrix* form of organization. This MMS structure ensures line responsibility for each of the functional MMS areas, such as purchasing and distribution, reporting to the director or manager of MMS. Simultaneously, this structure allows each user department to have a single individual responsible for all materials-management aspects relevant to that department's needs. Under this schema each departmental MMS manager

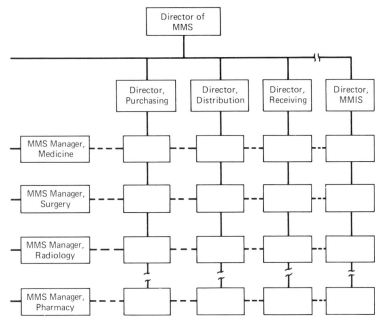

**Figure 2-8**. Matrix-Type Organization Structures

draws on the skills and expertise of specialists in each of the functional MMS areas. He or she has *functional* but not *line* responsibility over the specialists assigned to service the needs of that department.

It might be of interest to note that when the *horizontal* aspects of figure 2-8 are removed, the result is a traditional *hierarchical* organization. As indicated earlier, this is the most centralized MMS structure. On the other hand, when the *vertical* aspects are removed, the result is a depiction of a highly *decentralized* group of MMS teams.

The attributes of this form of organization are:

1. The matrix shows the vertical and horizontal lines of interrelated authority and responsibility.
2. It breaks away from the traditional pyramid type of management structure.
3. Each member of the team must answer to more than one boss—his traditional or functional boss plus the department MMS manager.
4. Some specialists may serve on more than one team.
5. It brings together many different disciplines, thus getting diverse types of people to work together as a team.

6. At its best a matrix organization reduces costs by using the time of each team specialist more efficiently while being more responsive to the provider departmental needs.
7. It demands excellent communication, both horizontally and vertically.
8. It requires a manager who is capable of getting results by acting as a general manager.

*Advantages of Matrix Organization*

1. Allows the organization to retain the advantages of centralization and decentralization at the same time.
2. Provides concentrated cost-effective materials management at the level where it is happening.
3. Forces decision making down to the immediately responsible levels.
4. Allows each provider or service function to have its materials managed in a way that is sensitive to "local" conditions.
5. Flexibility: Materials-management teams can be relatively quickly formed, abandoned, or adjusted in size as conditions warrant. (This is not of great consequence in stable, mature health institutions.)
6. Managers get broadened responsibilities and greater opportunity for personal growth.
7. Pragmatic: Responsive to immediate needs of the "marketplace" (characteristics of provider personnel)—can reorganize as desired.
8. Emphasizes knowledge, competence, and role rather than personal feeling and autocratic control as source of authority.
9. Promotes communication, cooperation, compromise, and teamwork in organizational behavior.
10. More knowledgeable decisions as two or more influences are brought to bear on negotiated solutions.
11. A deeper awareness in managers of the responsibilities and problems of others.

*Disadvantages of Matrix Organization*

1. Crossing over traditional vertical reporting lines confuses managers oriented to simple, vertical pyramidal structures.
2. The two-boss system sometimes causes severe emotional distress to the authoritarian personality put in an ambiguous reporting position.
3. Slowness in decision making can occur if managers check every direction before exercising any initiative.
4. Emphasis on teamwork and group problem solving can lead to excessive meetings.

5. The socially and politically skillful may prove ascendant over the knowledgeable and competent.
6. Conflict between function and business may often have to be resolved by a higher-level manager.
7. Requires excellent communication and participative management skills of all managers.
8. Can be costly if empire builders occur in both dimensions.
9. Is probably not appropriate to relatively static businesses in which control and efficiency are more important than problem solving, flexibility, and change.

## Materials-Distribution Structures

Closely associated with issues pertaining to the degrees of MMS centralization and MMS organizational structures are issues concerned with the systems and procedures of getting the right supplies in the proper quantities to the right locations at the right time. There are many approaches to accomplishing this. In fact, several actual scenarios contemplated by a large multifacility health center are discussed in a subsequent section. In general there are four basic distribution alternatives that were very compactly delineated by C.E. Housley [1], as shown in figure 2-9.

Distribution alternative number 1 in figure 2-9 represents a highly decentralized system, where the user departments purchase directly or through a central purchasing department, and receive and stock locally all materials so obtained. In this approach, requisitioning if not actual purchasing, receiving, inspection, and storage are locally administered functions. A radiology department's handling of X-ray film and other photoprocessing supplies has already been cited as an example of such a mode of procurement.

Distribution alternatives 2, 3, and 4 in figure 2-9 may be used in any one or any combination of at least three different basic modes of supply distribution. These are:

the fetch-and-carry system;

the PAR-level system;

the cart-exchange system.

### The Fetch-and-Carry System

In the fetch-and-carry system, someone on the nursing unit or in the user department is delegated the responsibility for maintaining adequate levels

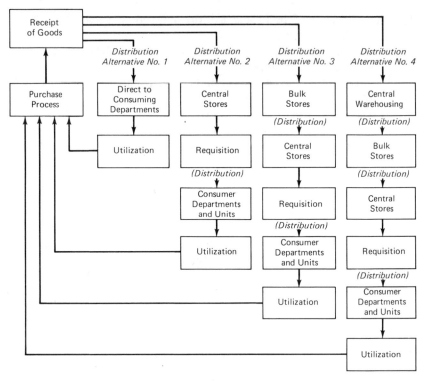

Reproduced with permission from C.E. Housley, "Distributing the Goods the Right Way," *Hospitals, JAHA*, June 16, 1977.

**Figure 2-9.** Distribution Alternatives

of supplies; filling out the required requisition forms, if any, for all the items needed; and getting the requisition to central stores for processing. Central stores in turn fills the order and delivers the requested items on a supply cart to its destination for proper disposition by the user-department personnel. Alternately, in some cases, the actual "picks" from the shelves are made by the requisitioner. This entire process may be repeated at regular intervals several times a week by all consumer units and departments.

According to Housley [2], the distinguishing advantage of this method of distribution is its simplicity. However, there are many disadvantages. Taking inventory before each requisitioning, if this is indeed done, is time consuming. As stated earlier, nursing and other user-department personnel must take time from their busy schedules to handle supply chores. They are not normally trained to do this in an enlightened way from an institutional point of view, and their salaries are generally somewhat higher than the salaries of those usually involved in the supply process. Furthermore, the entire burden of usage or demand forecasting is placed on user-department personnel. This method often results in expensive duplication of inventory that is rarely accounted for and that takes up valuable space and incurs high carrying costs. (Carrying or holding costs are discussed in chapter 4 and are defined in the glossary.)

## The PAR-Level System

In the PAR-level system, each department uses local storage space as when ordering from central stores. Supply quotas for each supply item are established in conjunction with each department, using—it is hoped—one of the decision rules discussed in chapter 4. To be effective, these quotas should be reviewed and updated at least quarterly, because dependability and system credibility from the user's perspective are of great importance with this supply system. The quotas are maintained by central stores. An attendant from central stores generally makes the rounds of all of the nursing units and user departments at sufficiently frequent intervals, approximately two to three times per week. Using a large transfer cart, the attendant replenishes all stock back to the preassigned "par" levels.

The essential differences between the PAR and the fetch-and-carry systems is that with the PAR-level system, user-department personnel are not involved once the quotas have been established. In essence it is an outreach program on the part of central stores: central stores comes to user departments rather than the other way around. This has a drawback, however. Since usage at the department level fluctuates, the attendant usually must return to central stores several times in the replenishment process to restock the transfer cart. This system also suffers from the drawbacks mentioned in connection with the fetch-cnd-carry system, such as space requirements at user-department levels and higher carrying costs, although these are more or less moderated by the PAR concept of replenishment.

## The Total-Supply-Cart-Exchange System

The newest mode of materials distribution is the total-supply-cart-exchange system. It appears to be gaining in acceptance within hospitals large and small, general and specialized, new and old, vertical and horizontal, as well as in clinics and, in a modified form (for examples, a tray versus a cart), even in private dental offices. The supply-cart-exchange system works best when carts include all items used by a nursing unit or user department, from paper clips to syringes, and when the quotas are, in principle, established as discussed in the previous case. Here too they need to be reviewed periodically to maintain service levels and hence system credibility.

One such system is depicted in figures 2-10 and 2-11. It appears to be practical, flexible, dependable, and uncomplicated. Its proponents claim that it saves time, paperwork, transportation or movement, personnel, inventory, and money. If set up and used properly, it provides for demand or usage forecasting, distribution, stocking, control, and patient-charge-

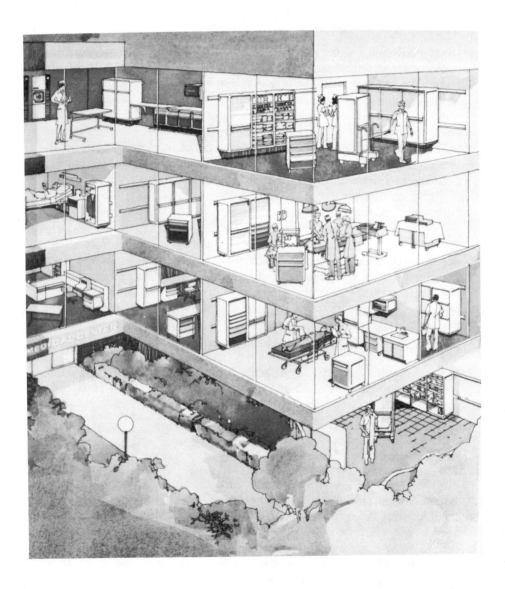

Reproduced with permission from Don Soth, director, Corporate Communications, American Sterilizer Company.

**Figure 2-10.** A General View of an Exchange-Cart System in Operation

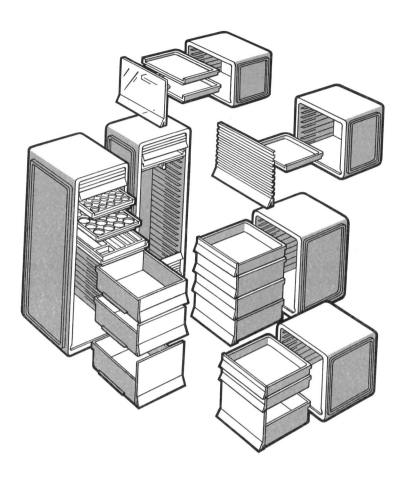

Reproduced with permission from Don Soth, director, Corporate Communications, American Sterilizer Company.

**Figure 2-11.** Physical Components of an Exchange-Cart System

accountability functions. Furthermore, according to Housley [2], this system is superior in forecasting usage. This is important, he states, because a supply shortage can be anticipated twenty-four hours in advance of the time the item is needed. Hence, the materials manager has adequate time to prepare and make the necessary steps to procure or substitute for an item. Parenthetically, in principle there is no reason that the PAR system could not have this same attribute. However, if the total supply-cart-exchange system is to work, accurate forecasting is imperative. In practice, accurate forecasting is aided in this system through the elimination of all other storage space, such as cabinets, drawers, and storage closets in the user departments.

In any nondecentralized MMS, dependability and reliability are essential if the system is to gain and maintain credibility with the various user-department personnel. According to Housley [2]:

> Ensuring reliability is the responsibility of the materials manager. Carts should be checked for quality and quantity before being distributed. The cart system also must operate on a 24-hour, seven-day-a-week basis. At least quarterly, there should be a conference between the materials manager and each of the respective using areas to adjust quotas and to discuss any problems either party is experiencing. A complete orientation to the purpose, functions, and benefits of the total supply cart exchange system should be given to all personnel, including the materials management department, at least twice annually.

> The size of carts should be carefully considered before purchasing them. A cart must have the capacity to hold approximately 200 different items and more than 1,000 items in total. Thus, the larger the cart the better, because the chances are good that there will be a need for more items than expected, not less. No more than two carts should be used per exchange, and they should be covered in storage and distribution to ensure clean, fresh supplies.

> There are many other applications for the cart exchange distribution system. It is an excellent system for supply and distribution of pharmaceuticals, linens, and dietary items. Isolation techniques and surgical care pack quotas also can be facilitated by the system.

The advantages and disadvantages of centralization and of decentralization of materials-management systems are further summarized in tables 2-1 and 2-2. Further ideas to be considered in connection with supply-cart-exchange systems are provided in appendix 2A in the form of a checklist.

### Examples of MMS Alternatives for a Multifacility HMO

During the course of a study concerned with the materials-management system in a multifacility HMO, three different feasible alternatives for requisitioning, stocking, deliveries, and transfers of materials were identified. These are:

A. Centralized ordering and inventory
   All or nearly all materials used in a facility are stocked in a central storeroom, say a CSR.
   All facility ordering and replenishing is done by CSR.
   All stocking locations are served by CSR personnel.

**Table 2-1**
**Advantages and Disadvantages of Centralization**

| Advantages | Disadvantages |
|---|---|
| Personnel efficiency:<br>Nursing personnel is solely in charge of patient care and supply functions are done by trained nonmedical personnel [3, 5]. | Management expertise:<br>This system "requires higher degree of management effort and expertise than a decentralized [one]" [4]. |
| Cost effectiveness:<br>Reduction in the number of personnel [5]; reduction in the duplication of expensive equipment; lower supply cost because of quantity discount [3]; reduction of space requirements. | Total organizational change:<br>It requires personnel retraining and re-orientation [5]; a redefinition of all the tasks and responsibilities; a completely new mentality toward materials management. |
| Functional and procedural uniformity:<br>The steps and procedures in each function are spelled out; therefore, a particular function is performed the same way regardless of its location. | Implementation:<br>These factors, coupled with resistance to change inherent in human beings, makes the initiation and afterwards implementation of this concept an extremely difficult process. |
| Unified management:<br>A single accountable person is in charge of the total system that cuts across all the departmental boundaries; policies governing each function are clearly stated, and responsibilities are carefully delineated to hospital materials-management personnel. | |
| Product standardization:<br>Ensures the quality of supplies and equipment; reduces the total number of items in inventory; reduces inventory levels. | |

Reproduced with permission from Javad Shahriar, "Multi-echelon Inventory Systems in Health Care Delivery Organizations" (unpublished Ph.D. dissertation, Case Western Reserve University, 1980).

Departmental personnel may obtain stock from the CSR.
Forms to be used:
 Revised standard-stock requisition form.
 Existing delivery record.
 Modified interdepartmental-stock-transfer form.
 Modified internal requisition form.

B. Departmental ordering with periodic stocking-location inventory surveys
 One nurse (per shift) is in charge of ordering for a department or a floor.

**Table 2-2**
**Advantages and Disadvantages of Decentralization**

| Advantages | Disadvantages |
|---|---|
| Speed:<br>Long lead times, elemental to the centralized systems, are avoided, for example, delivery lead times are eliminated. | Quality control [6]:<br>Since different procedures are practiced in different departments, it is difficult to establish a standard of performance and measure quality of patient care uniformly. |
| Maintenance of principle of asepsis [6]:<br>After sanitization and decontamination of supplies and equipment, it is immediately used in that department without further transportation. | Conflict of objectives [6]:<br>Departmental objectives might be in conflict with institutional objectives taken as a whole. |
| Lack of assembly-type production:<br>Since patient care is a personalized service, it is beneficial to let the physician have the supplies and equipment that he needs; where he needs it and when he needs it. | Lack of communication:<br>The kingdom phenomenon [7] intensifies the interdepartmental competition for scarce resources and causes the failure of formal communication channels and creation of informal communication channels. |
|  | Lack of economies of scale [4]:<br>With each department performining its own functions individually, the fixed cost of performing a job or running a machine is duplicated many times. |
|  | Lack of monitoring [4]:<br>Usage is hard to measure; obsolescence is abundant; pilferage and/or shrinkage are generally higher and are uncontrollable. |

Reproduced with permission from Javad Shahriar, "Multi-echelon Inventory Systems in Health Care Delivery Organizations" (unpublished Ph.D. dissertation, Case Western Reserve University, 1980.)

Ordering is generally from the warehouse with some items ordered from the CSR.

The nurse checks all department stocking locations for amounts of inventory on hand.

Periodically (say, once a month), a physical inventory is taken at all stocking locations to mitigate against overstocking.

Forms to be used:

Same as for scenario A, plus:

Periodic physical-inventory form.

C. Departmental ordering with ongoing inventory survey

The nurse orders as in scenario B except that each time an order is placed, all the inventories in all departmental stocking locations are checked.

Forms to be used:

Same as for scenario A except that a person in the department will be filling out the forms instead of a person in the CSR.

The effects of these alternatives on the CSR and the department were rated by the HMO administrators using a list of criteria for a good materials-management system. The results—how well the alternatives can meet these criteria—are indicated next.

*Effect of the Alternatives on the CSR*

| | Alternative | | |
|---|---|---|---|
| *Criterion* | *A* | *B* | *C* |
| Ability to rotate perishables in CSR | High | Med. | Med. |
| Preventing overstocking | High | Low | Low |
| Preventing stockouts and backorders | High | Med. | Med. |
| Ability to obtain the lead-time data | High | High | High |
| Security of materials | High | High | High |
| Ability to minimize space requirements in CSR | Low | High | High |
| Ability to minimize the taking of physical inventories | Low | Med. | Med. |
| Ease and quality of ordering rules for CSR | Med. | High | High |
| Availability of usage data for CSR | High | Med. | Med. |
| Availability of delivery-time data | High | High | High |
| Availability to minimize delivery and lead times to the CSR | High | High | High |
| Availability of processing-times data | High | High | High |
| Ability to minimize processing times | Low | High | High |
| Ability to minimize inventory levels | Low | High | High |
| Ability to minimize duplication of inventory | High | High | High |
| Information on inventory | High | High | High |
| Ability to minimize the number of people involved (at the CSR) | Low | High | High |
| Ability to minimize complexity of the mathematical model | Low | High | High |
| Ability to have less-complex computer programs | Low | High | High |
| Ability to minimize computer running time | Low | High | High |
| Ability to minimize computer memory needed | Med. | High | High |
| Ease of working with the paperwork | High | Med. | Low |
| Ability to minimize the authorizing | High | Med. | Med. |

| Criterion | Alternative | | |
|---|---|---|---|
| | A | B | C |
| Ease of implementation | High | High | Med. |
| Ability to minimize and schedule properly the ordering from the warehouse | High | Med. | Med. |
| Ability to minimize load on receiving clerk delivery items to CSR | Low | High | High |

### Effect of the Alternatives on the Departments

| | A | B | C |
|---|---|---|---|
| Ability to rotate perishables in departments | High | Med. | Med. |
| Preventing overstocking | Low | Med. | High |
| Preventing stockouts and backorders | Low | Med. | High |
| Ability to obtain the lead-time data | High | High | High |
| Security of materials | High | High | High |
| Ability to minimize space requirements | High | Low | Low |
| Ability to minimize physical inventories | High | Low | Low |
| Ease and quality of ordering rules | Low | Med. | High |
| Availability of usage data | High | High | High |
| Availability of delivery-time data | High | High | High |
| Ability to minimize delivery and lead times | High | Med. | Med. |
| Availability of processing-times data | High | High | High |
| Ability to minimize processing times | High | High | High |
| Ability to minimize inventory levels | High | Low | Low |
| Ability to minimize duplication of inventory | High | Med. | Med. |
| Information on inventory | High | Low | Med. |
| Ability to minimize the number of people involved (at the departments) | High | Med. | Low |
| Ability to minimize complexity of the mathematical model | Med. | Med. | Med. |
| Ability to have less-complex computer programs | Med. | Med. | Med. |
| Ability to minimize computer running time | Low | Med. | High |
| Ability to minimize computer memory needed | Med. | High | High |
| Ease of working with the paperwork | High | Med. | Low |
| Ability to minimize the authorizing | High | Med. | Med. |
| Ease of implementation | High | Med. | Low |
| Ability to minimize and schedule properly the ordering from the warehouse | High | Med. | Med. |
| Ability to minimize load on the receiving clerk delivering items to departments | High | Med. | Med. |
| Ability to minimize paperwork done by nurses | High | Med. | Low |

| Criterion | Alternative | | |
|---|---|---|---|
|  | A | B | C |
| Ability to obtain urgent items when stocked out | High | Med. | Med. |
| Ability to substitute items | High | Med. | Med. |
| Ease of finding transfers data | Low | High | High |
| Ease of recharging CSR stock to departments | Med. | High | High |

*Organizational Levels of MMS Accountability*

One of the key questions that must be asked and answered in designing or changing a materials-management system concerns the lowest organizational level to be used as the unit of responsibility and accountability for management of materials. Clearly, tradeoffs must be made between the increasing tightness of control the closer the responsibility lies to the ultimate user, and the correspondingly higher costs of administering such control.

In one such study the tradeoffs were between modules defined as the stocking locations and personnel that are served by one nursing station, one administrative suite or office, or a whole department—which may encompass one or more modules, suites, or offices. Moreover, this question was raised in connection with data collection for purposes of the study, for the conduct of future materials-management procedures, and for the proposed charging system. The findings of that particular study are shown next for purposes of illustration.

**Modules**: (1) stocking locations and personnel that are served by one nursing station (for most hospital areas and medical offices); or (2) one administrative suite or office, or (3) the whole stocking location for a department (for example, the CSR).

**Department**: The sum of the modules within the department (there might be only one, in which case the module and the department are the same).

Assume:

1. The existing departmental system is in effect.
2. In a module system, each module fills out a requisition. It is then routed to the department head if authorization is necessary.

Figures 2-12, 2-13, and 2-14 compare the results of data collection at the departmental level and at the module level.

**Management by Objectives**

The concept of *management by objectives* (MBO) [9] can be briefly described as a process whereby the superior and the subordinate jointly identify the common institutional goals and define each individual's major areas of

*Module better*

1. More precise data on usage. Replenishment, lead times, delivery times, processing times, inventory levels, stocking locations, and transfers are thus obtained.
2. It leads to ordering rules that optimize inventories at each module.
3. Stockouts and overstocking are minimized per module instead of per department.
4. It is easy to aggregate these data to department level if necessary.
5. Unnecessary duplication of inventory across modules within a department would be minimized.
6. Departmental personnel would have better information on what items were stocked in a particular module.
7. Departmental personnel would have better control over the individual modules.

*Department better*

1. Data on transfers is much easier to obtain than at the module level: one needs only to gather interdepartmental transfer data.
2. Fewer people need in-service training to assume responsibility for materials-management procedures within a department.
3. The mathematical models for decision rules are less complex than with modules.
4. The computer programs are less complex so that fewer manhours would be needed for design and less computer running time would be required.

**Figure 2-12.** Data Collection and Use

responsibility. This is done in terms of results expected. It can be applied within materials-management systems or subunits thereof. The measures established by the MBO process and extended to other staff members are used as guides for operating the unit and for assessing the contribution of each of its members.

*Attributes of an MBO System*

Management by objectives is a particular way of thinking about management. It goes beyond being a set of rules, a series of procedures, or even a set method of managing.

The basic organizational structure of the institution is often called a hierarchy. The formal hierarchy is depicted by the organizational chart, as shown in figures 2-7 and 2-8. Management by objectives is a means for making that structure work for the benefit of the institution and its staff, as well as for its clients—the patients. As a fringe benefit it normally brings about more vitality and personal involvement of the people in the hierarchy.

MBO provides for the maintenance, orderly growth, and containment of, and response flexibility to, changing conditions in the environment of the organization by means of operationally meaningful statements of what is expected of everyone involved, and measurement of what is actually

*Module better*
1. Same as the "module better" items for data collection.
2. Tighter procedures for routing items delivered to the individual modules.
3. Urgent items are found more easily when they are needed because of better information availability.
4. Substitutable items are found more easily for the same reason as (3) above.

*Department better*
1. Same as the "department better" items (1) — (3) for data collection.
2. The computer programs would be less complex so that less running time would be required and fewer manhours to provide data would be required.
3. There are fewer forms to fill out since the whole department is treated as one stocking location.
4. Delivery procedures within facilities do not have to be changed (deliveries would have to be split up into modules with the other system).
5. Possible shorter lead times in the requisitioning process because of less routing of materials and forms.
6. Department heads need to authorize a fewer number of orders.

**Figure 2-13.** Materials-Management Procedures

achieved. It assigns risks to all responsible leaders and makes their progress—even their tenure—dependent on results. It stresses the ability and achievements of leaders rather than their personalities.

MBO is particularly applicable to professional and administrative employees. It can extend to first-line supervisors and can also cover many staff and technical positions. The same basic system, such as measuring results against standards, can be used to manage hourly rated or clerical employees as well. However, the methods of setting standards and measuring results in the latter cases are significantly different.

It is claimed that MBO, when skillfully implemented, helps overcome many of the chronic problems of managing administrators and some professionals. For example:

It defines the major areas of responsibility for each person in the organization, including joint or shared responsibilities.

It provides a means for determining each manager's span of control.

It provides a means of assessing the contributions of individual administrators.

By defining the common goals of people and organizations and assessing the individual contributions toward achievement of such goals, it enhances the probability of achieving coordinated effort and teamwork without eliminating personal risk taking.

| Module better | Department better |
|---|---|
| 1. Tighter inventory control could be obtained and maintained if charging were done at the module level. | 1. Since current charging system is at the department level, it would not have to be changed. |

**Figure 2-14.** Charging System

Its processes are geared to achieving the results desired, both for the organization as a whole and for the individual contributors.

It offers an answer to some key questions of salary administration, especially where merit increases are practiced.

It aids in identifying potential for advancement and in finding the promotable people.

It eliminates the need for individuals to alter their personalities to fit the mold.

*Major Premises of an MBO System When Applied to MMS*

The major premises of MBO can be stated as follows:

A. Health-services administration takes place within the socioeconomic system that provides the environment for the individual institution. This environment has changed drastically over the past ten years, imposing new expectations and new constraints on institutions and on individual administrators.

B. MBO is an approach to meeting these ever-changing developments. It presumes that the first step in management is to identify the goals and the objectives of the institution in general and of the MMS in particular. All other management methods, systems, and procedures follow this preliminary step.

C. Once institutional MMS goals have been identified, orderly procedures for distributing authority and responsibility among individual workers are set so that their individual and combined efforts are directed toward achieving those preset goals.

D. MBO assumes that managerial behavior and therefore the outcomes of such behavior are more important than manager personality. This behavior, MBO presumes, must be defined in operationally meaningful terms so that the results can be measured against the individually established goals, rather than in terms of common goals for all managers, or common methods of managing.

E. It regards the successful administrator as a manager of situations, most of which are best defined by identifying the purpose of the institutional MMS and the managerial behavior best suited to achieving that purpose in that institutional setting. Clearly, the best form of management for one setting may not be suitable in another.

## Installing an MBO System

In installing a system of management by objectives, it is absolutely necessary to have the support, endorsement, or permission of the principal manager of the organizational unit in which the system is to be used. MBO is based on the premise that success for every subordinate "helps the boss to succeed." Furthermore, the boss must be in accord with the goals of the subordinate and in accord with the methods the subordinate uses to achieve such goals.

The place to begin an installation of MBO is therefore at the highest possible level of an MMS hierarchy, or above. Any manager whose boss is not opposed to his or her using the MBO system can go ahead and install it in that department or unit, as long as he or she has discretionary power over methods of managing. Usually the installation proceeds through the following phases:

1. Familiarization of the top unit administrator and key subordinates with the MBO system and how it operates.
2. Following the decision to install the system, the top administrator, working with subordinates, establishes measures of organization performance.
3. Goal-setting methods are then extended through the organization down to the first-line supervisory level via a successive series of meetings between the various organizational units and their superiors.
4. The necessary changes are made in such areas as the appraisal system, the salary and bonus procedures, and the delegation of responsibility. Ambiguous policies are clarified and procedures that may be blocking effective operation of the system are amended. Other changes, such as the installation of a system of "responsibility accounting" by the cost department, can also be made.
5. At the beginning of each budget cycle, each manager and each subordinate, meeting in pairs, agree on the subordinate's targets and measures of performance for that budget cycle. Clearly, the results are guideposts for use during the budget-cycle period.

6. At the end of the budget cycle they jointly review the subordinate's performance against these targets.

Appendix 2C provides a checklist for determining whether an MBO program exists, and another for evaluating an MBO program that is claimed to exist. Finally, the appendix provides audit procedures that might be used to establish the efficacy of any and all MBO processes.

**MMS Control Indexes**

MMS systems and procedures must always be monitored and controlled by management on an ongoing basis and at all institutional levels—facility, department, module, and so on. No matter how well-conceived the MMS, unless control mechanisms are in place some or all of the following will result:

1. Excessive stockpiling of items at the various locations and levels.
2. Nonuniformity of stocking policies at stocking points.
3. Unavailability, noncurrency, or unreliability of vital cost, physical inventory, usage and shrinkage data.
4. Frequent stockouts of items at some use locations despite excessive inventory levels of these items within the institution or the region.
5. Deterioration of systems and procedures. This is especially significant for the costwise significant and the nonstandard-stock items.

Such negative consequences often result from institutional growth in terms of size and complexity, over a period of time, without institutional management carefully watching the MMS and its corresponding growth needs.

*Inventory Turns Ratio*

One of several measures of the effectiveness with which inventory is managed is the so-called *turns ratio*. The turns ratio measures the number of times inventories are turned over within a given budgetary cycle, often a year. Thus if 1,000 units is the annual usage of a given item, and its maximum inventory during the year is 500, then the turns ratio for this item can be said to be two. On the other hand, if the maximum inventory of this item is 3,000, then the turns ratio can be said to be one-third, or 0.33. As indicated earlier, one of the major components of the total cost of materials management is the cost of monies tied up in inventories. For example, a hospital having a $1-million annual total budget is likely to spend $270,000 on consumables, disposables, and reusables. If it is assumed that the average inventory turns ratio in this institution is unity, then it could be further assumed that the average dollar value of inventory carried by this institution is $135,000 or one half of the $270,000 maximum. For the sake of argument, if the cost of capital is 10 percent per year, then $13,500 must be paid for the use of the money tied up in keeping materials on the shelves. If the turns ratio could be increased to two, the average inventory in this example would drop to 67,500, and therefore the cost of monies tied up would be reduced to about $6,750. In this illustrative example, therefore, the difference between $13,500 and $6,750, or $6,750, is saved by replenishing the inventory approximately twice as often. This saving, however, must be balanced against the additional costs involved in reordering and restocking of inventory. However, unnecessarily large stocks tend to increase the costs of deterioration, depreciation, and shrinkage. In fact, according to R.C. Mitchell [10], the total annual cost of carrying inventory was 32 percent of the average value of inventory carried in 1978.

## Other Indexes

Although the turns ratio is a popular index, it is not the only ratio used as an index for inventory-management control. In fact, if the turns ratio exclusively is used by top management, it can result in *counterproductive* behavior. Monitoring of *service levels*, such as the percentage of transactions *not* experiencing stockout conditions, is often a good index to use in order to provide checks and balances.

Other useful indexes relate inventory to some *unit of capability* such as inventory per bed, or to some *unit of service provided*, such as inventory per occupied bed. Since a typical health-care institution encompasses a large set of rather different and disparate services, it is often desirable to monitor inventory, and especially usage, on a more deaggregated basis than the entire institution. Specifically, it is desirable to focus on the emergency room (ER), the operating room (OR), the intensive-care unit (ICU), or on, say, internal medicine. Under these conditions one can always find capability or service-rendered parameters that are more specific to the given functions and thus provide a more meaningful index. Several such parameters have been suggested in the literature for each of the typical health-care-provider functions. These are enumerated in tables 2-3 and 2-4.

Appendix 2D provides a checklist for materials-management-system audits and evaluations.

## Systems and Procedures

Relationships between various systems and procedures within institutions are complex and difficult to control. Many organizations have therefore

**Table 2-3**
**Suggested Base-Statistic Parameters for Clinical Departments**

| Department | Jankowski [11] | Ruchlin [12] |
|---|---|---|
| Emergency room | Occasions of service | — |
| Laboratory | Number of procedures by type of units of service by type | — |
| Operating room | Length of operation, minutes or man-minutes | Number of operations, man-minutes, Relative Valve Unit, RVU |
| Radiology | Number of procedures by type and units of service by type | |
| Clinic | Occasions of service | — |
| Recovery room | Length of stay (hours) | — |
| Anesthesia | Length of operation (minutes or man-minutes) | Number of patients served, RVU |
| Physical therapy | Number of modalities by type, weighted units by type | Length of treatment, number of treatments, number of treatments by modality, RVU |
| Nuclear medicine | Number of procedures by type and units of service by type | — |
| Blood bank | Number of procedures by type and units of service by type | Number of procedures by type |
| Inhalation therapy | Number of procedures by type, weighted units by type | |
| ECG, EEG, and so on | Number of procedures by type, weighted units by type | Number of procedures by type, RVU |
| Cardiac catheter | Number of procedures by type | — |
| Speech therapy | Number of sessions | — |
| Occupational therapy | Number of sessions (individual and group); total number of patients in attendance | Length of treatment, number of treatments, number of treatments by modality, RVU |
| Recreation therapy | Number of sessions (individual and group); total number of patients in attendance | Minutes of treatment, number of patients treated, number of patient days of treatment |
| CSR | — | Costed requisitions, number of line items sold per patient day |
| Social services | — | Hours of service, number of discharges, number of personal contacts |

**Table 2-4**
**Study by a Task Force of Hospital Financial Management Association on Shur Statistics**

| Department | Standard Unit of Measure per Manual [13] | More Appropriate Unit of Measure if Available |
|---|---|---|
| Skilled nursing care | Number of patient days | — |
| Intermediate nursing care | Number of patient days | — |
| Residential care | Number of patient days | — |
| Emergency room | Number of visits | Emergency-room minutes or man-minutes |
| Lab—clinical | RVU | — |
| Lab—pathology | RVU | — |
| Operating room | Number of surgical man-minutes | — |
| Labor and delivery | Number of procedures; normal surgical man-minutes; Caesarean sections | — |
| Dietary | Number of patient meals | — |
| Cafeteria | Number of meals served | — |
| Radiology | RVU | — |
| Medical records | Number of inpatient admissions plus one-eighth of total ER services | Average number of medical-records sheets processed for each department serviced |
| Clinic services | Number of visits | Minutes or man-minutes |
| Surgery | Number of surgical minutes | Number of minutes of patient in OR |
| Recovery room | Number of recovery room minutes | — |
| Anesthesia | Number of anesthesia minutes | — |
| Pharmacy—inpatient | Number of inpatient days | Line-item issues |
| Pharmacy—outpatient | Number of line items sold | — |
| Physical therapy | RVU | — |
| Medical-surgical | Number of patient days | — |
| Pediatrics | Number of patient days | — |
| Psychiatry | Number of patient days | — |
| Obstetrics | Number of patient days | — |
| Ambulance service | Occasions of service | Mileage and/or time of round trip to hospital |
| Home health services | Number of residential visits | Mileage and/or time of round trip to hospital |
| Medical-surgical supplies | Number of line items sold | — |
| Blood bank | RVU | — |

**Table 2-4** *(continued)*

| Department | *Standard Unit of Measure per Manual [13]* | *More Appropriate Unit of Measure if Available* |
|---|---|---|
| EKG, EEG, and so on | RVU | — |
| Nuclear medicine | RVU | — |
| CAT scanner | Number of procedures | Should be related to time and resources required |
| Cardiac catheter | Number of procedures | Should be related to time and resources required |
| Inhalation therapy | RVU | — |
| Renal dialysis | Number of hours of treatment | — |
| Occupational therapy | RVU | — |
| Speech pathology | Number of treatments | Should relate to time and resources |
| Recreation therapy | Number of treatments | Should relate to time and resources |
| Electromyography | Number of treatments | Should relate to time and resources |
| Organ acquisitions | Number of acquisitions | Should relate to time and resources |
| Cast room | Number of casts applied | Should relate to time and resources |
| Research projects | Number of research projects | Should relate to time and resources |
| Education | Full-time-equivalent students | — |
| Laundry and linen | Number of dry and clean pounds processed | — |
| Social services | Number of contacts | Should relate to time and resources |
| Purchases | Number of gross square feet | Number of PSs processed: By capital items By supplies |
| Plant operation | Number of gross square feet | — |
| Plant maintenance | Number of gross square feet | Should use direct work orders |
| Security | Number of gross square feet | — |
| Parking | Number of parking spaces | Breakdown by inpatient and outpatient, indoor and outdoor |
| Housekeeping | Number of square feet surfaced | — |
| CSR | Number of inpatient days | Line-item issues, amount of priced requisitions |
| Central transportation | — | Based on time and hours and charged to using department |

**Table 2-4** *(continued)*

| Department | Standard Unit of Measure per Manual [13] | More Appropriate Unit of Measure if Available |
|---|---|---|
| General accounting | Total hospital operating expenses | Should include totals of revenues and expenses |
| Patient accounting | Total gross patient revenue | Patient discharges or days |
| Data processing | Number of minutes of CPU time | — |
| Communications | Number of full-time-equivalent hospital employees | Number of telephone outlets |
| Admitting | Number of inpatient admissions | — |
| Hospital administration | Number of full-time-equivalent hospital employees | — |
| Management engineering | Number of full-time-equivalent employees | Hours of service by department served |
| Personnel | Number of W2 and 1099 forms issued | W2 forms issued |
| Medical library | Number of physicians on active staff | Should be related to number of books and subscriptions handled |
| Medical-staff administration | Number of physicians on active staff | — |
| Medical-care review | Number of inpatient admissions | — |
| Nursing administration | Average number of nursing service personnel or FTE's | — |
| Inservice education | Average number of hours of instruction | — |
| Medical photography and illustration | Number of original prints rendered | Weighted value for originals and reprints |

established specialized functional units for the purposes of analyzing and developing cost-effective systems and procedures. Such units are at times called, for example, management-engineering or systems departments. These are normally staff functions reporting to upper levels of management, reflecting the role that systems development and analysis plays within the entire organization.

*Planning and Analysis of Organizations*

The management-engineering or systems department can be given the responsibility for examining the formal organization of the institutional

MMS and for recommending changes that would improve the cost effectiveness of its services. Clearly, in such an endeavor the systems staff must work closely with administration and with the health providers. As discussed in [11], not to do so in a meaningful way could lead to disaster.

### Analysis and Design of Systems

Systems analysis in health-care settings is discussed in [14] and summarized later in chapters 5 and 6. At this juncture it must be emphasized that the functioning of the entire organization in terms of its activities as it strives to achieve its materials-management and ultimately health-provider goals is very much dependent on the systems and procedures in place.

### Systems Description or Audits of Management

Systems description, or a management audit, is a survey and documentation of the ways in which certain activities of the institution are performed or the manner in which certain departments or even the entire organization goes about its work. Essentially, this is a cost-effectiveness study to measure how well the organization, or parts of it, are being managed.

### Preparation of Written Procedures

A detailed description of the manner in which things are to be done, the policies that are to be enforced and how, and other matters of day-to-day operations fall within the responsibilities of the systems department. These descriptions often employ flow charts. Some are shown in chapter 5 and will be further discussed later.

### Design and Control of Forms

Transmission of information wihtin the organization is usually effected through the use of business forms. The design of these forms and the procedures by which they are transmitted is a field of endeavor that can pay off handsomely in terms of improved cost effectiveness of the materials-information system, the entire materials-management system, and hence the institution.

### Report Analysis

"Business" reports, which are used by the institution to transmit information internally to decision makers and externally to third-party payers, regulatory and government agencies, and the like, are analyzed by the systems department for ways to increase their usefulness. Removing unnecessary and redundant information from a report and adding relevant information are major steps in improving the quality of decisions made by the users of such reports, because these procedures save time and provide decision makers with pertinent information.

## Management of Records

The form in which records are kept and whether they are stored in a way that makes them available when needed and, at the same time, minimizes the cost of their maintenance are other factors that affect efficiency. In fact, management of records has become so important in the last few years that a specialized area within systems work has developed to meet its needs. This area is often called *information retrieval* and is discussed in [15, 16, 17, 18].

## Simplification of Work

Work measurement and simplification is an area of professional expertise that has its roots in the efforts and writings of Fred W. Taylor [19], Frank and Dr. Lillian Gilbreth [20], and so on. Management engineering or the systems department should not limit this activity to production-work measurements in the laundry or dietary departments, but should expand its scope to the evaluation and improvement of the performance of office, clerical, and logistical-support tasks. The same techniques can be employed for all these groups to achieve the same ends—more efficient or cost-effective work methods through simpler and more effective procedures.

Work simplification involves the use of scientifically based methods to analyze business work procedures and to develop more effective ways to get work done. Several basic tools are used in work simplification. These include process flow charts, procedure flow charts, work measurement, work sampling, and time-and-motion studies. Some of these will be discussed later in this book.

Work measurement is a technique of determining the time required to complete a unit of work in comparison with time standards that serve as a basis of control. Work measurement usually involves breaking down the job under study into its most fundamental elements and analyzing these with a view toward increasing the efficiency with which the job is accomplished. Such analysis is familiar to industrial engineers who perform time-and-motion studies in analyzing the repetitive types of work done in manufacturing processes [21, 22]. This type of work analysis has found its way into the office, where clerical procedures are analyzed using the same techniques [22].

*Layout of Equipment and Facilities*

The physical arrangement of service-facility space and data-processing equipment, as well as the general layout of facilities, is often delegated to the management-engineering or the systems department. Once again, this illustrates the close relationship between the providing of health services, on the one hand, and systems on the other, and the procedures involved in the orderly flows of people, information, materials, and so on within any given institution.

*Implementation of Systems and Procedures*

One of the most difficult responsibilities of the systems function is implementing new systems and procedures. It is one thing to design a better way to do things and quite another to persuade others to adopt and properly use these ways. Most systems analysts will acknowledge that the hardest part of their job is dealing with people within the institution and enticing them to change their modus operandi—the way they have been doing things. Yet no matter how well the system is designed, no matter how much more effectively the job will be accomplished with the new system, unless that system is properly implemented, all the effort put into its design is wasted. Systems personnel must always keep in mind that the people in the organization are there primarily to satisfy their own personal goals. Some of these personal goals may at times conflict with those of the institution. For this reason it may be impossible to persuade people to change their methods with the argument of increased organizational efficiency alone. Systems personnel must also be sales personnel in the sense of selling the "product" (a new system or procedure) by appealing to the personal needs and goals of those who must adopt the new system. However, selling the product, as discussed in *Systems Analysis in Health Care Delivery* [14], is infinitely easier if the ultimate "consumer," the client or the user of the systems effort, has been *meaningfully involved* in the development of the new system from inception to completion.

The position of the management-engineering or systems department within the organization, because of its characteristic crossing of functional areas within the organization's systems network, is, as indicated earlier, a staff position by nature. These personnel are typically not line decision-makers, although they have the ability, because of the services they perform for decision makers, to wield a powerful influence over the decisions that are made. Since the advent of automated data processing and its highly technical aspects, decision makers frequently are at the mercy of their data-processing and systems advisors. Thus systems personnel may advise a decision maker that certain types of information are impossible to obtain with the information system available when, in fact, it is perfectly feasible to gather and present the information required by the decision maker. The decision maker, because of his or her lack of technical knowledge of the field, has no way of knowing this and will make do with what he or she has, perhaps making decisions of much lower caliber than would be possible if such additional information were provided.

## Purchasing

The purchasing function is the interface between a health-provider institution and its suppliers. From the supplier side of the interface, the health center is viewed as a customer. Accordingly, the health center is called on by the sales or vendors' personnel and is susceptible to their various marketing strategies. On the other side of the interface, purchasing monitors or acts as a clearinghouse and a pipeline to supplies needed to maintain or provide health-care services. The health provider and support units generate their requisitions, the requests are reviewed and converted to orders, and the filled orders flow back to restock supplies in the operating units of the health center.

Purchases, as indicated earlier, are roughly divided into three categories: maintenance supplies, raw materials, and finished products such as ready-to-use products. The main question is how much to keep on hand; a temporary shortage of styrofoam cups has far less impact on providing services to patients, especially if plastic or paper cups are on hand, than does the absence of X-ray film or heart valves.

### Purchasing Function

Purchasing is a service function that supports the activities of the other health-provider and support functions. In turn, it receives assistance from other operating units. Effective functioning requires a steady and reliable flow of information between concerned departments. The relationship of the purchasing structure to other parts of the institutional system is displayed in figure 2-15.

Health-service providers and support functions are the terminal points for most materials flow and are the initiating points for most materials requests. Two age-old customs color the dealings between purchasing and, especially, the health-provider functions. The first is the "squirrel" or "cover-your-rear-end" complex which causes allied and paraprofessionals to hoard supplies. This protective policy certainly limits the chance of work

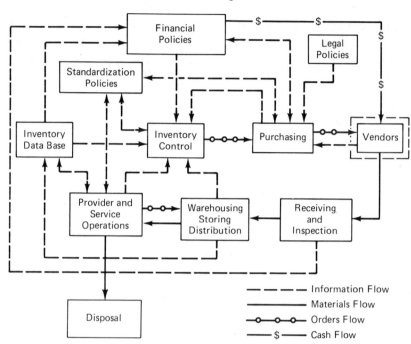

**Figure 2-15**. Interaction of Purchasing with Other Organizational Units

delays occurring owing to a shortage of supplies or materials, but it builds up a big inventory throughout the institution that is subject to damage, loss, obsolescence, and, most importantly, to the cost of the monies tied up. The second custom is a "brand-X" complex, a preference for a particular brand that has previously provided good service or has been used by the doctor or nurse at the place where he or she trained. Again, there are legitimate bases for such feelings because past performance is an indicator of future satisfaction. The troublesome aspect is that new products are continually being developed; a loyalty to one brand eliminates the chance to recognize equal or even higher quality at a lower price.

When these types of actions lead to competent product selection and competitive prices, they are eminently acceptable. When they represent a path of least resistance for writing specifications, they are questionable. Purchasing agents, as contacts for the health center with salesmen from prospective suppliers, often learn about new, lower-cost materials sooner than physicians or nurses. The agents usually do not have the technical knowledge to evaluate new-material developments; therefore, they should have them appraised by those who do. Distribution of appropriate literature or meetings of standardization or quality-evaluation committees, health providers, and suppliers can produce new use patterns and lower procurement costs.

Legal aspects require attention whenever binding agreements are made between the health center and the supplier. Standard forms, already checked for legality, are available for most routine purchases. The larger, longer contracts that incorporate special conditions rate a thorough legal review to ensure that both sides understand their responsibilities. Health-center lawyers can also assist purchasing by the interpretation of new legislation or existing laws applicable to fair pricing, misrepresentation, rebates, freight rates, and similar subjects.

*Receiving* personnel report the quantity and quality of supplies received. Purchasing uses this information to appraise the supplier's performance: When shipments are late, purchasing initiates contacts with vendors to determine the state of progress and to expedite matters. Reimbursements or allowances are negotiated for shipments damaged in transit. After a shipment is accepted by receiving, it is moved to the requisitioning department or to inventory-storage areas.

*Accounting*, at times through a data-processing system, pays for the shipments after receiving notification of their arrival and acceptance. Prompt notification is often necessary to take advantage of cash discounts awarded for quick payments. Actions taken to speed deliveries and to secure reimbursement for damaged shipments should be reported because either accounting or the materials-management information system also handles the internal paperwork of inventory records, invoicing checking, and other financial details for material transactions.

Purchasing functions are usually coordinated by a purchasing department. There appears to be a trend in industry, and more recently in various kinds of health centers, toward grouping purchasing along with other materiel-oriented functions within a single materials-management department; and I am in sympathy with this trend. The intricate network of information channels and the high dollar volume of activity make purchasing a prime candidate for system coordination. By combining material procurement with control, many communications lines are shortened and purchasing policies are likely to achieve greater strategic effectiveness.

Centralized purchasing, as practiced by most health institutions, indeed by some regional hospital associations, is a step toward systematization. Passing all orders through one office allows consolidated purchasing. Buying in greater quantities may lead to cash discounts. Purchasing agents can specialize in certain accounts and negotiate more effectively with suppliers. However, centralization tends to reduce flexibility and may be less sensitive to local needs or peculiarities of individual physicians. Frequently, these disadvantages are reduced by central purchasing of high-cost, high-volume supplies while allowing local control of small nonstock items. Decentralization of authority for some purchases does not necessarily dilute the principles of centralization if the wielders of such authority follow the institutional objectives.

In summary, purchasing does the following:

It receives information from:
    Vendors regarding
        Availability of materials
        Price (price breaks)
        Lead times
        Shipping costs
    The financial functions regarding
        Cash-flow consideration
        Lease-versus-buy policy
        Make-versus-buy policy
        Vendor-handling policy

    Inventory Control regarding
        Requisitions
            Specifications
            Quantities
            Due dates

Purchasing transmits information to:
    Inventory Control regarding
        Availabilities
        Lead times
        Price information, including price breaks
        Shipping costs
        Reorder costs

Purchasing should:
    Find the vendors who will supply the items at
        A. Least cost
        B. Equal or better quality than specified
        C. The right time
            Early deliveries are not always appreciated because of
            Cash-flow considerations
            Storage considerations
        D. Endeavor to maintain multiple sources of supply
        E. Endeavor to guarantee uninterrupted supply
        F. Make enlightened tradeoffs between A, D, and E

Purchasing requires different decision rules for:
    Consumables

        For manufacturing or processing
           Raw materials
           Components
           Subassemblies
        For services
           Repair parts
           Supplies
    Durables (capital goods)
        Plant
        Equipment

Decision rules for purchasing of:
    Durables (capital goods)
        Payback period
        Discounted cash-flow analysis
           Present worth
           Equivalent annual cost
           Rate-of-return method
    Consumables
        Economic lot-size formulas
        Requirements planning
        Min-max
        Reorder point-economic order quantity (EOQ)
        Break-even analysis

Purchasing is a service function.
    It serves
        Operations
        Health-care delivery
        Dietary
        Pharmacy
        Central Processing
        Laundry
        Maintenance
        Housekeeping and so forth

    It should not control operations
        By design
        By happenstance
        Overtly
        Covertly

Purchasing often serves the double duties of Purchasing and of Inventory Control. In such organizational structures control of operations through materials control is quite proper if the double function is recognized and accepted, and appropriate compensating controls are clearly understood and applied.

*Example of a Purchasing-Policy Statement*[a]

*Areas Affected*: All divisions, services and departments of the Cleveland Clinic Foundation

*Effective Date*: January, 1977

*Policy Responsibility*: Administrative Council

*Policy*: The Purchasing Department is to provide centralized procurement and control of all supplies, equipment, and materials used in the Foundation; and to assure that there is an uninterrupted flow of these items in order that the Foundation's efficiency may be maintained. It is recognized that there are certain commodities or services that, because of their unique nature, must be acquired in a decentralized manner.

*Procedural Guidelines*:
1. The Director of Purchasing shall direct the activities of the department in accordance with the job description for that position.
2. Inventoried items must be acquired as a result of competitive bidding, and will be resubmitted for new quotations in a time frame no greater than that of a year. Non-inventoried items must have competitive bids obtained from at least three suppliers for all acquisitions. The following exceptions will apply:
   a. When limited by an existing standardized system.
   b. When previous bidding has resulted in standardizing on one brand which is available from one vendor.
   c. When there is only one source of supply.
   d. When there is an emergency order and the time required for the bidding process would be detrimental.
   e. Whenever practical, all requisitions valued in excess of $500.00 shall have competitive quotes.
3. A regular review of inventoried items shall be conducted in order to prevent loss through obsolescence and/or deterioration. Inventory investments are to be kept at minimum in order to preclude the unnecessary use of cash assets.
4. All orders are to be awarded on the basis of the most advantageous cost to the Foundation. All considerations being equal, preference should be given to local companies in support of community relations and good will.
5. As a matter of policy we will support the Greater Cleveland Hospital Association and other group purchasing organizations. Group purchasing, where applicable, should be considered since it may be advantageous in obtaining economies and controlling price increases.

---

[a]I am indebted to Mr. Paul Widman, director of operations, Cleveland Clinic Foundation, for permission to reproduce this material.

6. The Purchasing Department shall insure that the Foundation's name is not used for an endorsement of any commercial commodity or organization.
7. Purchases of goods and services for the personal use of the employees will not be made by the Purchasing Department.
8. A record keeping and retention system shall be maintained for all requisitions, bids and purchases. Cross referenced must be achieved and retention shall be for a period of seven years. These records are subject to review and audit on a periodic basis.
9. A formal automatic expediting system shall be established to insure that items are delivered within a reasonable period of time.
10. Purchasing will assist, on an advising basis in the disposal of surplus or scrap material in accordance with the following priority: All sales must be made at current fair market value for the goods.
    a. Sale of items
    b. Gifts to charitable organizations
    c. Removal at no cost
    d. Payment to have items removed
11. Purchasing will participate in all standardization programs which are essential to quantity procurement. This program is to include generic name pharmaceuticals and form controls.
12. Purchasing will subcontract for services that are beyond the resources of the Foundation and negotiate leasing agreements, when it is determined that this is the most advantageous means of making acquisitions.
13. Procedures shall be developed for the filing of transportation claims which will insure speedy recovery of losses which result from damage in shipment.
14. All orders will be issued by the Purchasing Department and these orders are to be sent directly to the vendor. Cancellations or alterations are to be done through the Purchasing Department. Normally, orders will be issued only after a firm price has been determined.
15. All Leases and Contracts will be submitted to the Legal Department for review prior to committing to any agreement.
16. All Purchasing Department activities shall be in accordance with the "Principles and Standards of Purchasing Practice" issued by the National Association of Purchasing Management or the basic Code of Ethics.

The Purchasing Department is to be a product information resource for the Foundation and the following is considered necessary to insure that this service meets with the requirements of the various using departments.

1. Developing alternate materials that can be used as a substitute when necessary.
2. Market study and cost analysis should be an ongoing activity.
3. Keep abreast of the factors that regulate supply and demand and thus the price and availability of materials. Additionally, this requires a constant search for better values that yield the best combination of price, quality and service.
4. The need to have a current, broad based, product information library is recognized.

The using department will comply with the following:

1. Initiate all requisitions in writing on a "Purchase Requisition Form" and plan their requests in such a manner that will allow for the most economical acquisition.
2. All requisitions require the personal signature of specified authorized personnel.
3. The Purchasing Department will consult with the requisitioning department in order to obtain information on the items to be purchased. They may suggest alternatives that would more appropriately meet the department's needs or that of the Foundation.
4. Matters that cannot be resolved between the Purchasing Department and using department will be referred to the appropriate Administrative Director for his decision.
5. Purchases of a capital equipment which are $500.00 or greater will be referred to the Equipment Committee and the using department will be notified of this action.

In order for the full potential of the purchasing policy to be realized, the following should be observed:

1. All requests for samples or product information should be channeled through the Purchasing Department.
2. All interviews with company representatives are to be coordinated through the Purchasing Department.
3. Negotiations, commitments and expressions of opinion of a binding nature on the merit and acceptability of a product are not to be considered in the discussion between vendors without prior concurrence and discussion with the Purchasing Department.
4. No individuals will divulge any information regarding the source of supply of any product, competitive performance or past prices paid for such products and/or services.
5. Purchasing Department will check quantities ordered for conformance with manufacturers standard packaging and quantity discounting.
6. Items that are placed in inventory by a particular department must be completed prior to the replacement of that item.
7. Inventories within individual departments are to be kept at a minimum. These storage areas are subject to periodic audit by the Internal Auditor and/or the Purchasing Department.
8. Request for equipment on a trial basis will be made through the Purchasing Department and this should be contracted for on a formalized purchase order.
9. The Purchasing Department upon specific authorization will utilize electronic data processing systems in order to more efficiently conduct their operation.

Appendix 2E provides a checklist that includes questions one might ask to establish the extent to which the purchasing department promotes competition between vendors and suppliers. Moreover, audit procedures, for institutional measures to develop vendor competition, are also provided in appendix 2E.

*Purchasing Processes and Procedures*

Purchasing responsibilities begin with a decision to buy certain materials, and they end when the material is received and accepted by the institution. Many procedures are involved in this process.

A requisition for acquisition or replenishment of materials at user locations typically represents the beginning of a purchasing cycle. The cycle ends with payment to the vendor for goods or services received and delivered in acceptable form to the original requisitioner. The purchasing function includes some but clearly not all responsibilities throughout the cycle. Some of the more important responsibilities and procedures are discussed next.

**Receipt of Requisitions.** Purchase and replenishment requisitions, depending on the MMS structure, can be made out by personnel from many if not all functional areas of the health center. The requisition forms include information as to what and how many items are wanted and which unit or who is making the request and, in some cases, when materials requisitioned should be available. A column for "quantity on hand" can be included to force the requisitioner to check whether this replenishment is truly needed at this time.

The elapsed time between placing an order and its receipt is known as lead time. It plays a significant role in purchasing and in inventory control. Many purchasing departments urge requisitioners to anticipate materials demands well ahead of actual need, or they keep buffer inventories in the warehouse or central supply room. Early requests act as buffers against the consequences of unexpected delivery delays. Allowing a long lead time also means that larger inventories must be kept in order to cover the anticipated needs during the longer wait between ordering and receiving. Requisitioners certainly should be award of a minimum lead time. The purchasing department should attempt to correct suppliers' delivery delays instead of automatically increasing allowed lead times.

**Reviews of Requisitions.** *Value analysis* is performed to study the functions materials are supposed to accomodate. Value analysis represents a relatively recent trend for the purchasing function. This technique refocuses attention from obtaining the *best price* for a certain item to finding the *lowest cost* for any item that will satisfy an intended function. The analysis answers such questions as: Could a less-expensive product serve the same function? Is the function necessary? Could it be eliminated? Could other items serve the same function? Can they be simplified? Could the supplier reduce the price by a cooperative redesign or by revised specifications? Incentive clauses promoting the use of value analysis are widely included in U.S. government contracts. Savings from the value program are split at a given rate, such as 90 percent to the government and 10 percent to the vendor.

Purchasing generally does not have the authority to substitute or modify the materials designated by the health providers or even by the service units. It does have the responsibility, especially for the high-dollar-value items, to question requistions and to suggest alternatives available at better prices. When the original requisitioners know that their requests will be scrutinized, they will pay more critical attention to such decisions.

Value analysis usually identifies three types of value, each having a distinct relationship to cost and function:

*Use value*—a monetary measure of the qualities of an item that contribute to its performance.

*Esteem value*—a monetary measure of the properties that contribute to its acceptability or desirability.

*Exchange value*—a monetary measure of the qualities and properties of an item that enable it to be exchanged for something else.

Use of the value-engineering approach should be guided by the following equation:

$$\text{exchange value} = \text{use value} + \text{esteem value}$$

When applied to the purchasing of, say, stationery, this equation would require first assigning a dollar value for any writing materials and then placing a price on the worth of options or accessories, such as fancy letterheads or colored paper. The exchange value, then, is the amount that must be paid to satisfy the other functions: It is a value established by comparison and not by any other means.

In applying this equation, the emphasis clearly must be on the *use* value. One way to focus on the use function is to force a description by two words, a *verb* and a *noun*. For instance, the primary function of packaging boxes is to "protect contents." A secondary function could be to "create impressions" or to "explain contents." This value analysis focuses attention on the primary issue of *use* as opposed to the inadvertent (but not common) focus on the frivolous or secondary functions that may unnecessarily increase cost.

Purchasing employees have the knowledge of suppliers' offerings and competitive prices. Medical and technical personnel have the knowhow for technical comparisons. Health providers and supporting-function personnel know what services they need and the practical limitations for substitutions. It takes a creative, questioning attitude in a cooperative effort to identify new ways to do something, to evaluate these innovations, and to get them accepted by users. Standardization committees, including representatives from the ranks of physicians and surgeons, administrators, nurses, technologists, pharmacists, and so forth, are excellent sponsors of value analysis and implementation. It should be recognized, however, that some practices tend to discourage the recognition and acceptance of change. According to Riggs [25] these are; (1) inability or refusal to gather all the facts; (2) failure to explore all possible ways to perform a function; (3) decisions made based on what is believed to be true rather than on facts; and (4) habits that were formed in the past and attitudes that keep them from changing.

**Selection of Suppliers.** Sources of supplies originate with the vendor's sales-personnel contacts; advertisements in trade or professional journals; descriptions of products in buyer's guides, mailers, or correspondence; inspection tours of plants; and experience with a supplier's products. From combinations of such sources, an *approved-supplier list* is developed. The list results from rating the vendors according to such criteria as quantity of product, price schedules, services offered, and delivery reliability. An approved list is usually developed for each class of supplies. Thus a purchasing agent merely has to contact a few acceptable suppliers to obtain quotes on price and delivery.

An up-to-date and complete list of suppliers is helpful in getting better prices and services. New sources should be continually sought and developed. The performance of existing vendors should be continually monitored to see if the poor performances have improved or if the better vendors have become careless. Some suppliers offer exceptional technical assistance, training programs, equipment-borrowing privileges, and other inducements. When such services are helpful, the appropriate vendor should be known.

Shipping costs may at times swing the total cost advantage from a distant vendor with low prices to a nearby vendor with somewhat higher prices. Most institutional buyers distribute large orders among two or more suppliers to provide a competitive check on the major supplier. In this case, one supplier often receives 50 to 75 percent of the orders. This policy also helps protect against delivery defaults stemming from mismanagement, strikes, fire, or natural catastrophes. However, a trend toward what is known in the trade as prime-vendor contracts is beginning to be discernable [23].

A checklist for the existence and use of a value-analysis program, as well as audit procedures for applications and use of value analysis in product selection, are both provided in appendix 2F.

*Placement of orders.* Purchasing procedures for nonstandard-stock- or individual-item requisitions clearly differ from procurement of standard-stock items or continuous purchases. Moreover, procedures for very large purchases differ from those for very small purchases.

The purchase price of low-cost, infrequently needed items may be less than the cost of processing a purchase order. Such processing costs may range from $10 to $100 per order or higher. The absurdity of incurring processing costs greater than the amount of the order is evident. Institutions often have a petty-cash account for purchases of less than a certain dollar value. Typically, an open account is established with a vendor who inventories many minor but occasionally required items. The vendor keeps track of direct orders and periodically bills the buyer. Purchasing negotiates the original open contract and monitors payments to keep the practice from getting out of control.

Individual purchase orders are avoided for standard-stock or continuous-demand items by blanket purchase orders. Such contracts differ from open contracts in that the orders are generally predictable and are for relatively homogeneous items such as X-ray film, antibiotics, or food supplies. A price for such materials may be negotiated annually, with deliveries made on request during the year. The list price is changed for each delivery, but a discount based on total annual quantity is usually obtained at the end of the year. Both the buyer and the seller receive benefits from the agreement. The buyer can negotiate at one time for a substantial portion of annual supplies, thus reducing order-processing costs. The seller, assured of a market for his products, can reduce his advertising and other promotional expenses. Blanket purchasing often is applied to only a portion of annual demand, say 60 percent, in order to maintain a competitive bargaining position for future transactions.

*Monitoring of orders.* Important, involved, or extensive orders should be checked on an ongoing basis by purchasing personnel to establish whether delivery schedules will be maintained. Production and shipping difficulties owing to labor unrest or materials shortages at the supplier or at his vendors, or due to change orders from within the supplier's own firm, can occasionally put the purchasing agent in an uncomfortable position. The original requisitioners will blame late delivery on purchasing personnel's lack of followup. The supplier blames order changes requested by the agent's colleagues within the provider institution for the delays. The purchasing agent replies to both that there is not enough time to monitor every order with every vendor, especially when so many end up marked "CHANGED-RUSH."

Such sensitive issues emphasize the need for coordination in material management, as they are not uncommon. Open channels of communication are the key to cooperation. Purchasing acts as the communication conduit between the institution and its vendors.

*Receipt of materials ordered and arrangements for payment.* Receipt of a contract for a quantity of supplies in an acceptable condition triggers the completion of the purchase transaction. Records of the purchase are consolidated and payment is made. Depending on the contract, the final price may be subject to a trade, quantity, or cash discount. In some contracts, however, escalation clauses may increase the final price.

Questions one might ask in evaluating purchasing procedures, as well as purchasing-accounting procedures, are delineated in two checklists provided in appendix 2F. Audit procedures for purchasing-department accounting functions are also provided in appendix 2F.

### Supplier-Performance Evaluation

In their pamphlet "Evaluation on Supplier Performance" (New York, 1963), the National Association of Purchasing Agents outlined a plan for numerically rating suppliers. The plan attaches a dollar value to each of four major procurement factors: price, quality, delivery, and service. Thus the supplier who consistently provides the required material at the lowest net-value cost is, in theory at least, most frequently selected. The net-value-cost evaluation procedure is summarized as follows:

*Step 1.* Net delivery price = list price − discounts + freight cost + insurance, taxes, and so on.

*Step 2.* Quality/cost ratio = $\dfrac{\text{material quality costs}}{\text{total value of purchases}}$

The material quality costs are taken from past quality reports on purchases made from each supplier. These expenses include the cost for laboratory tests, incoming inspections, processing inspection reports, handling and packaging rejects, spoilage and waste, and manufacturing losses. The yearly trend of the ratio indicates whether quality levels are being maintained or improved by the supplier.

*Step 3.* Acquisition cost ratio = $\dfrac{\text{acquisition and continuity costs}}{\text{total value of purchases}}$

The denominator of the equation is the same as in step 2. The numerator is derived by the purchasing department from the cost of sale negotiations, communication tools, surveys, premium transportation, monitoring, and progress reporting.

$$\textit{Step 4.}\ \text{Delivery cost ratio} = \frac{\text{acquisition cost ratio}}{+\ \text{promises} = \text{kept penalty}}$$

The cost of deliveries later than promised is expressed as a percentage of the total value of purchases delivered.

$$\textit{Step 5.}\ \text{Service cost ratio} = \frac{\text{maximum possible rating} - \text{supplier rating}}{\text{maximum possible rating}}$$

(A supplier rating below a given level, such as 60, automatically makes the ratio = 1.0.) Service costs are determined from absolute ratings of special considerations that suppliers offer with products and services. These ratings are converted to a penalty percentage and charged against the supplier lacking the considerations. The following list illustrates how a supplier-service cost ratio of $(100 - 75)/100 = 0.25$ could be obtained.

| Maximum Points | Category | Supplier Rating |
|:---:|:---|:---:|
| | Competence and ability: | |
| 15 | Product development and advancement | 10 |
| 15 | Product leadership and reputation | 10 |
| 10 | Technical ability of staff | 8 |
| 10 | Capacity for volume production | 9 |
| 10 | Financial solvency and profitability | 8 |
| | Attitudes and special considerations: | |
| 5 | Labor-relations record | 4 |
| 10 | Business approach | 8 |
| 5 | Field service and adaptability to changes | 3 |
| 10 | Warranty conditions | 6 |
| 10 | Communication of progress data | 9 |
| 100 | Total points | 75 |

*Step 6.* Net value cost = net delivery price + (net delivery price × sum of ratios from steps 2, 4, and 5)

The comparison of suppliers is based on their present net delivery price modified by additional costs expected from the history of their past performance. For instance, a net-value cost for one supplier could result in the following price and penalty pattern:

Step 1: Price quote ($100,000) − discount (10% × $100,000) + freight ($500) = net delivery price ($90,500)

Steps 2-5: Sum of ratios = quality cost (2.2%) + delivery cost (1.2%) + service cost (0.3%) = 3.7%

Step 6: Net value cost = $90,500 + $(90,500 × 0.037) = $93,848.50

Such ratings are then compared for each order to identify the preferred supplier.

A checklist for supplier-performance evaluation is provided in appendix 2F and audit procedures for supplier-performance evaluation are also provided in appendix 2F.

## *Types of Contracts and Unit Prices*

One of the major aids available to a buyer in search of fair, reasonable, or lowest unit prices consistent with adequate standards of quality is the contract-type option. The type of contract selected for any purchase directly affects the unit prices. In determining the best type of contract in any given purchase, the buyer must consider all available contract types and the factors influencing the use of each. Some of the more important factors influencing contract-type selection are:

1. The number of potential vendors and the competition among them.
2. The vendor's cost and production experience in manufacturing these or similar items.
3. The availability, accuracy, and reliability of pricing data in general.
4. The extent of the business risk involved for the vendor.
5. The extent to which inflation is expected to affect the items under consideration.

Selection of contract type would not be a problem if it were always possible to purchase on a fixed-price basis. However, purchasing many items on a fixed-price basis is costly and wasteful in a rapidly changing economic and technological environment.

There are two basic types of contracts: *fixed-price* contracts and *cost-type* contracts.

Fixed-price contracts include:
    firm fixed price
    fixed price with escalation clauses
    fixed price with redetermination clauses

> maximum price
> flexible price
> fixed-price incentive
> firm fixed-price level of effort

Cost-type contracts include:
> cost plus a percentage of cost
> cost plus fixed fee
> cost plus incentive fee
> cost without fee
> cost sharing
> time and materials
> letter contracts

*Fixed-Price Contracts*

**Firm Fixed Price.** Such contracts are most preferred by buyers. There is an agreement for the buyer to pay a specified price when the seller delivers what was purchased if a fair, reasonable, and/or lowest price can be arrived at either by competition or by adequate price or cost analysis. A firm fixed-price contract requires minimum administration; it gives the seller the maximum incentive to produce efficiently; and all financial risks are borne entirely by the seller.

**Fixed Price with Escalation.** In contracts extending over long periods and involving large sums of money, vendors do not prefer to quote firm fixed prices, especially during an inflationary period. If forced to make a commitment in such situations, vendors will include in their quotations contingencies for increases in labor and materials costs, but not in overhead. Such contingencies may not materialize. Thus, to avoid paying for something not received, the buyer should negotiate escalation clauses. These clauses provide for either upward or downward price changes reflecting material- and/or labor-rate changes. Upward adjustments are either limited to some percentage figure or are tied directly to reliable and timely price indexes. The two most commonly used indexes are the Bureau of Labor Statistics' Wholesale Price Index (for materials) and the Wage and Increase Series by Standard Industrial Classification (for labor).

**Fixed Price with Redetermination.** In escalation-type contracts the amounts of labor and material required to complete the contract are known, but wages and material prices are unknown. Price redetermination is used when the amounts of labor and material (and in some cases their prices also) are unknown at the time the contract is negotiated but are expected to become known with some production experience. This, then, is a temporary or estimated fixed-price contract.

However, the earlier in the life of a contract that price redetermination can be made, the more effective is this type of contract. (Thirty-percent completion is a typically satisfactory redetermination point.) *Maximum price redetermination* provides that prices can only be adjusted downward at the time of redetermination. *Flexible price redetermination* means that price adjustments can be made upward or downward; however, an upward limit of some percentage is usually imposed.

**Fixed-Price Incentive.** This type of contract is used when a reasonable target price can be established but the exact pricing cannot be initially established. This is a variant of the redetermination type of contract. It provides for a *target price*, a *ceiling price*, and a *variable-profit* formula, depending on the type of contract for which it is used. Although this type of contract is now used routinely by industry, it is still basically involved in high-cost capital acquisitions as opposed to materials purchases.

**Firm Fixed-Price Level of Effort.** This type of contract is primarily used for research and development, that is, when the work cannot be precisely described in advance but the quality and quantity of effort required to accomplish it can be both described and agreed on. Under this type of contract, the seller is obligated to a specified level of effort, for an agreed-on time and for an agreed-on fixed price.

**Cost-Type Contracts.** These types of contracts should only be used when any of the fixed-price types of contracts cannot be invoked, as in a case of having to develop some new material, process, or instrument. *Under cost-type pricing, the buyer assumes almost all the financial risks.* Generally, sellers are guaranteed reimbursement for all their allowable costs up to a predetermined figure, regardless of performance. Beyond this figure they do no additional work unless the buyer agrees to provide more money. Typically, sellers are also guaranteed a fee in addition to their costs. Therefore, under a cost contract, a seller has no effective incentive to keep down costs, and therefore prices. In addition to the obvious disadvantage to a buyer, cost-type contracts are very expensive to administer. All costs that are allowable must be agreed on in advance and subsequently must be audited and reconciled. This requires a rather elaborate accounting system in order to be workable.

**Cost Plus Percentage of Cost.** From a buyer's perspective, this is the most undesirable of all types of contracts. Despite the obvious fallacy of the concept, "the higher the cost the greater the profit," this type of contract is used mostly by the construction industry.

**Cost Plus Fixed Fee**. This contract type stipulates that the seller shall be paid for all allowable costs up to a maximum, plus a fixed fee. The fixed fee is usually a percentage of the estimated cost. For example, if the estimated cost of the contract is $3,000 and a 10-percent fee is agreed on, the fee is $300; the fee remains fixed at $300 even if the cost rises to $4,000 or more or if, on the other hand, it is kept below $3,000. This type of contract is used primarily in research or exploratory studies where the level of effort required to achieve success, if this is at all possible, is unknown.

**Cost Plus Incentive Fee**. Under this variant of the fixed-price incentive contract, the buyer and seller agree on a tentative fee based on estimated costs and then establish target costs. If the seller can keep his costs below the target, then both seller and buyer share in such reduction. Under this type of contract, a seller can lose all or part of his fee; but all his costs must be paid by the buyer. This type of contract is used in development work where successful results are reasonably certain. Target costs are not exact but are considered close enough to provide a basis for rewarding, with incentive fees, any and all management efficiencies.

**Cost Without Fee**. Nonprofit institutions, such as teaching and research hospitals and clinics, usually do research work under government, industry, or foundation grants and contracts without the objective of making a profit. Such research is done under cost-type contracts without a fee. Naturally, the research institution recovers all overhead in addition to any direct personnel or materials costs which, in most cases, include remuneration for faculty, staff, and graduate students for their work on such contracts.

**Cost Sharing**. In some situations an institution doing research under a cost type of contract stands to benefit if the product developed can be used in the services it provides or if the institution wants to benefit society in general. Under such circumstances, the buyer and seller agree on what they consider to be a fair basis to share the costs.

**Time and Materials**. In contracts requiring instruments, equipment, or building repairs, the precise work to be done cannot be predicted in advance. For instance, it cannot be known exactly what must be done to a malfunctioning diagnostic instrument until it is opened and examined. It may have a faulty electrical contact, or it may need the replacement of an entire circuit board. One method of pricing this type of work is the time-and-materials contract, in which the parties agree on a fixed rate per labor hour that includes overhead and profit, with materials supplied at cost.

**Letter Contracts**. Letter contracts should be used rarely. However, they may be used in situations of high urgency requiring work to start immediately on a complex project or a portion of some materials to be sent expeditiously. Letter contracts are preliminary authorizations so that the seller can commence work immediately. He can prepare drawings, obtain required materials, and start actual production. Under letter contracts, the seller is reimbursed for his costs up to a specified amount. Letter contracts should be converted to definite contracts at the earliest possible date.

*Single-Source-Supplier Concepts*

The preceding section discussed various forms of contracts that health-provider institutions may draw on in dealing with suppliers. Also discussed were the attributes of multiple sources of supplies, especially in a competitive environment. Inasmuch as recent practice and the literature are showing an interest in the single-source supplier concept [23], it is imperative to give some attention to this notion as it need not be totally inconsistent with the multiple-source theory and that could entail any one of the contract forms discussed.

Under this concept of buying, the single-source supplier, in consideration of a long-term contract, promises to supply the institution in a timely fashion with all its needs for the range of products under contract. The supplier undertakes to stock all items in its warehouse, thus minimizing the need for one or more stocking echelons within the institution, such as central stores or CSRs. According to Paul Neuman [23], some "single suppliers" involve many distributors or dealers around the country organized and incorporated as a profit-making cooperative, owned equally by each participating dealer.

The system entails an initial storeroom evaluation of a year's purchases. The dealer would actually request to see every purchase order issued during the prior year for the range of supplies being considered for contract. He would analyze how the institution's stockroom is set up and operating. He would look for quantities of repeat items, duplications, and obsolete merchandise.

The dealer then draws up a requisition list of standard supplies that the company will stock for immediate availability. The system also provides for special orders. The dealer will also redesign the stockroom layout, since the requisition list (see figure 2-16) under this system is actually broken down according to stockroom location of each item to facilitate inventory-control inspection.

This form is used by the buyer to draw supplies once a month. Keypunched by the dealer, it generates computer reports each month. These reports give the buyer such information as a list by item showing cost, year-to-date usage, inventory balance, a list of items consumed by each department, and a list of dollars charged to each department.

## OSOS OFFICE SUPPLIES REQUISITION

| DEPARTMENT NUMBER |
| --- |

| ACCT. NO. | DATE | REQUISITIONER | DEPARTMENT NAME |
| --- | --- | --- | --- |

**Instructions:** This requisition will be key punched and, in turn, the information will be used to print-out the stockroom reorder and departmental charge back. Write only in the quantity column. Correct errors with liquid correction fluid. Do not cross out or make check marks in this column. Please order in multiples of "unit pack" only, no fractions or decimal changes of any kind. Example: a dozen pens which have a unit pack of "each" must be ordered as "12" and not as "1 doz". This form is part of a copyrighted and patented program of Office Supply Order Systems · Corporate Headquarters 22 Okner Parkway, Livingston, New Jersey 07039.

| CODE | QUANTITY NO. OF UNITS | UNIT PACK | LOC. | DESCRIPTION | CODE | QUANTITY NO. OF UNITS | UNIT PACK | LOC. | DESCRIPTION |
| --- | --- | --- | --- | --- | --- | --- | --- | --- | --- |
| 1000 | | XX | | **OFFICE SUPPLIES** | 1290 | | ea. | C-17 | Pencils Colored Yellow Omega 804 |
| 1005 | | ea. | 31 | Add Tape 2¼" | 1295 | | ea. | C-22 | Push Pins |
| 1010 | | ea. | 31 | Add Tape 2½" | 1300 | | box | C-23 | Reinforcements TD909 |
| 1015 | | ea. | 31 | Add Tape 3" | 1305 | | ea. | 34 | Ribbons Selectric 71 3330-09200 |
| 1020 | | ea. | Bulk | Blotter 20x34 Blue | 1310 | | ea. | 34 | Ribbons Marathon 3222-08805 |
| 1025 | | bx/100 | 32 | Carbon Paper Letter Type 7-40 | | | | | |
| 1030 | | pad | 32 | Carbon Marathon Film Blk. 8½x11 | | | | | |
| 1035 | | ea. | C-1 | Cement Best Test 4 oz. | 1450 | | XX | | **LOOSE LEAF SUPPLIES** |
| 1040 | | bx/100 | C-2 | Clips Paper No. 1 | 1455 | | ea. | 35B | Binders Acco Press BF3007 Red |
| 1045 | | bx/100 | C-3 | Clips Paper Giant | 1460 | | ea. | 35C | Binders Acco Press BF2507 Red |
| 1050 | | ea. | C-4 | Clips Binder No. 20 Small | 1465 | | ea. | 35C | Binders Acco Press BG1702 Black |
| 1055 | | ea. | C-4 | Clips Binder No. 50 Medium | 1470 | | ea. | 35B | Binders Data 11¾x8½ 14-128NJ Blue |
| 1060 | | ea. | C-4 | Clips Binder No. 100 Large | 1475 | | ea. | 36 | Binders Ring Black 1" Cap. 68-989 |
| 1065 | | ea. | C-5 | Correction Fluid Liquid Paper White | 1480 | | ea. | 36 | Binders Ring Black 1½" Cap. 68-985 |
| 1070 | | ea. | C-5 | Correction Fluid Liquid Paper Canary | 1485 | | ea. | 36 | Binders Ring Black 2" Cap. 68-982 |
| 1075 | | ea. | C-5 | Correction Fluid Liquid Paper Goldenrod | 1490 | | ea. | 37 | Covers DuoTang 1258 Yellow |
| 1080 | | ea. | C-5 | Correction Fluid Liquid Paper Green | 1495 | | ea. | 37 | Covers Duo Tang 1258 Grey |
| 1085 | | ea. | C-5 | Correction Fluid Liquid Paper Buff Ledger | 1500 | | ea. | 37 | Covers DuoTang 1258 Green |
| 1090 | | ea. | C-5 | Correction Fluid Liquid Paper Green Ledger | 1505 | | ea. | 37 | Covers DuoTang 1258 Black |
| 1095 | | ea. | C-5 | Correction Fluid Liquid Paper Thinner | 1510 | | ea. | 37 | Covers DuoTang 1258 Dk. Blue |
| 1100 | | ea. | C-6 | Erasers Pink Pearl No. 100 | 1515 | | ea. | 37 | Covers DuoTang 1258 Lt. Blue |
| 1105 | | ea. | C-6 | Erasers Type No. 1087 | 1520 | | ea. | 37 | Covers DuoTang 1258 Red |
| 1110 | | ea. | C-7 | Fasteners Paper No. 2 1/2" | 1525 | | ea. | 38 | Folders VPD 9½x14¾ KS-4 Clear |
| 1115 | | ea. | C-7 | Fasteners Paper No. 3 3/4" | 1530 | | box | C-29 | Index Tabs Aico 1/3" clear |
| 1120 | | ea. | C-7 | Fasteners Paper No. 5 1¼" | 1535 | | set | 39 | Index 11x8½ P 1-213-8 color |
| 1125 | | 100 | 32 | Index Cards 3x5 white ruled | | | | | |
| 1130 | | 100 | 32 | Index Cards 5x8 white ruled | | | | | **SPECIAL ORDER ITEMS** |
| 1135 | | ea. | C-7 | Ink Stamp Pad Black 2 oz. | | | | | |
| 1140 | | ea. | C-7 | Ink Stamp Pad, Red 2 oz. | | | | | |
| 1145 | | ea. | C-7 | Ko-Rec-Type White | | | | | |
| 1150 | | sheet | 32 | Labels Avery Address 5275 | | | | | |
| 1155 | | sheet | 32 | Labels Avery 1-1½ S-1624 | | | | | |
| 1160 | | sheet | 32 | Labels Avery 4x2 S-6432 | | | | | |
| 1165 | | sheet | 32 | Labels Avery 1½x3 S-2448 | | | | | |
| 1170 | | 10 | 32 | Labels Assoc. Gum 4x2½ No. 2008 | | | | | |
| 1175 | | ea. | C-8 | Markers Fine Tipped No. 30 Black | | | | | |
| 1180 | | ea. | C-8 | Markers Fine Tipped No. 30 Red | | | | | |
| 1185 | | ea. | C-8 | Markers Fine Tipped No. 30 Blue | | | | | |
| 1190 | | ea. | C-9 | Markers Fine Tipped No. 30 Green | | | | | |
| 1195 | | ea. | C-10 | Markers HiLiter Yellow Carter No. 774 | | | | | |
| 1200 | | ea. | C-11 | Markers Markette 680 Black | APPROVED BY: | | | | |
| 1205 | | ea. | C-11 | Markers Markette 680 Red | | | | | |

Reprinted with permission from Office Supply Order Systems, Livingston, N.J.

**Figure 2-16.** Office-Supplies Requisition Form

The promoters of this system say that these reports are management-information tools that allow the administrator to account for pilferage, waste, and obsolescence. They claim that studies show that 20 percent of stationery stock generally goes home, 10 percent is repairable (but un-repaired and consigned to the wastebasket), and 5 percent of obsolete items are returnable but gather dust on stockroom shelves. Since the dealers participate on a cooperative basis, they are able to service national accounts as readily as can neighborhood institutions or firms.

Other systems offer a "stockless" type of system in which the dealer says, in essence, "Let us be your stockroom." The buyer issues an open purchase order, with the dealer having a contract on certain items. Dealers provide catalogs of items from which buyers order directly (this is how the previously discussed concept handles special orders). This system is computerized; buyers receive a monthly inventory report by department or cost center, plus a usage report.

Other single suppliers offer half-and-half stockless/stocked inventory concepts that include furniture items, such as files, in addition to consumables. They may also utilize preprinted requisition forms that can be filled out as often as every day. This approach, it is claimed, is economical wherever the volume is large enough. A computerized printout breaks out products by kind and dollars expended, charging them to ordering departments.

Single-supplier enthusiasts claim that the buyer organization can thus obtain supplies at low prices while reducing carrying and reorder costs and minimizing exposure to pilferage, damage, and/or obsolescence.

In contemplating a single-source contract, consideration must be given to the potential loss of buyer advantage when sellers are constantly in competition and to the requirements for auditing the vendor's reporting performance.

Clearly this approach to buying must be considered, when available, as one of a number of alternatives or options. The choice should be based on an analysis in terms of benefits and costs, including risks, performed on each alternative approach before a contract is written, signed, sealed, and delivered.

A checklist for evaluating purchasing functions, as well as audit procedures for the same, are provided in appendix 2F.

## Purchasing-Department Ethics

### General Statement of Ethics

As indicated earlier, the purchasing department in general, and the buyers in particular, are the link between a health-provider institution and its outside materials and equipment vendors. Specifically, institutional purchases involve substantial dollar volume. No discussion of the purchasing functions would be complete without addressing and encouraging a code of ethics. Many health-care institutions have embraced the principles and standards of the purchasing practice, as advocated by the National Association of Purchasing Management. This statement is as follows:

> To consider the interest of the institution in all transactions and to carry out and believe in its established policies.

> To be receptive to competent counsel from colleagues and to be guided by such counsel without impairing the dignity and responsibility of the office.

> To buy without prejudice, seeking to obtain the maximum ultimate value for each dollar of expenditure.

> To strive consistently for knowledge of materials and processes of manufacture, and to establish practical methods for the conduct of the purchasing office.

> To subscribe to and work for honesty and truth in buying and selling, and to denounce all forms and manifestations of commercial bribery.

> To accord a prompt and courteous reception, so far as conditions will permit, to all who call on a legitimate business mission.

> To respect his obligations and to require that obligations be respected, consistent with good business practice.

> To avoid sharp practice.

> To counsel and assist fellow purchasing agents in the performance of their duties, whenever occasion permits.

> To cooperate with all organizations and individuals engaged in activities designed to enhance the development and standing of purchasing.

*Conflict of Interest and Employee Purchases*

In addition to subscribing to the Code of Ethics of the Purchasing Management Association, many health centers provide statements of policy regarding conflict of interest as well as that of employee purchases. The following paragraphs represent one such policy statement. (reproduced with permission from the Materials Management Manual, Cleveland Clinic Foundation (CCF), 1977).

*Conflict of Interest*

1.  Any C.C.F. employee who has any financial or other interest in a C.C.F. supplier or potential-supplier company either directly or indirectly through members of immediate family, and has direct or indirect input into C.C.F. Specifications and/or price negotiations with that supplier's or potential supplier's products shall so report such financial or other interests, in writing, to his Department Head or Administrative Director for immediate submission to the C.C.F. Vice Chairman, Board of Governors responsible for Operations.
2.  The Vice Chairman, Board of Governors responsible for Operations will decide whether the interest in question is of sufficient magnitude to warrant the disqualification of the employee concerned from becoming involved with the C.C.F. Specifications and/or pricing for the products in question.

*Employee Purchases*

1.  Purchases of goods and services to be paid for by C.C.F. or C.C.F. employees and for the personal use of the employees will not be made by the Purchasing Department. Exceptions to this policy may possibly exist for uniforms and/or materials and clothing such as safety shoes, goggles, gloves, etc. worn by employees to promote their safety and health or to improve their working conditions. The exception items will be so designated by the Director of Purchasing, approved by the Director of Materials Management and Director of Administrative Services, and will be available for review in the Purchasing Department.
2.  Whenever surplus obsolete machinery, tools, furniture, supplies, or equipment becomes available for disposition, such items may be sold to employees, by the Director of Capital Equipment Control, only at prices at least equal to those attainable through normal outlets. Accurate records of such transactions including, item specifications, price, the employee buying the item, the date of transaction, etc. will be maintained by the Director of Capital Equipment Control and the Accounting Department.

A checklist of questions for evaluating purchasing ethics, as well as audit procedures for the same, are provided in appendix 2F.

## Receiving and Central-Stores Activities

Receiving and central-storage functions constitute one of the important phases in the materials-management cycle. Regardless of the efficiency with which requisitioning, purchasing, and the other inventory-management activities are conducted, the health providers will be supplied satisfactorily only if the receiving and stores functions are effectively coordinated with the other aspects of the MMS.

*Responsibilities of Receiving and Central Stores*

Receiving and central-stores operations perform service and control functions. From a managerial viewpoint, they exist for three reasons. First, they provide a service for the "mainline" operations, namely the health-provider and related activities. The physicians, nurses, physiotherapists, and so on can better perform the functions for which they are best qualified if someone else is specifically designated to organize and control the physical flow of needed materials. Second, the receiving and stores organization acts as a custodial and controlling agency. It is responsible for the physical status and control of a substantial portion of the institution's "lifeblood,"—its supplies. Third, the existence of stores permits quantity or volume purchasing and the attendant cost savings in price, paperwork, and handling.

*Specific Responsibilities*

The receiving function or unit is responsible for receipt, logging in, expeditious identification, and general inspection of all incoming materials. Receiving also is responsible for notifying all interested parties of the receipt and of the condition of incoming material in a timely and effective fashion through the established materials-management information system (MMIS) procedures directly or on a by-exception basis.

The central-stores department bears responsibility for safe and accessible, technically sound physical storage of all materials prior to their distribution to ultimate user locations.

The central-stores department must protect materials in its custody against shrinkage, unauthorized usage, and unnecessary damage or deterioration. It must also adequately classify, mark, and locate all materials so as to maximize their accessibility for distribution to user locations when and as needed. Finally, the central-stores function must control the physical issuance of all items in a manner that provides effective service for the mainline operations.

*Cost Implications*

Receiving and central-stores activities indirectly influence costs of running a health-service facility in several ways. Costs owing to deterioration and pilferage of materials, as well as costs of stores labor, clearly depend on the way these activities are organized and managed. An alert central-stores organization along with a good MMS can help reduce costs of obsolescence by developing check systems to detect inactive materials. Similarly, efficient use of scarce storage space can further reduce costs.

The stores operation can also exert a direct influence on labor costs. Timely service for "production" personnel, such as laboratory technicians and dietary workers, can help reduce the unproductive time of such workers. Workers and facilities waiting for materials delivery add nothing to the productive effort of an institution.

### Receiving of Materials

Receiving is basically a clerical activity but is nonetheless important. It is at the receiving desk that paperwork directing the flow of purchased materials meets the actual materials as they first enter the system at the receiving dock. Thus any discrepancy, problem, or error (shortage in quantity, damaged materials, wrong items shipped) in a specific transaction should become evident during the receiving operation. If the problem is not detected and acted on during the receiving operation, the cost of correcting the mistake later will be much higher. For example, if a shortage in quantity is not discovered at the time of receipt, any combination of departments can be drawn into the problem later. Many hours are frequently spent in resurrecting what happened and in rectifying the situation. Hours are required to correct an error that could have been corrected at the receiving dock in minutes.

The report completed by the receiving clerk upon receipt of a shipment is the only document an institution possesses detailing the materials actually received. The document is the basis for invoice payment, for continued purchasing negotiation, and for closing the order. Therefore, accuracy in this activity cannot be overemphasized. Since poor receiving performance can have costly consequences, receiving should be supervised by personnel who are reasonably familiar with the physical characteristics of the materials purchased and capable of exercising sound judgment in situations where a choice of alternatives must be made.

Receiving is an important control point in a materials-management system. Receiving records show which suppliers are consistently late in their deliveries, which have the maximum number of rejects, and which deliver the greatest number of split shipments. Any of these supplier failures is costly to the buyer. Close coordination between purchasing and receiving is thus essential; however division or segregation of responsibilities is desirable wherever possible in order to minimize opportunities for inappropriate, collusive action between the purchaser and the receiver.

### Receiving Procedures

A typical receiving procedure consists of four steps:
1. Unloading and checking shipments for:

a.  The number of containers and/or units unloaded by the shipper.
b.  The number of containers and/or units on the freight bill.
c.  Comparison of a and b.
d.  Inspection of containers or units for any externally visible damages.
e.  Notifying the shipper regarding any discrepancies or problems in the above.
2.  Unpacking and inspecting the shipment.
a.  Verification of the materials received, with the seller's packing slip, and with the corresponding purchase order.
b.  Verification of the quantity of the shipment.
c.  Inspection of the general condition of the materials received.
3.  Completion of the receiving report. Notification of material received is typically sent to the requisitioner—the ultimate user in some cases but most generally the central supply room and/or inventory-control activity; the purchasing department; the accounting department; and, where appropriate, the technical-inspection department. This report should indicate:
a.  Items and quantities received.
b.  Items and quantities on purchase order not received.
4.  Delivery of the material. Depending on the institution's systems and procedures, the receiving unit must either direct or deliver the materials to the proper stocking location. This may be:
a.  A warehouse, a central supply room, or the ultimate user location. The recipient of the materials signs off on the receiving report upon delivery of the material, thus relieving the receiving clerk of any further responsibilities.

Appendix 2G provides a checklist for evaluating materials-receiving functions, followed by recommended audit procedures for the receiving function.

## Materials Storage

Physical storage and movement of materials might be considered analogous to the operation of filing systems. As with a filing system, the objective is to place and to withdraw materials as rapidly and economically as possible. The following are some of the more-efficient ways of locating materials in storage spaces.

### Systematic Storage Procedures

**Storage by Part Number**. In this procedure, the units are stored in the sequence of their stock numbers.

In general, this system of storing by part numbers is suitable for small items and units of issue having similar characteristics and a fairly uniform quantity on hand. Tongue depressors, syringes, sutures, and similar items that are used in small quantities can be stored very conveniently by this method. For large cartons of such items, however, there are better storage systems.

**Storage by Coordinate-Index Number.** In this procedure the storage area is laid out in a coordinate-index system, and a cross-reference is established between the stock part number and the index. One way of setting up the index is to number the storage spaces as in figure 2-17. The aisles are numbered in sequence, as are the rows and levels of bins. A number, such as 4-2-4, would indicate the bin in the fourth aisle, second column, at the fourth level. A number designating the particular storage area could have been added as another digit.

However, since many stock-number systems in health institutions focus on the category or family of the item, instead of locating material by stock number, the location of the material is shown on the inventory record or on a special index sheet. This requires a little more time in the record keeping but permits greater flexibility and more efficient utilization of space. If

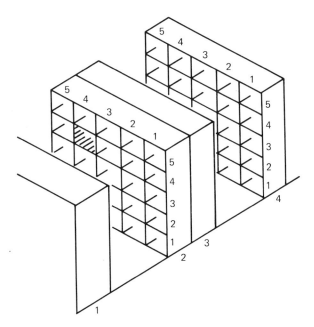

**Figure 2-17.** Storage by Coordinate Index

there are excess items for a certain area, they can overflow into another space as long as the cross-reference is made. When the inventory is reduced, the space can be utilized for other purposes.

**Storage by Serial Index Number.** Rather than establish the index number by coordinates, some storerooms prefer to number storage spaces in sequence. This has some advantage for areas that are not perfectly rectangular. Personnel unfamiliar with the locations might take longer to find any particular item. There is also some advantage in this system since the numbers need not be in blocks as in the coordinate system.

**Storage by Frequency of Use.** Some storerooms, especially pharmacies, have made extensive studies to determine their most frequently used material. Those products that are withdrawn most often are located near storage-area exits. Other organizations, in particular pharmacies, place some of these materials near the point of use and maintain additional material in remote storage areas. This latter method is likely to make the record keeping somewhat more complicated. The index-number method is still quite suitable for frequency-of-use storage procedures.

*Complicating Aspects of Storage*

There are many reasons why storage of materials becomes more complicated than would appear necessary. In attempts to conserve space, institutions often allocate less-than-prime space to storerooms. Inconvenient and undesirable space is often used. Frequently the space is not symmetrical, so it becomes difficult to install standard racks and nearly impossible to lay out the space in order to take advantage of a uniform indexing system. Often the space provided is in out-of-the-way locations, with inadequate access for materials-handling equipment.

Often city ordinances and fire-insurance policies require that inflammable materials be placed in remote locations. Some materials have disagreeable or corrosive characteristics that make it desirable to have them located away from the usual storage area.

Heavy items and materials that have to be handled by materials-handling equipment should be placed near corridors with sufficient access for the moving equipment necessary.

As indicated earlier, at times material can be stored at the point of use, as is often the case with X-ray film. This can save money by reducing the warehouse-supervision costs. However, this should be done only if the value of the material is so small as to be unimportant, or its size and shape such that it cannot be carried out without being detected—neither of which is true of X-ray film. The latter consideraton is especially important for items having a high "street value," such as syringes and even linen.

Audit procedures for the central stores in an institution are delineated in appendix 2G.

## Charging and Billing

Charging and billing for supplies used or consumed are two interrelated functions. Patients have traditionally been billed for certain items used by them or in their behalf, such as specialized medications. Most housekeeping supplies, on the other hand, cannot now be billed to the patient. They are often charged to the using department. Current trends, however, indicate that patients or their insurers will be presented with itemized bills that will include an ever-increasing variety of consumables and even of reusable supply items.

To decide which categories of items are to be billed requires some good cost-benefit analysis, on the one hand, and often negotiation with the third-party payers on the other. Clearly, it would be folly for anyone to insist that institutions keep records on how many tongue depressors were used on a given patient on a given day. The quantity and the type of intravenous (IV) solution consumed or the number and type of sterile-instrument packs opened, used, and returned are yet another matter.

To an ever-increasing extent, institutions in the future will rely on "charging" committees working closely with "standardization" committees within the institution and with representatives of the third parties, such as health insurers, Blue Cross, Blue Shield, government, and so on for decisions about which items can be billed directly to the patient. These committees will be further discussed in chapter 4.

Regardless of whether a given item can be billed if it is stocked in a given department or module, then it must be charged to that organizational unit at the time of delivery. Deciding what is the lowest organizational level to be used for charging purposes, for example, a department or a module, is again clearly a matter of cost effectiveness. As indicated earlier, in this chapter it is a matter of tradeoffs between better more-detailed control, which is offset by the greater need for paperwork and record keeping. Inasmuch as issues of billing and also of charging are matters of concern to several functional and administrative functions of the institution, the materials-management information system must therefore meaningfully interface with the other management information systems such as accounting. Materials-management information systems will be discussed in greater detail in chapter 3.

The appendix 2H to this chapter provides some further food for thought regarding the charging functions in the form of a checklist for evaluation of materials-charging functions and in terms of suggested audit steps for charging procedures.

## References

1. Housley, C.E. "Distributing the Goods the Right Way." *Hospitals, JAHA* 51, no. 12, June 16, 1977.
2. Housley, C.E. *Hospital Materiel Management*. Germantown, Md.: Aspen Systems Corporation, 1978.
3. Housley, C.E. "The Case for Centralized Purchasing." *Dimensions in Health Service* 54 (March 1977).
4. Lammers, L. "Facilities Design and Equipment." *I.M.M.S. Hospital Material Management Seminar*. Los Angeles: Loyola Marymount University, January 27-28, 1976.
5. Housley, C.E. "Materiel Management Means Savings and Space." *Dimensions in Health Service* 54 (January 1977).
6. Bregande, B.J. "Unit Management Techniques and the Interface between Material Management and the Nursing Staff." *I.M.M.S. Hospital Material Management Seminar*. Los Angeles: Loyola Marymount University, January 27-28, 1976.
7. Rose, G.W. "Objectives of Hospital Material Management." *I.M.M.S. Hospital Material Management Seminar*. Los Angeles: Loyola Marymount University, January 27-28, 1976.
8. Javad, S. "Multi-echelon Inventory Systems in Health Care Delivery Organizations." Unpublished Ph.D. thesis, Case Western Reserve University, 1980.
9. Carroll, Stephen J., Jr., and Tosi, Henry L., Jr. *Management by Objectives: Applications and Research*. New York: Macmillan, 1973.
10. Mitchell, R.C. "Hospital-Wide Inventory Turnover Gives Hospitals Positive Results." *Hospitals, JAHA*, July 1, 1978.
11. Jankowski, Teresa E. "Do Your Rates Reflect Costs?" *Hospital Financial Management* (May 1977).
12. Ruchlin, H.S. "Problems in Measuring Institutional Productivity." *Topics in Health Care Financing* 4, (Winter 1977).
13. SHUR Statistics. *System for Hospital Uniform Reporting*. Washington, D.C.: U.S. Department of Health, Education, and Welfare, Office of Policy and Research, September 29, 1978.
14. Reisman, Arnold. *Systems Analysis in Health Care Delivery*, Lexington, Mass.: Lexington Books, D.C. Heath and Company, 1979.
15. Schmitz, Homer H. *Hospital Information Systems*. Germantown, Md.: Aspen Systems Corporation, 1979.

16. Voich, Dan, Jr.; Mottice, Homer J.; and Shrode, William A. *Information Systems for Operations and Management*. Cincinnati, Ohio: Southwestern Publishing Company, 1975.
17. Bocchino, William A. *Management Information Systems: Tools and Techniques*. Englewood Cliffs, N.J.: Prentice-Hall, 1972.
18. Garrett, Raymon D. *Hospital Computer Systems and Procedures*. New York: Petrocelli/Charter, 1976.
19. Taylor, Fred W. *Scientific Management*, New York and London: Harper and Brothers, 1947.
20. Gilbreth, Frank, and Gilbreth, Lillian. *Applied Motion Study; A Collection of Papers on the Efficient Method to Industrial Preparedness*. New York: Sturgis and Walton Company, 1917.
21. Harold B. Maynard, ed. *Industrial Engineering Handbook*. New York: McGraw-Hill, 1971.
22. Barnes, Ralph M. *Work Sampling*. Dubuque, Iowa: W.C. Brown Company, 1956.
23. Neuman, Paul. "New Systems for Controlling Supplies." *Administrative Management* (April 1979).
24. Barnes, Ralph M. *Motion and Time Study: Design and Measurement of Work*. New York: John Wiley and Sons, 1968.
25. Riggs, James L. *Production Systems: Planning, Analysis, and Control*. New York: John Wiley and Sons, 1970.
26. Cantor, Jerry. "Evaluating Purchasing Systems." American Management Association, 1970.
27. Leenders, Michiel R. "Improving Purchasing Effectiveness Through Supplier Development." Boston, Mass.: Division of Research, Graduate School of Business Administration, Harvard University, 1965.
28. Bolton, Ralph A. "Systems Contracting: A New Purchasing Technique." American Management Association, 1966.

# Appendix 2A: Checklist for an Effective Supply-Cart-Exchange System

|  | Comments<br>*(Provide data on "yes" answers. Explain "no" answers.)* | |
| :--- | :---: | :---: |
| *Questions* | *Yes* | *No* |
| A. Does the exchange cart contain all supplies needed by a user location? | _____ | _____ |
| B. Does the exchange cart contain a twenty-four-hour supply? | _____ | _____ |
| C. Is the exchange cart totally inventoried every twenty-four hours? | _____ | _____ |
| D. Is the cart covered at all times? | _____ | _____ |
| E. Is the cart wiped clean daily? | _____ | _____ |
| F. Is the cart replenished by a responsible trained attendant? | _____ | _____ |
| G. Is there an effective way to charge using departments? | _____ | _____ |
| H. Are supplies "charged off" of inventory at times of replenishment? | _____ | _____ |
| I. Are there individualized unit quotas? | _____ | _____ |
| J. Are quotas reviewed quarterly? | _____ | _____ |
| K. Are the carts tagged at the time of inspection? | _____ | _____ |
| L. Are the exchange carts cultured at least quarterly? | _____ | _____ |
| M. Are the exchange carts distributed manually? | _____ | _____ |

*Comments*
*(Provide data on*
*"yes" answers.*
*Explain "no"*
*answers.)*

| *Questions* | *Yes* | *No* |
|---|---|---|
| N. Are carts restocked and distributed on the right shifts? | ____ | ____ |
| O. Are the carts restocked and distributed in an assembly-line process? | ____ | ____ |
| P. Is an evaluation conducted as to the effectiveness of the program at least semi-annually? | ____ | ____ |
| Q. Does the cart system provide the nursing units and departments with a total medical-surgical supply system? | ____ | ____ |
| R. Does the supply-cart system provide the right supply item at the right place at the right time and in the right quantities? | ____ | ____ |
| S. Does the supply-cart system relieve the nursing units and other related departments of all of the non-nursing functions of inventory, requisitioning, recording, delivery and processing of supplies? | ____ | ____ |
| T. Does the supply-cart system effectuate a practical system of control of "unofficial inventory" that had already been expensed and dispensed to the various units? | ____ | ____ |
| U. Does the supply-cart system place full responsibility and accountability in the Materials Management Department for the functions of supply, process and distribution? | ____ | ____ |
| V. Does the supply-cart system help in implementing a system of accountability for patient charges? | ____ | ____ |

# Appendix 2B: Checklist for Evaluating a Materials-Management Infrastructure

This appendix is based on "Checklist and Guidelines for Evaluating Purchasing and Materials Management Functions in Private Hospitals: Opportunities for Improving Hospital Purchasing, Inventory Management and Supply Distribution" part II, U.S. General Accounting Office, PSAD 79-58B, April 1979.

*Comments*
*(Provide data on*
*"yes" answers.*
*Explain "no"*
*answers.)*

*Questions*

|  | *Yes* | *No* |
|---|---|---|
| A. Does one department or official, such as a materials manager, centrally manage and supervise purchasing, inventory, and supply distribution? | _____ | _____ |
| B. If yes, is that department or official responsible for: | | |
| 1. All supplies and equipment including food and pharmaceuticals? | _____ | _____ |
| 2. All contract services? | _____ | _____ |
| C. Is there a written policy statement: | | |
| 1. Describing objectives for purchasing, inventory management, and supply distribution? | _____ | _____ |
| 2. Centralizing management of purchasing, inventory and supply distribution? | _____ | _____ |
| 3. Delegating purchasing, inventory, and supply-distribution functions to other departments, and monitoring and controlling delegated functions? | _____ | _____ |
| 4. Covering a code or standard of conduct governing the performance of purchasing and supply personnel as well as contractors | _____ | _____ |

| *Questions* | *Yes* | *No* |
|---|---|---|
| D.  Does one department control institutional inventories, including departmental "floor" stocks? | _____ | _____ |
| E.  Is there a central storeroom from which departments requisition supplies? | _____ | _____ |
|    1. Are there written procedures for the organization and operation of central stores (including requisitioning and distributing stock items)? | _____ | _____ |
|    2. Is access to the storeroom area restricted to supply personnel? | _____ | _____ |
|    3. Are properly authorized requisitions required for obtaining items from central stores? | _____ | _____ |
|    4. Is there a stock-numbering system? | _____ | _____ |
|    5. Is there a catalog of centrally stored items? | _____ | _____ |
|    6. Are major items such as intravenous solutions, X-ray film, and sutures stocked in central stores? | _____ | _____ |
|      a. If not, are inventories of these items controlled by a central manager | _____ | _____ |
|    7. Is there a list of inventory items that have expiration dates, and are these items reviewed regularly? | _____ | _____ |
|    8. Is the inventory reviewed periodically to remove static, slow-moving, or obsolete items? | _____ | _____ |
|    9. Is the stock properly rotated? | _____ | _____ |
|   10. Are there controls against pilferage? | _____ | _____ |
|   11. Is there adequate storage space? | _____ | _____ |
| F.  Are annual physical inventories reconciled with accounting-department control accounts? | _____ | _____ |

*Comments*
*(Provide data on*
*"yes" answers.*
*Explain "no"*
*answers.)*

| *Questions* | *Yes* | *No* |
|---|---|---|
| 1. Is the physical inventory taken or supervised by a member of another department (such as the accounting department)? | _____ | _____ |
| 2. Is the physical inventory verified by the hospital's external auditors? | _____ | _____ |
| G. Does a central manager have responsibility for the inventory—determining safety stock levels, reorder points (or review periods), and order quantities (maximum quantities) of each item (The parameters in parentheses correspond to a periodic review policy.) | _____ | _____ |
| H. Is there a product evaluation and standardization committee? | _____ | _____ |
| 1. Does a written statement define its responsibilities, membership, and functions? | _____ | _____ |
| 2. Are formal minutes of the meetings filed? | _____ | _____ |
| 3. Are medical staff, administration, pharmacy, nursing, materials management, and fiscal management all represented? | _____ | _____ |
| 4. Are acceptable product standards and specifications obtained or written for each item considered? | _____ | _____ |
| 5. Are value-analysis techniques used? | _____ | _____ |
| 6. Are the committee's decisions communicated to the hospital staff? | _____ | _____ |
| I. Is there a pharmacy-and-therapeutics committee responsible for standardizing pharmaceuticals? | _____ | _____ |
| 1. Does a written statement define its responsibilities, membership, and functions? | _____ | _____ |

|  | *Comments (Provide data on "yes" answers. Explain "no" answers.)* | |
| :-- | :--: | :--: |
| *Questions* | *Yes* | *No* |
| 2. Are formal minutes of the meetings filed? | _____ | _____ |
| 3. Does the committee consider and endorse generically equivalent items unless it has evidence for not using them? | _____ | _____ |
| 4. Has the committee developed specific criteria to guide its brand selections? | _____ | _____ |
| 5. Are the committee's brand selections communicated to the medical staff? | _____ | _____ |
| J. Do centralized distribution systems, such as PAR-level or exchange-cart systems, control medical-surgical supplies issued to nursing stations and other units? | _____ | _____ |
| K. If materials replenishment is accomplished by departmental requisitions: | | |
| 1. Are departmental inventory levels and reorder points established by a central manager? | _____ | _____ |
| 2. Are floor stocks monitored for stockpiling, obsolescence, and waste? | | |
| 3. Are floor stocks included in periodic physical inventories? | _____ | _____ |
| L. Is a PAR-level or exchange-cart system used for distributing linen? If so: | _____ | _____ |
| 1. Are department quotas based on usage? | _____ | _____ |
| 2. Are additional requests for linen monitored? | _____ | _____ |
| M. Where requisitions are used: | | |
| 1. Are units monitored for excess linen? | _____ | _____ |
| 2. Has management considered use of PAR-level or exchange-cart system for linen distribution? | _____ | _____ |

|  | Comments<br>*(Provide data on<br>"yes" answers.<br>Explain "no"<br>answers.)* | |
|---|---|---|
| *Questions* | *Yes* | *No* |
| N. Are periodic physical inventories taken of all linen in the hospital? | _____ | _____ |
| O. Are records maintained of linen usage by department? | _____ | _____ |
|    1. Is department usage monitored for potential misuse of linen? | _____ | _____ |
| P. Does management periodically compare the quantity issued with linen returned by departments? | _____ | _____ |
| Q. Is new linen kept in central stores before use? | _____ | _____ |
| R. Are there procedures to control requisitions received after regular working hours? | _____ | _____ |
| S. If pharmacy staff purchases pharmaceuticals, does the hospital have written instructions for use by the pharmacy? | _____ | _____ |
| T. If so, are there specific instructions that: | | |
|    1. Cannot be changed without review by the purchasing chief or central manager and approval by top management? | _____ | _____ |
|    2. Restrict the pharmacy's purchases to pharmaceuticals, requiring it to requisition capital items and supplies through purchasing? | _____ | _____ |
|    3. Promote maximum use of competition? | _____ | _____ |
|    4. Encourage the pharmacy to purchase generic drugs that are less expensive than brand-name drugs? | _____ | _____ |
|    5. Permit purchases from local retail pharmacies in emergencies only? | _____ | _____ |

|  | *Comments (Provide data on "yes" answers. Explain "no" answers.)* | |
|---|---|---|
| *Questions* | *Yes* | *No* |

U. Do the pharmacy's written instructions require:

   1. Issuing purchase orders for all purchases, including those from local pharmacies and other hospitals?     \_\_\_\_\_     \_\_\_\_\_

   2. Prenumbering and controlling purchase orders?     \_\_\_\_\_     \_\_\_\_\_

   3. Controlling and monitoring emergency purchases?     \_\_\_\_\_     \_\_\_\_\_

   4. Separating the duties of purchasing, receiving, storing, and charging (preparing the charge sheet)?     \_\_\_\_\_     \_\_\_\_\_

   5. Sending copies of the purchase orders and receiving reports to the accounting department for invoice verification?     \_\_\_\_\_     \_\_\_\_\_

   6. Preparing a return goods memo, which states the amount of credit expected for all goods returned to the vendor for credit, and sending a copy to the accounting department?     \_\_\_\_\_     \_\_\_\_\_

V. Is the dietary department responsible for controlling inventories of food and other supplies?     \_\_\_\_\_     \_\_\_\_\_

   1. Are there written procedures for the organization and management of the dietary inventory?     \_\_\_\_\_     \_\_\_\_\_

   2. Is the inventory reviewed periodically to remove static, slow-moving, or obsolete items?     \_\_\_\_\_     \_\_\_\_\_

W. If food purchases are made by the purchasing department, do the written instructions require:

   1. Issuing purchase orders for all purchases, including those from local retail stores?     \_\_\_\_\_     \_\_\_\_\_

| | *Comments (Provide data on "yes" answers. Explain "no" answers.)* | |
|---|---|---|
| *Questions* | *Yes* | *No* |

2. Prenumbering and controlling purchase orders? _____ _____

3. Controlling and monitoring emergency purchases? _____ _____

4. Separating the duties of purchasing, receiving, and storing? _____ _____

5. Sending copies of the purchase orders and receiving reports to the accounting department for invoice verification? _____ _____

6. Preparing a return-goods memo, which states the amount of credit expected, for all goods returned to the vendor for credit, and sending a copy to the accounting department? _____ _____

X. If food service is provided by contract or other arrangement, does the hospital:

1. Compare the costs and benefits with those of providing the service in house? _____ _____

2. Audit the contractor's periodic billings for food service and determine the reasonableness of the charges? _____ _____

3. Examine the contractor's records? _____ _____

4. Compare the contractor's charges for food purchases with prices available under group-purchase agreements and other sources? _____ _____

# Appendix 2C: Checklist for Determining if an MBO Program Exists

|  | Comments (Provide data on "yes" answers. Explain "no" answers.) | |
| --- | --- | --- |
| *Questions* | *Yes* | *No* |
| A. Do clear and concise statements of goals and objectives exist? | _____ | _____ |
| B. Are there realistic action plans to obtain these objectives in a set specific time? | _____ | _____ |
| C. Is there a systematic monitoring and measuring of performance and achievement? | _____ | _____ |
| D. Are corrective actions taken when necessary to achieve planned results? | _____ | _____ |

## Checklist for Evaluating an Existing MBO Program

|  | Yes | No |
| --- | --- | --- |
| A. Does the chief executive encourage managerial practices consistent with the MBO program? | _____ | _____ |
| B. Do subordinates participate with their superiors in making certain managerial decisions? | _____ | _____ |
| C. Are objectives expressed in tangible, operationally meaningful, measurable or verifiable terms? | _____ | _____ |
| D. Are written objectives and perceived benefits derived from the MBO program clearly communicated throughout the hospital staff? | _____ | _____ |

| Questions | Comments (Provide data on "yes" answers. Explain "no" answers.) | |
|---|---|---|
| | Yes | No |
| E. Is there a procedure for reducing paper-work? | _____ | _____ |
| F. Is there a formal training program for those not familiar with the MBO program? | _____ | _____ |
| G. Do all employees with authority participate in the training of MBO procedures? | _____ | _____ |
| H. Are there well-defined lines of authority? | _____ | _____ |
| I. Are objectives at all levels in the institution compatible? | _____ | _____ |
| J. Have all MMS departments implemented the MBO program? | _____ | _____ |
| K. Are the objectives of the different departments mutually reinforcing? | _____ | _____ |
| L. Are there both monetary *and* non-monetary rewards for employees? | _____ | _____ |
| M. Do objectives include employee's personal-development considerations? | _____ | _____ |
| N. Are objectives prioritized? | _____ | _____ |
| O. Are objectives set high enough to assure better-than-average performance? | _____ | _____ |
| P. Are time-limit objectives used? | _____ | _____ |
| Q. Do procedures ensure that those involved in objective achievement participate in their formulation? | _____ | _____ |
| R. Do procedures specify compliance standards in terms of accountable performance? | _____ | _____ |

| *Questions* | *Yes* | *No* |
|---|---|---|
| S. Do procedures ensure that there is an understanding concerning the manner in which the achievements of those involved in the objective-achieving process are weighed and measured? | _____ | _____ |
| T. Are action plans formulated to achieve objectives? | _____ | _____ |
| U. Are objectives integrated at all management levels? | _____ | _____ |
| V. Does the system ensure that objectives are reviewed periodically by the manager and his or her superiors? | _____ | _____ |
| W. Are objectives and objectives-standards revised as situations change? | _____ | _____ |
| X. Does the administrations' understanding of materials MBO include:<br>   1. Management and control of the flow of supplies from acquisition to disposition? | _____ | _____ |
|    2. Applying management methods to the supply, processing, and distribution of materials; that is, value-analysis, cost-analysis, and product-utilization studies? | _____ | _____ |
|    3. Centralization of all purchasing functions for control and cost effectiveness? | _____ | _____ |
|    4. Providing the mechanism whereby an atmosphere will prevail to ensure an improved level of patient care through product standardization and evaluation, with emphasis on the quality of care and the containment of costs? | _____ | _____ |

|  | Comments (Provide data on "yes" answers. Explain "no" answers.) | |
| :--- | :---: | :---: |
| *Questions* | *Yes* | *No* |
| 5. Providing for a unified supply, processing, and distribution of goods and services under the same area and supervision? | _____ | _____ |
| 6. Reduction of costly inventories to cost-effective minimums? | _____ | _____ |
| 7. Keeping administration, department heads, and other appropriate parties informed and abreast of changes in equipment, products, and supply methods? | _____ | _____ |
| 8. Meeting or exceeding all the requirements of the prudent-buyer concept? | _____ | _____ |
| 9. Controlling the amounts of unofficial inventory by quarterly physical inventories and/or stockless purchasing? | _____ | _____ |
| 10. Relieving nursing and other departments of all supply functions—inventory, requisitioning, recording, delivery, and processing of supplies and equipment? | _____ | _____ |
| 11. Providing all consumer departments with a total supply system (always having the right supply at the right place at the right time in the right quantities)? | _____ | _____ |
| 12. Purchasing all supplies and equipment prudently with consideration for cost, service, and quality? | _____ | _____ |
| 13. Improving vendor relations through centralized contacts and sales-representative orientations to the hospital materials-management philosophy? | _____ | _____ |

|  | Comments (Provide data on "yes" answers. Explain "no" answers.) | |
|--|--|--|
| Questions | Yes | No |
| 14. Reducing and containing all direct and indirect operating costs of the total materials function? | _____ | _____ |

## Audit Procedures for MBO Processes

*Objective*: To determine if MBO functions are properly implemented.

*Audit Steps*

1. Ask each department manager
   a. If he (she) has set specific goals for his (her) department and if these goals are written.
   b. How he (she) has arrived at these goals (and ask for supporting data for that decision).
   c. If he (she) has relayed this information to other managers and how was it relayed.
   d. If he (she) has discussed these goals with other involved employees.
2. Obtain a set of written goals and objectives.
   a. Verify that the reasons behind these goals are documented.
   b. Verify that these are updated and revised when needed.
   c. See that all managers have a set that is easily accessible.
   d. Verify that the goals are assigned a specific time in which to be accomplished.
3. Observe the procedures used in trying to achieve the set goals and objectives.
   a. Determine whether the procedures are clear cut to everybody concerned.
   b. Verify that lines of authority are being followed.
   c. Check managers' files for adequate documentation on how procedures are implemented.
   d. Check for a written description of who has what authority.
4. Review the objectives and goals of all of the departments.
   a. To determine whether they are compatible.

    b.   To determine that they have all been reviewed and approved by the top hospital-management staff.

    c.   To see whether there is a procedure for assigning priorities to goals.

5.  Hold a periodic meeting for the MBO staff.

    a.   If new problems are identified, check the method in which this problem is documented and how it is followed up on.

    b.   Check on the method in which achieved results are compared with desired goals.

    c.   If progress toward a goal is too slow, take steps to correct this.

6.  Review the flow of paperwork.

    a.   To determine if communication is satisfactory.

    b.   To check on whether important documents and authorizations are properly filed.

    c.   To determine whether some of the paperwork is unnecessary to accomplish the task.

    d.   To determine whether all paperwork is delivered on a timely basis to the designated person.

7.  If there is a training program for new staff:

    a.   Check to see if there are texts available for the introduction of the MBO program and procedures.

8.  Verify that there is a monitoring system for.

    a.   Analyzing overall institutional goals in the context of individual department goals.

    b.   Evaluating employee performance.

    c.   Determining a long-range plan along with short-run goals.

    d.   Reviewing overall costs of obtaining specified goals.

# Appendix 2D:
# Checklist for MMS
# Audits and Evaluations

This section is based on "Checklist and Guidelines for Evaluating Purchasing and Materials Management Functions in Private Hospitals: Opportunities for Improving Hospital Purchasing, Inventory Management and Supply Distribution," part II, U.S. General Accounting Office, PSAD 79-58B, April 1979.

| *Questions* | *Comments (Provide data on "yes" answers. Explain "no" answers.)* | |
| --- | --- | --- |
| | *Yes* | *No* |
| A.  Is there an audit to evaluate the effectiveness or economy of the various materials-management functions, such as purchasing, inventory management, and supply distribution? | _____ | _____ |
| B.  Does the central manager or top management periodically evaluate the procedures of the various departments involved in materials-management functions: | | |
|     1. Assure consistency with hospital policy? | _____ | _____ |
|     2. Evaluate efficiency of operations? | _____ | _____ |
| C.  Are the hospital's purchasing practices and inventory controls monitored by any of the following indexes: | | |
|     1. Inventory per bed? | _____ | _____ |
|     2. Inventory-turnover rate? | _____ | _____ |
|     3. Purchasing cost per $1,000 of procurement? | _____ | _____ |
|     4. Purchasing cost per purchase order issued? | _____ | _____ |
|     5. Out-of-stock condition? | _____ | _____ |

|  | *Comments (Provide data on "yes" answers. Explain "no" answers.)* | |
|---|---|---|
| *Questions* | *Yes* | *No* |
| 6. Dollar value of inventory? | _____ | _____ |
| 7. Emergency purchase? | _____ | _____ |
| 8. Any other ratios? | | |
| | _____ | _____ |
| D. Does the hospital use an index to track changes in the cost of cross sections of all major-commodity purchases? | _____ | _____ |

# Appendix 2E: Checklist and Audit Procedures for Vendor Competition

## Checklist for Vendor Competition

|  | *Comments (Provide data on "yes" answers. Explain "no" answers.)* | |
| --- | --- | --- |
| *Questions* | *Yes* | *No* |
| A. Is there a written inquiry and quotation practice? | _____ | _____ |
|    1. If so, is the request for quotation the recognized method of securing competitive bids from qualified suppliers of goods and services? | _____ | _____ |
|    2. Are there established dollar limits for requirements of a quote? | _____ | _____ |
|    3. Is a formal inquiry necessary on low-total-cost standard catalog, or emergency purchases? | _____ | _____ |
|    4. Are requests for quotation issued to three or more qualified suppliers a reasonable amount of time prior to execution of the purchase order, contract, or agreement? | _____ | _____ |
|    5. Are inquiries issued only by authorized purchasing personnel, and to vendors that meet proper qualification standards, including credit rating, ability and capacity to produce, and other standards? | _____ | _____ |
|    6. Are periodic requotes (annually, as a maximum) provided as a basis for evaluating the competitive status of an established supplier and for discovering qualified new sources? | _____ | _____ |

|  | Comments (Provide data on "yes" answers. Explain "no" answers.) | |
| :--- | :---: | :---: |
| *Questions* | *Yes* | *No* |

7. Are suppliers who are asked to submit quotations or to develop an improved design normally given an opportunity to "participate in the available business" if they submit the most favorable (best-total-value) bid or design?                    _____          _____

8. Is consideration given to the supplier who provides the initial value-improvement concept?                    _____          _____

9. Are inquiries clearly written and concise, and do they contain adequate information for accurate vendor bids?                    _____          _____

10. Are quotation requests and supporting records and information retained for management review and company or government audit, as appropriate?                    _____          _____

11. Where a purchase is not placed with the bidder having the lowest price, are written explanations filed describing factors supporting the purchase decision?                    _____          _____

12. Particularly on single-source quotations, is there an intensive effort made to establish the value for an item by comparison, cost analysis, or value studies?                    _____          _____

13. Is each set of costs submitted by vendors and evaluated by purchasing as specified in the inquiry, including such cost considerations as transportation point, price breaks, cost and rate analysis, tooling, quality levels, discount terms, and special instructions?                    _____          _____

|  | *Comments (Provide data on "yes" answers. Explain "no" answers.)* | |
| :--- | :---: | :---: |
| *Questions* | *Yes* | *No* |

14. Are specific supplier prices, costs, and other data submitted on quotations generally considered as restricted or confidential information?      _____      _____

15. Are stringent precautions taken not to reveal such information to competitors or unauthorized persons?      _____      _____

B. Is there a written procedure for supplier evaluation and selection?      _____      _____

   1. Before a purchase commitment is made, are prospective suppliers evaluated for their ability to deliver a product or service as scheduled, representing the best combination of required quality, lowest price and final cost, and added service values necessary for customer satisfaction?      _____      _____

   2. Does each purchasing organization have a continuing system for evaluating suppliers and recording supplier performance and qualifications, in order to ensure a top purchasing job?      _____      _____

   3. Does this record cover performance in meeting delivery schedules, quality performance, price and quotation performance, rejection rates?      _____      _____

   4. Does it also evaluate credit and financial data, before-and-after-sales service, research contribution, special design features, supplier facilities, and so forth?      _____      _____

|  | *Questions* | *Yes* | *No* |
|---|---|---|---|

    5. Are new suppliers encouraged to contribute whenever they can to the effectiveness and efficiency of the institution? _____ _____

    6. Are surveys of facilities and business operations conducted by experienced personnel from the several functions to provide a valuable basis for a supplier evaluation? _____ _____

C. Is there a program for verifying the authenticity of vendors and maintaining an approved vendor master file? _____ _____

    1. Does the vendor master file include evaluations of competitive vendors? _____ _____

D. Are there specific routines for approving use of other than low-quoting vendors? _____ _____

E. Are there routines requiring specific authorization for nonstandard purchases ("no-charge")? _____ _____

F  Are there procedures for adequate review and approval of major-project quotations, especially those with high risk factors (such as long cycle, new technology, or nonstandard terms)? _____ _____

    1. Is appropriate approval authority obtained in line with the risk value of the purchase? _____ _____

G. Is there a routine for securing sealed bids, opening sealed bids, and informing bidders of outcome? _____ _____

**Audit Procedures for Institutional Measures
to Develop Vendor Competition**

This section is based on "Checklist and Guidelines for Evaluating Purchasing and Materials Management Functions in Private Hospitals: Opportunities for Improving Hospital Purchasing, Inventory Management and Supply Distribution," part II, U.S. General Accounting Office, PSAD 79-58B, April 1979.

*Objective*: To appraise the hospital's measures to obtain competition.

*Audit Steps*

1.  Obtain the list of prospective vendors and locate the competitive solicitation files for each department with purchasing authority.
    a.  If the institution has a set dollar limit above which competition is required, identify any purchases of the walkthrough items exceeding this limit that have not been competitive.
        i.  Ask the purchasing agent why competition was not obtained.
        ii. If a noncompetitive purchase was necessary, evaluate the procedures followed to assure that a reasonable price was negotiated.
    b.  For each high-dollar-volume walkthrough item available from more than one vendor (but not from the institution's purchase group), review the competitive solicitation files.
        i.  Through discussion with the purchasing agent, users, and other hospitals, identify any vendors not included in the solicitation.
        ii. Determine the reasons for excluding these vendors.
        iii. Examine the contracts covering these items and determine the contract period for each. If the contracts are less than a year, evaluate the department's justification for the shorter period.
    c.  For walkthrough items not bought from the lowest bidder, evaluate the reasons for selecting a higher bid.
        i.  If the purchase was justified as emergency, determine whether the "emergency" could have been avoided with better planning and scheduling.
        ii. If the purchase was justified with other reasons, substantiate them. For example, "better service" is a weak justification if the low bidder provides adequate service.
2.  Determine by discussion with the purchasing agent whether any of the institution's policies, such as a "buy-local" policy, restrict competition.

3.　Where competition has been inadequate, attempt to obtain competitive prices from some of the excluded vendors or from nearby hospitals that use competitive procedures. With this information, estimate the savings obtainable through competitive procedures.
4.　Discuss your observations with the purchasing manager and resolve any questionable areas.

# Appendix 2F:
# Checklist and
# Audit Procedures
# for Purchasing

## Checklist for Evaluating Purchasing Procedures

|  | Comments *(Provide data on "yes" answers. Explain "no" answers.)* | |
|---|---|---|
| *Questions* | *Yes* | *No* |
| A. Are routines established for approving, modifying, and issuing purchase orders? | _____ | _____ |
| B. Are approval limits established for various types of purchases? | _____ | _____ |
| C. Is there periodic independent verification of purchase authorizations? | _____ | _____ |
| D. Is there a program for qualifying and selecting vendors? | _____ | _____ |
| E. Are purchasing employees involved in determining material specifications and vendor capabilities? | _____ | _____ |
| F. Are there routines for obtaining and evaluating competitive quotes? | _____ | _____ |
| G. Is there a routine established for approving use of other than low-quoting vendors? | _____ | _____ |
| H. Is there a program for verifying the authenticity of vendors? | _____ | _____ |
| I. Is an approved vendor master file maintained? | _____ | _____ |

## Checklist for Evaluating Purchasing Accounting Procedures

A.  Is there a procedure for:

| | Comments (Provide data on "yes" answers. Explain "no" answers.) | |
|---|:---:|:---:|
| *Questions* | *Yes* | *No* |
| 1. Investigation of price, quantity, sales terms or other discrepancies between purchase orders and vendor invoices? | _____ | _____ |
| 2. Precluding and detecting duplicate payments? | _____ | _____ |
| 3. Investigating vendor debit balances? | _____ | _____ |
| 4. Control of input to mechanized systems and reconciliation with associated output? | _____ | _____ |
| 5. Inspecting incoming material and routines for filing, recording, and following shortage, damaged, and rejected-material claims? | _____ | _____ |
| 6. Control of advance payment to vendors? | _____ | _____ |
| 7. Ensuring that all cash discounts offered by vendors are taken? | _____ | _____ |
| 8. Determining that all checks are prenumbered and accounted for? | _____ | _____ |
| 9. Control of check usage and verification of disposition of spoiled or voided checks? | _____ | _____ |
| 10. Letting supporting details accompany checks presented for signature? | _____ | _____ |
| 11. Controlling and issuing replacement checks? | _____ | _____ |
| 12. Prohibiting of drawing checks payable to "cash" or "bearer"? | _____ | _____ |
| 13. Proper approval of retainer agreements or special payments? | _____ | _____ |

**Audit Procedure for Purchasing-Department
Accounting Functions**

*Objective*: To evaluate accounting controls over the purchasing operations.

*Audit Steps*

1. Observe and evaluate
   a. Routines established for approving, modifying, and issuing purchase orders.
   b. Routines for obtaining and evaluating competitive quotations.
   c. Program used for qualifying and selecting vendors.
2. Select several purchase orders and
   a. Verify that they have been properly authorized.
   b. Check whether approval limits have been complied with.
   c. Verify that they involve only properly authorized vendors.
3. Select several vendor payment records and determine whether
   a. There was independent approval of checks.
   b. Vendor payments were made on time.
   c. Checks were made out to the proper vendors and prenumbered.
   d. Only authorized personnel issued vendor payments.
4. Check for written procedures on
   a. How to control and record the return of inactive or undeliverable checks.
   b. How to document any special payments.
   c. Issuing replacement checks.
5. When materials are received, observe the procedures for
   a. Verifying and written documentation on the materials received from authorized personnel.
   b. Follow-up routines on any discrepancies in material ordered and material received.
6. Select some vendor invoices and determine whether they were processed for
   a. Arithmetical accuracy.
   b. Cash discounts offered by vendors.
   c. Prompt recording.
7. Evaluate the controls and procedures on
   a. Precluding and detecting duplicate payments.
   b. Investigation of vendor debit balances.

    c.  Input to mechanized systems and reconciliation with associated output.

    d.  Advance payments to vendors.

    e.  Investigation of price, quantity, sales-terms, or other discrepancies between purchase orders and vendor invoices.

**Checklist for Existence and Use
of a Value-Analysis Program**

|  | *Comments (Provide data on "yes" answers. Explain "no" answers.)* | |
| --- | --- | --- |
| *Questions* | *Yes* | *No* |
| 1. Is there a formal procedure for analysis of alternative services, products, and/or supply items? | _____ | _____ |
| 2. Does that procedure require the following information for each alternative: | | |
|   a.  A listing of all alternatives/products? | _____ | _____ |
|   b.  The cost per unit or total cost of each alternative/product? | _____ | _____ |
|   c.  The expected use span of each alternative/product? | _____ | _____ |
|   d.  The possible versatility of each alternative/product? Can the alternative be used by other departments? | _____ | _____ |
|   e.  The possible flexibility of each alternative/product? | _____ | _____ |
|   f.  Does the alternative/product meet the desired standards? | _____ | _____ |
|   g.  Does the alternative/product meet the required standards? | _____ | _____ |
|   h.  Is the alternative/product compatible with the present systems and procedures? | _____ | _____ |
|   i.  Will the use of this alternative/product require employee training? | _____ | _____ |

|  | *Comments (Provide data on "yes" answers. Explain "no" answers.)* | |
| --- | --- | --- |
| *Questions* | *Yes* | *No* |

j. Is purchase the only alternative? _____  _____

k. Will the use of this alternative/ product require additional capital investment? _____  _____

l. Can the alternative/product become a standard for the institution? _____  _____

3. Is the aim of the procedure to choose the most cost-effective alternative/product? _____  _____

4. Are alternatives derived from brainstorming sessions? _____  _____

**Audit Procedures for Applications and Use of Value Analysis in Product Selection**

This section is based on "Checklist and Guidelines for Evaluating Purchasing and Materials Management Functions in Private Hospitals: Opportunities for Improving Hospital Purchasing, Inventory Management and Supply Distribution," part II, U.S. General Accounting Office, PSAD 79-58B, April 1979.

*Objective*: To determine whether the hospital seeks cost reductions by modifying, replacing, or eliminating the materials it buys.

*Audit Steps*

1. Select some of the high-dollar-volume walkthrough items for value analysis. The selection should include routine items, as well as nonstock supplies purchases.
   a. Interview users of each item and determine whether:
      i. The item is necessary.
      ii. Inessential features can be eliminated or other modifications made to reduce cost.
      iii. The item could be made in house at less cost.

    iv. Lower-cost substitutes would satisfactorily serve the same purpose.

  b. Observe the items used by other departments for similar purposes. If different items are used for the same purpose, compare prices to identify a lower-cost alternative.

  c. Contact nearby institutions and determine whether they have been able to eliminate, modify, or substitute for these items.

  d. If the institution has a product evaluation committee, determine whether it has evaluated these items and with what results.

  e. Where potential exists for modifying, replacing, or eliminating an item, calculate the annual savings.

  f. Discuss observations with the purchasing-and user-department managers. If the institution does not have a product-evaluation committee, suggest forming one.

2. If the hospital has a product evaluation committee, review its minutes to determine the extent of value analysis.

  a. Determine how the committee identifies opportunities for value analysis.

  b. Identify some specific items that have been evaluated by the committee, including routine as well as nonstock supplies. Determine for each item the extent to which the committee questioned:

    i. The need for the item and its usefulness.

    ii. Special features included in the specifications.

    iii. The item's cost in proportion to its usefulness and the cost to make it in house.

    iv. The availability of lower-priced alternatives or substitutes.

  c. If the committee did not fully evaluate an item, apply audit step 1 to assess the accuracy of the committee's evaluation.

### Checklist for Supplier-Performance Evaluation

|  | *Comments (Provide data on "yes" answers. Explain "no" answers.)* | |
|---|---|---|
| *Questions* | *Yes* | *No* |
| A. Does the supplier deliver per schedule? | _____ | _____ |
| B. Does the supplier market a product that meets the required quality specifications? | _____ | _____ |

|  | *Comments (Provide data on "yes" answers. Explain "no" answers.)* | |
| --- | --- | --- |
| *Questions* | *Yes* | *No* |

C. Is the supplier active in cost reducing the products and services he supplies to benefit the cost position of his customers? _____ _____
  1. Does the supplier consciously improve packing and handling costs? _____ _____
  2. Does the supplier use standardization of items or sizes to reduce costs? _____ _____
  3. Does supplier utilize substitute materials when applicable? _____ _____

D. Can supplier deliver per routing instructions? _____ _____

E. Does the supplier assist the purchaser by performing the following important acts? _____ _____
  1. Advises of potential trouble? _____ _____
  2. Acts on correction-action requests? _____ _____
  3. Furnishes necessary technical data? _____ _____
  4. Provides adequate technical representation? _____ _____
  5. Maintains technical service in the field? _____ _____
  6. Provides prompt assistance in time of emergencies? _____ _____

F. Does the supplier replace rejections promptly and without undue inconvenience? _____ _____
  1. Are credit memos issued punctually? _____ _____
  2. Does the supplier work with the purchaser to keep rejections at an acceptable minimum? _____ _____

G. Does the supplier invoice correctly? _____ _____

H. Does the supplier accept and honor purchaser routines, for example:

|  | *Comments*<br>*(Provide data on*<br>*"yes" answers.*<br>*Explain "no"*<br>*answers.)* | |
|---|---|---|
| *Questions* | *Yes* | *No* |

|  |  |  |  |
|---|---|---|---|
| | 1. Does not ask for special consideration<br>from purchasing? | _____ | _____ |
| | 2. Does not ask for special financial<br>consideration? | _____ | _____ |
| | 3. Answers questions readily? | _____ | _____ |
| I. | Does the supplier respond to inquiries for<br>quotation promptly? | _____ | _____ |
| J. | Is there little or no need to follow up and<br>expedite delivery? | _____ | _____ |
| K. | Does the supplier submit prompt test<br>reports, drawings, and so on? | _____ | _____ |

## Audit Procedures for Supplier Performance Evaluation

*Product Performance*

*Objective*: To determine that suppliers provide products that meet or exceed performance requirements.

*Audit steps*:

1. Verify from receiving reports that the supplier delivers per schedule.
2. Verify that records are maintained to test required quality specifications.
   a. Verify that supplier quality meets or exceeds specifications. Review incoming inspection procedures and records to validate information kept on supplier quality performance.
   b. Determine whether supplier submits prompt test reports, drawings, and so on.
   c. Verify that the supplier works with the purchaser to keep rejections at an acceptable minimum.

d.  Verify from shipping and receiving records that the supplier replaces rejections promptly.


*Supplier Credibility*

*Objective*: To determine that the supplier not only provides a quality product but does so in an efficient, effective manner.

*Audit steps*:

1.  Determine by reviewing selected supplier invoices that:
    a.  Credit memos are issued punctually.
    b.  Invoices are correct.
    c.  There is little or no need to follow up and expedite corrected invoices.
2.  Review supplier's ability and willingness to cost improve his product.
    a.  Review amount of technical service provided in the field.
    b.  Review records for action on correction requests, assistance in time of emergencies, and advice of potential trouble.
    c.  Determine that records are maintained to validate that the supplier consciously improves package and handling costs, uses standardization of items or sizes to reduce costs, and utilizes substitute materials when applicable.
    d.  Verify that the company properly evaluates and approves supplier changes.
    e.  Verify that written routines are established and written forms are provided to capture these items so that valid judgments regarding credibility can be made. In addition, verify that forms and documents are retained for specified periods of time.
3.  Review terms of invoices and quotes to ensure that supplier does not ask for or receive special financial consideration.
    a.  If special consideration is granted, is proper approval obtained?
    b.  Review that inquiries for quotes are responded to promptly.


**Checklist for Evaluating Materials-
Purchasing Functions**

This section is based on "Checklist and Guidelines for Evaluating Purchasing and Materials Management Functions in Private Hospitals: Opportunities for

Improving Hospital Purchasing, Inventory Management and Supply Distribution," part II, U.S. General Accounting Office, PSAD 79-58B, April 1979.

|  | Comments (Provide data on "yes" answers. Explain "no" answers.) | |
| --- | --- | --- |
| *Questions* | *Yes* | *No* |
| A. Are there written instructions for central and departmental purchasing? | _____ | _____ |
|    1. If so, do they specify procedures for purchases of supplies, equipment, and contract services? | _____ | _____ |
| B. Do the written instructions require: | | |
|    1. Issuing purchase orders for all purchases? | _____ | _____ |
|    2. Prenumbering and controlling purchase orders? | _____ | _____ |
|    3. Purchasing nonstock items only after receipt of properly authorized departmental requisitions? | _____ | _____ |
|    4. Controlling and monitoring emergency requisitions and purchases? | _____ | _____ |
|    5. Separating the duties of purchasing, receiving, storing, and charging (preparing the charge sheets)? | _____ | _____ |
|    6. Sending copies of the purchase orders and receiving reports to the accounting department for invoice verification? | _____ | _____ |
|    7. Preparing a return-goods memo, which states the amount of credit expected, for all goods returned to the vendor for credit, and sending a copy to the accounting department? | _____ | _____ |
| C. Do the written instructions: | | |
|    1. Promote maximum use of competitive procedures? | _____ | _____ |
|    2. Provide for the receiving, controlling, opening, and evaluating of bids? | _____ | _____ |

| | *Comments (Provide data on "yes" answers. Explain "no" answers.)* | |
|---|---|---|
| *Questions* | *Yes* | *No* |

3. Specify that purchases (capital and noncapital) over a certain dollar amount be advertised for competitive bids? _____ _____

4. Require evaluations to determine whether it is more economical to perform services in house than to contract? _____ _____

5. Stipulate conditions under which blanket purchase orders may be used? _____ _____

6. Provide special procedures for noncompetitive purchases? _____ _____

D. Does the central manager or purchasing department:

1. Maintain a list of prospective vendors? _____ _____

2. Maintain written product and performance criteria for prescreening vendors? _____ _____

3. Award contracts for at least a one-year period to obviate frequent rebidding? _____ _____

4. Maintain a bid record to help identify collusion among bidders? _____ _____

5. Control all contracts and warranties? _____ _____

6. Maintain records of purchase-order or contract numbers, vendors, quantities, and prices? _____ _____

E. Does the central manager or the purchasing department:

1. Monitor departmental purchase requisitions for opportunities for consolidation, substitution, standardization, and so forth? _____ _____

| | Comments (Provide data on "yes" answers. Explain "no" answers.) | |
|---|---|---|
| *Questions* | *Yes* | *No* |
| 2. Monitor usage histories for changes in demand? | _____ | _____ |
| 3. Forecast future needs? | _____ | _____ |
| 4. Monitor the purchases made by departments such as dietary, pharmacy, laboratory, and radiology? | _____ | _____ |
| 5. Purchase directly from manufacturers when possible? | _____ | _____ |
| 6. Take advantage of volume discounts? | _____ | _____ |
| 7. Monitor outstanding purchase orders? | _____ | _____ |
| 8. Initiate and monitor cost recovery programs, (for example reclamation on silver from X-ray-film processing? | _____ | _____ |
| F. Does the hospital participate in group purchasing? If so: | | |
| 1. Does purchasing decide whether to buy independently or under group agreements? | _____ | _____ |
| 2. Are specific criteria available for determining which items will be purchased under group agreements? | _____ | _____ |
| 3. Are savings and other benefits from group purchasing evaluated? | _____ | _____ |
| 4. Are group prices periodically compared with those of other sources? | _____ | _____ |
| 5. Where the hospital has a choice of purchasing groups, are potential savings compared for representative items? | _____ | _____ |
| 6. Is there a list of group contracts and the items offered under them? | _____ | _____ |
| G. Does the hospital participate in group pharmaceutical purchasing? | _____ | _____ |
| 1. Must the pharmacy justify in writing independent purchases of items available through the group? | _____ | _____ |

|  | Comments *(Provide data on "yes" answers. Explain "no" answers.)* | |
|---|---|---|
| *Questions* | *Yes* | *No* |

2. Are these justifications periodically reviewed by management and considered before the group-purchasing agreement is renewed? _____ _____

3. Are group prices periodically compared with other sources? _____ _____

4. Where the hospital has a choice of purchasing groups, are potential savings compared for representative pharmaceuticals? _____ _____

5. Is there a list of group contracts and the items offered under them? _____ _____

6. Do the documents (for example, purchase-record form or traveling requisition form) used to record individual purchases indicate the contract (if any) under which the item was purchased? _____ _____

H. Does hospital policy require the pharmacy to competitively contract for its high-dollar-value pharmaceuticals and product groups? _____ _____

1. Does purchasing supply technical assistance to the pharmacy in developing competitive procedures and assure that they are consistent with hospital policy? _____ _____

2. Does the pharmacy maintain a list of prospective vendors? _____ _____

3. Has the pharmacy established written product and performance criteria for prescreening vendors? _____ _____

4. Is the prescreening based on objective evidence instead of subjective preference (such as that generated by vendor advertising), and documented for future reference? _____ _____

|  | Comments *(Provide data on "yes" answers. Explain "no" answers.)* | |
| :--- | :---: | :---: |
| *Questions* | *Yes* | *No* |

5. Are the contracts for at least a one-year period to obviate frequent rebidding? _____ _____

6. Does the pharmacy have written procedures for receiving, controlling, opening, and evaluating bids? _____ _____

7. Does the pharmacy maintain a record (such as a bid history) to help identify collusion among bidders? _____ _____

8. Is a complete file maintained of current pharmaceutical contracts? _____ _____

9. Is there a formal program for identifying vendors not previously solicited? _____ _____

I.   If the hospital participates in group purchasing,
1. Is there a list of group contracts and food supplies offered? _____ _____
2. Must the dietary department justify in writing independent purchases of items available through the purchasing group?
3. Are these justifications periodically reviewed by management? _____ _____
4. Are group prices periodically compared with those of other sources? _____ _____
5. Where the hospital has a choice of purchasing groups, are potential savings compared for representative food supplies? _____ _____

J.   Does hospital policy require the dietary department to contract competitively for its high-dollar-value food supplies? _____ _____
1. Does purchasing supply technical assistance to the dietary department

in developing competitive procedures
and assure that they are consistent
with hospital policy?                                    \_\_\_\_\_        \_\_\_\_\_
2. Does the dietary department maintain
a list of prospective vendors?                       \_\_\_\_\_        \_\_\_\_\_

## Audit Procedures for Purchasing Functions

This section is based on "Checklist and Guidelines for Evaluating Purchasing
and Materials Management Functions in Private Hospitals: Opportunities for
Improving Hospital Purchasing, Inventory Management and Supply
Distribution," part II, U.S. General Accounting Office, PSAD 79-58B,
April 1979.

The auditing steps described in this section should also be applied to
other departments, such as pharmacy and dietary, if they are making their
own purchases.

### Authority and Responsibility

*Objective*: To assess adherence to the hospital's central purchasing policies,
where all or some portion of the purchasing is centralized, and to gauge the
effect where the responsibility is decentralized.

### Audit steps:

1. Select invoices and the related purchase orders for the most recent purchases of each walkthrough item.
   a. Examine these documents to determine if the purchases were
      authorized and completed by the responsible departments.
   b. If purchases were completed outside established authority, obtain
      an explanation from the individuals involved.
2. Where more than one department is purchasing the same items:
   a. Compare prices paid by the departments.
   b. Discuss with the hospital purchasing agent and vendors the prices
      obtainable by consolidating and centralizing these purchases.
   c. Discuss price differences with the purchasing and other department
      managers involved.

### Planning

*Objective*: To determine whether the purchasing department has maintained
and used the data needed to manage its purchasing functions effectively.

*Audit steps*:

1. Interview the department manager and determine the extent of detailed records (vendor files, purchase-history cards, usage summaries, and so on) maintained for the department's purchases.
   a. If the department has accumulated usage data, determine the extent and frequency of analysis.
   b. Determine (1) whether the department has ranked its purchases to identify potential for competition and (2) what use has been made of this information.
   c. Review the department's forecasts of future needs. Determine how the forecasts were prepared and whether they are used in soliciting competition.
   d. Ascertain (1) what records are maintained on the individual line items and (2) whether these records show each purchase's source, quantity, date, and price.
   e. Review the department's documentation of vendor and product performance and assure that this information is sufficiently detailed.
2. Select invoices for the most recent purchases of each walkthrough item.
   a. Compare the department's detailed records with the vendor invoices to assure that they agree and that all purchases are recorded.
   b. Follow up on significant discrepancies by observing procedural weaknesses in record keeping. Discuss discrepancies and related procedural weaknesses with the persons responsible.

*Purchasing*

*Objective*: To determine whether the department's purchase orders are prepared and processed properly.

*Audit steps*:

1. Interview the department manager and determine who prepares the purchase orders. Observe the preparation and determine whether:
   a. The purchase order is filled in completely, including the price and terms, at the time the order is prepared.
   b. The purchase order is prepared by someone other than the person responsible for receiving and storing the goods.
   c. A copy of the purchase order is sent promptly to the accounting department and a copy is retained for receiving the goods.
2. Select invoices for the most recent purchases of each walkthrough item and determine whether:
   a. Orders are issued for all purchases.
   b. Purchase orders are prenumbered and controlled.

c. Nonstock items are purchased only with a properly authorized departmental requisition.

d. Emergency requisitions are controlled and monitored.

*Group Purchasing*

*Objective*: To determine whether the hospital effectively uses group-purchasing agreements.

*Audit steps*:

1. Through discussion with the purchasing manager, determine what purchasing groups are available. If necessary, contact other institutions in the area to identify purchasing groups.
2. If the institution belongs to a purchasing group, ascertain how the group was selected. If more than one group was available, determine what factors influenced the selection. If the institution did not compare costs, savings, and other benefits among groups, make this comparison. The savings should be projected on the basis of annual purchases for each item.
3. Evaluate the institutional monitoring of group prices.
   a. Determine how frequently group prices are compared with those offered by other sources.
   b. Examine the most recent price comparisons to assure that they included all high-dollar-volume items as well as a representative selection of other items.
   c. If the group vendor is unsatisfactory or higher priced than other sources, determine whether those conditions have been brought to the purchasing group's attention.
4. Obtain the group's current price list.
   a. Identify the walkthrough items covered by the group, including equivalent generic as well as brand-name products.
   b. Examine recent invoices to ascertain whether all purchases of the walkthrough items available through the group were made from the group's vendors. For items that were not purchased from the group's vendors, compare the prices paid with the group prices; discuss these departures with the purchasing manager; and evaluate their reasonableness.
      i. If the purchases were justified as emergencies, determine whether the "emergency" could have been avoided with better planning and scheduling.
      ii. If the purchases were justified with other reasons, substantiate them. For example, "better service" is a weak justification if the group's vendor provides adequate service at lower prices.

**Checklist for Purchasing Ethics**

|  | Comments (Provide data on "yes" answers. Explain "no" answers.) | |
|---|---|---|
| Questions | Yes | No |

A. Is the purchasing of goods and services initiated on the basis of appropriate authorization?
    1. If so, are routines established for approving, modifying, and issuing purchase orders?
    2. Are approval limits established for various types of purchases?
    3. Are approval limits established for various amounts of purchases?
    4. Are there periodic independent verifications of purchase authorizations?

B. Is there a written policy manual that is prepared under the authority of the director of purchases and published over the signature of the chief executive officer?
    1. Does this statement include broad policy outlines affecting corporate relationships, vendors, and interdepartmental relations?
    2. Is the policy manual available to all interested employees and vendors?
    3. Is there a routine for written procedures that covers the use and flow of records handling of orders, inventory control, receiving reports, scrap disposal, and internal management controls.
    4. Is maximum use of competitive procedures promoted?

C. Is there a written practice for employees engaged in purchasing and other transac-

|  | *Comments (Provide data on "yes" answers. Explain "no" answers.)* | |
| --- | :---: | :---: |
| *Questions* | *Yes* | *No* |

tions with suppliers and subcontractors that details moral and legal obligations to serve their institution with undivided loyalty and high ethical standards?

1. Because purchasing personnel maintain wide associations and have authority to commit funds, is there a formally or informally stated code of behavior?

2. In the case of business affected by government procurement, are instructions established by law detailed and specific?

D. Are employees who deal with supplies expressly restricted from the following types of activities, which may result in divided loyalty or in a conflict with the responsibility for discharging assigned purchasing duties?

1. Investing directly or indirectly in supplier companies, except for those whose securities are listed on a national exchange.

2. Making security purchases of a listed stock of a supplier for which the employer is an important customer if this might reasonably influence purchasing decisions.

3. Engaging in outside financial or other business interests to such an extent as to occupy a considerable portion of one's time.

4. Acting as a subcontractor or supplier to the employer in a part-time business enterprise; or accepting

|  | *Comments (Provide data on "yes" answers. Explain "no" answers.)* | |
|---|---|---|
| *Questions* | *Yes* | *No* |

    salaries, fees, or other compensation from such suppliers or subcontractors.      \_\_\_\_\_     \_\_\_\_\_

  5. Holding a position as director, partner, or officer of another corporation except with executive-office approval of the employer.     \_\_\_\_\_     \_\_\_\_\_

  6. Having an assigned responsibility involving the placement, with close relatives or personal friends.     \_\_\_\_\_     \_\_\_\_\_

  7. Transacting business with former employees of the employer, who have acquired knowledge that could give them a competitive advantage, except after managerial approval or until a year has elapsed since termination of their employment.     \_\_\_\_\_     \_\_\_\_\_

  8. Do exceptions to the restrictions indicated here have authorized managerial or executive approval?     \_\_\_\_\_     \_\_\_\_\_

E. Are the facts concerning solicitation or acceptance of gifts or gratuities from suppliers clearly communicated to employees in writing as being forbidden by law and company policies?     \_\_\_\_\_     \_\_\_\_\_

F. Are there recommended written practices for proper information disclosures?     \_\_\_\_\_     \_\_\_\_\_

  1. If so, are instructions clear stating that specific supplier product and price information is not to be revealed or discussed with competing suppliers or other persons except (1) in-house personnel having a proper functional interest in this information; (2) the supplier's

*Questions*                                          *Yes*          *No*

authorized representatives; or
(3) others with the supplier's express
approval?

2. Although the details of bids must not
be revealed, are unsuccessful bidders
given an opportunity to learn the
reasons for an adverse decision on
their proposal if they initiate a request?

3. Are there procedures for in-house information intended for internal use
only to be released to outside
only with prior managerial approval?

4. Are visits to in-house facilities or to
supplier facilities, where operations or
installations are of a restricted nature,
approved by similar managerial
and/or legal clearance?

5. Are outside requests for factual information on dollar purchases, material
usage, suppliers, employment, and so
on handled with caution and cleared
with finance or other appropriate
functions?

6. Will such data be supplied (1) if the
information is a matter of public
knowledge and not of a restricted
nature; or (2) if appropriate data are
requested by a government agency,
trade association, or other organization of national reputation?

7. Is recommended practice to decline
an answer whenever in doubt, or to
restrict the information supplied?

8. Are requests for opinion-poll information, for example, from chambers

*Comments*
*(Provide data on*
*"yes" answers.*
*Explain "no"*
*answers.)*

*Questions*                                    Yes              No

of commerce or universities, completed if a reply (1) will be good
public or business relations for the
institution; (2) will not expend any
appreciable amount of time;
and (3) will not divulge any restricted,
competitive, or otherwise improper
information?                              _____          _____

G.  Are there recommended written practices
for related functions and work since
employees responsible for purchases
act as the legal agent and representatives
of the institution in business relations
with outside suppliers?                  _____          _____

   1. Do purchasers exhibit a responsibility
for reviewing, consolidating, and
evaluating the purchase requisitions
and requirements submitted to them;
and, further, for questioning and
recommending revisions that may
bring improvements in cost, quality,
and service to customers?                _____          _____

   2. Do purchasers enlist the technical
knowledge and assistance of
employees in other functions in their
purchasing decisions and business
relations with suppliers?                _____          _____

   3. Do purchasers provide purchase
analysis of products and market conditions, so as to assure full competition and timely buying, as well as the
usual information from supplier
literature, catalogs, and contacts?      _____          _____

   4. Is full use made of the multifunc-
tional or team approach in planning

|  | *Comments (Provide data on "yes" answers. Explain "no" answers.)* | |
| --- | --- | --- |
| *Questions* | *Yes* | *No* |

and negotiating important purchases and in cost-improvement or value-planning projects? _____ _____

5. Are purchasing's internal work relationships and procedures reviewed periodically and the results incorporated in written instructions? _____ _____

6. Whenever purchasing relationships with other functions cause duplication of effort, preventable delays in ordering, excessive material costs, or losses in product quality, is the situation brought to the attention of functional representatives affected and, as necessary, of higher management—with recommendations for solution? _____ _____

H. Are there stringent procedures that eliminate coercion, force, threat, bribe, and other forms of leverage to induce a customer-supplier to deal with the purchaser on a reciprocal basis? _____ _____

I. Are there stringent procedures to prevent agreements or arrangements to buy from a customer-supplier if, because, or on the condition that the customer-supplier buys from us, or vice versa? _____ _____

J. Are there stringent procedures to prevent purchasing from a customer-supplier at a premium or for special considerations, unless the premium can be clearly shown to be due to reasons entirely apart from any element of reciprocity? _____ _____

**Audit Procedures for Purchasing Ethics**

*Authorization*

*Objective*: To assess adherence to routines detailing the purchasing of goods and services on the basis of appropriate authorization.

*Audit steps*:

1. Verify that there is a written routine for approving, modifying, and issuing purchase orders.
2. Select invoices for a recent period and verify that proper purchasing routines support these invoices. Resolve differences with manager.
3. Note that approval limits have been established and verify by following step 2.
   a. Examine documents to determine whether the purchases were authorized and completed by the responsible departments.
   b. If purchases were completed outside established authority, obtain an explanation from the individuals involved.

*Ethical Standards*

*Objective*: To determine that employees engaged in purchasing and other transactions follow institutional policies that detail moral and legal obligations.

*Audit Steps*:

1. Verify that there is a formally written policy stating the institution's ethical standards.
2. Verify that purchasing employees have agreed to this policy by presence of their signature on forms stating understanding of and compliance with policies. Verify that the following relationships have been covered:
   a. Investing directly or indirectly in supplier companies, except for those whose securities are listed on a national exchange.
   b. Making security purchases of a listed stock of a supplier for which the employer is an important customer if this might reasonably influence purchasing decisions.

c. Engaging outside financial or other business interests to such an extent as to occupy a considerable portion of one's time.

d. Acting as a subcontractor or supplier to the employer in a part-time business enterprise; or accepting salaries, fees, or other compensation from such suppliers or subcontractors.

e. Holding a position as director, partner, or officer of another corporation except with executive-office approval of the employer.

f. Having an assigned responsibility involving the placement, with close relatives or personal friends.

g. Transacting business with former employees of the employer, who have acquired knowledge that could give them a competitive advantage, except after managerial approval or until a year has elapsed since termination of their employment.

h. Facts concerning solicitation or acceptance of gifts or gratutities from suppliers are clearly communicated to employees in writing as being forbidden by law and institutional policies.

3. Determine whether there is an existing routine that captures exceptions to restrictions indicated in items 2a-h. Determine that employees list potential exceptions.

4. Determine whether proper management authorization is required for exceptions to institutional policies.

5. Test that policies are being followed by performing the following types of audit procedures:

a. With employee's permission, verify security purchases of stock for companies with which the employer is an important customer.

b. Check that employee does not hold a position in another company (particularly a supplier or competitor) without executive approval of the employer.

c. Check to determine if employees, relatives, or close personal friends are involved as purchasing agents representing vendor companies.

d. These items would be carried out in conjunction with determining that purchases are made on the basis of price, quality and delivery. In the event that purchasing decisions are not consistently made on this basis, it will be necessary to do some checking of the employees as described in items 5a-c. This type of inquiry will require more extensive investigation than normal audit practices, with accompanying additional costs.

e. Establish that disclosure of gifts is being done in connection with laws.

6. Discuss and resolve discrepancies to curtail future occurrences.

7. Follow up at a later date to ensure that compliance with policies has been accomplished.

*Information Disclosures*

*Objective*: Determine existence of written instructions clearly stating supplier product and price information. Determine that such information is not revealed or discussed except with (1) in-house personnel having a proper functional interest in this information, (2) the supplier's authorized representatives, or (3) others who have supplier's express approval.

*Audit Steps*:

1.  Verify that documents are retained to indicate that quotes have been secured based on institutional policies and dollar limits of purchases.
2.  Select specific invoices within dollar requirements of quote routine and determine that proper quotes have been obtained.
3.  Additionally, check that unsuccessful bidders have been notified if they initiate a request.
4.  Verify that proper approval procedures are in existence for releasing information of a proprietary nature. Determine that the procedure is being followed by checking documentation of procedures. Discuss discrepancies with employees and management.
5.  Follow up at a later date to ensure compliance.

*Purchasing Relationships*

*Objective*: Determine existence and following of recommended practices with related functions to achieve cost improvements and value analysis.

*Audit Steps*:

1.  Verify that there is a routine for reviewing, consolidating, and evaluating the purchase requisitions and requirements.
2.  If a committee or team for evaluating purchased items among different functions is not established, recommend that one be established for questioning and recommending revisions that may bring improvements in cost, quality, and service to customers.
    a.  Review minutes of meetings to determine actions that are being taken.
    b.  Verify documented cost improvements resulting from functional cooperation.
    c.  Review results with managers.

3. Determine that purchase analysis of products and market conditions are being performed to assure full competition and timely buying.
   a. Verify that documented analyses are maintained.
   b. Review that decisions are made as a result of these analyses.
   c. Verify that exceptions are documented and possess proper approval.
4. Review purchasing relationships with other functions to ensure that the following situations do not exist:
   a. Duplication of ordering.
   b. Delays in ordering.
   c. Losses in product quality.
   d. Excessive material costs.
   e. Review with functional representatives and, as necessary, higher-management recommendations to eliminate situations of items a-d.

*Restraint of Competition-Collusion*

*Objective*: To determine that trade is carried on under lawful conditions and that purchasing is carried on in an unrestricted environment.

*Audit Steps*:

1. Verify that stringent procedures prohibit coercion, force, threat, bribe, or other unlawful forms of leverage to induce a customer-supplier to deal with the purchaser on a reciprocal basis.
   a. Determine that those procedures have been communicated to employees.
   b. Determine that offenders will be dealt with in proportion to the seriousness of the act.
2. Review purchase agreements and sales agreements to determine that agreements or arrangements do not exist to buy from a customer-supplier if, because, or on the condition that the customer-supplier buys from us or vice versa.
   a. Review findings with management.
   b. Determine that documentation exists for agreements that appear to fall in a questionable area.
   c. Review findings in 2b with legal personnel of the institution if this has not already been done.

# Appendix 2G: Checklist and Audit Procedures for Receiving

## Checklist for Evaluating Materials-Receiving Functions

|  | *Comments (Provide data on "yes" answers. Explain "no" answers.)* | |
|---|---|---|
| *Questions* | *Yes* | *No* |
| A. Is there a central receiving area? | _____ | _____ |
| B. Are all incoming materials and supplies required to pass through the central receiving area? | _____ | _____ |
| C. Are copies of the purchase orders furnished to the receiving department? | _____ | _____ |
| D. If so, are the ordered amounts deleted from the document in order to ensure an actual physical count of amounts received? | _____ | _____ |
| E. Are approved receiving reports completed for all materials received? | _____ | _____ |
| F. Are receiving reports prenumbered? | _____ | _____ |
| G. Is a duplicate of the report kept in the receiving department? | _____ | _____ |
| H. Is there an inspection of the specifications and quality of the materials received? | _____ | _____ |
| I. Are all pharmaceutical purchases brought directly to the pharmacy receiving area unopened? | _____ | _____ |

|  | Comments *(Provide data on "yes" answers. Explain "no" answers.)* | |
|---|---|---|
| *Questions* | *Yes* | *No* |
| J.  Are the pharmaceuticals received and a complete receiving report prepared by someone other than the person who placed the order? | _____ | _____ |
| K.  Are all food supplies brought directly to the receiving area unopened? | _____ | _____ |
| L.  Are the food supplies received and a complete receiving report prepared by someone other than the person who placed the order? | _____ | _____ |

**Audit Procedures for the Receiving Functions**

This section is based on "Checklist and Guidelines for Evaluating Purchasing and Materials Management Functions in Private Hospitals: Opportunities for Improving Hospital Purchasing, Inventory Management and Supply Distribution," part II, U.S. General Accounting Office, PSAD 79-58B, April 1979.

*Objective*: To determine whether the receiving department inspects and accounts for the goods it receives.

*Audit steps*:

1.  Ask the department manager who prepares the receiving reports. If the size of the institution does not permit separate purchasing and receiving departments, determine whether it has segregated these responsibilities by assigning them to different individuals.
2.  Observe the receiving-report preparation to determine whether:
    a.  The receiving reports are prenumbered.
    b.  A receiving report is prepared for all incoming items, including "free" goods.
    c.  The completed receiving reports are sent promptly to the accounting department.

d. Credit memos are prepared for all returned goods, showing the amount of credit due.
3. Select invoices for the most recent purchase of each walkthrough item and determine whether:
   a. The paid invoices are supported by signed receiving reports.
   b. The amounts shown on the invoices and receiving reports agree, and any discrepancies have been investigated and resolved.
   c. Credits shown on the invoices agree with the amounts shown on the hospital's credit memos.

**Audit Procedures for Central Stores**

This section is based on "Checklist and Guidelines for Evaluating Purchasing and Materials Management Functions in Private Hospitals: Opportunities for Improving Hospital Purchasing, Inventory Management and Supply Distribution," part II, U.S. General Accounting Office, PSAD 79-58B, April 1979.

*Objective*: To determine whether the hospital effectively controls its materials inventories.

*Audit steps*:

1. Inspect storerooms (central stores, pharmacy, food, and so on).
   a. Observe whether all patient-chargeable items have been priced and dated.
   b. Check the expiration dates to determine whether any expired stock is in inventory.
   c. Identify items that appear obsolete, unusable, excessively stocked or slow moving. (Such items may be dust covered or stored in remote or hard-to-reach locations.)
   d. Determine whether unofficial or "floor" stocks exist that unnecessarily duplicate supplies in central stores.
2. Perform the following examination for the walkthrough items.
   a. If the items have been dated and priced, compare the prices on the items with applicable invoice prices.
   b. If there is a catalog, or formulary in the case of pharmaceuticals, determine if the listing of items accurately reflects current inventory.
   c. Compare the perpetual-inventory balance with the amount actually in stock.
3. Observe perpetual-inventory-keeping procedures and determine whether perpetual inventories are:

    a. Kept by people other than those who have access to the actual inventory.

    b. Periodically compared to the physical count, with discrepancies recorded separately and explained.

4. Discuss observations with the department manager and resolve any discrepancies.

5. Discuss your observations with the central-stores and central-supply managers. Determine how they monitor user departments for evidence of stockpiling, obsolescence, pilferage, and waste.

# Appendix 2H: Checklist and Audit Procedures for Distribution

**Checklist for Evaluating Distribution Functions Medical-Surgical Supplies**

This section is based on "Checklist and Guidelines for Evaluating Purchasing and Materials Management Functions in Private Hospitals: Opportunities for Improving Hospital Purchasing, Inventory Management and Supply Distribution," part II, U.S. General Accounting Office, PSAD 79-58B, April 1979.

|  | *Comments (Provide data on "yes" answers. Explain "no" answers.)* | |
|---|---|---|
| *Questions* | *Yes* | *No* |
| A. Does the storeroom distribute all medical-surgical supplies directly to user departments? | _____ | _____ |
| B. If not, | | |
| 1. Are medical-surgical supplies stocked and distributed by central-supply or other departments? | _____ | _____ |
| 2. Has the hospital considered consolidating inventories and distribution functions of central-supply and central-stores departments? | _____ | _____ |
| 3. Has management considered establishing a centralized distribution system? | _____ | _____ |

**Checklist for Safeguarding in the Distribution Process**

A. Are records and unused documents (checks, vouchers, check requests, and so on) protected from theft, misuse, destruction, or misappropriation by the following procedures:

1. Access to purchase orders; invoices; receiving reports; and unused, signed and returned checks are restricted to authorized employees. _____ _____

2. The use of a designated receiving area with restricted access. _____ _____

3. There is a designation of authorized receivers and procedures for receiving material during off-shift periods. _____ _____

4. Receiving reports forwarded directly to accounts payable and voucher detail are cancelled to preclude reuse. _____ _____

5. A comparison is made of facsimile-signature usage with check-usage records. _____ _____

6. There is a review of unclaimed items for proper disposition and authorization. _____ _____

B. Are records, operating systems, processing areas, and physical assets protected from misuse or destruction by the following:

1. There is restricted access to storage and distribution areas; accounting records; and shipping, billing, and cash-receipt forms. _____ _____

2. There are periodic test counts of unused forms and prompt investigation of discrepancies identified. _____ _____

3. There are secured storage areas at the various distribution and chain levels. _____ _____

4. Notes or negotiable instruments received from vendors or customers are secured. _____ _____

**Checklist for Evaluation of Materials-Charging Functions**

This section is based on "Checklist and Guidelines for Evaluating Purchasing and Materials Management Functions in Private Hospitals: Opportunities for Improving Hospital Purchasing, Inventory Management and Supply Distribution," part II, U.S. General Accounting Office, PSAD 79-58B, April 1979.

|  | *Comments (Provide data on "yes" answers. Explain "no" answers.)* | |
| --- | --- | --- |
| *Questions* | *Yes* | *No* |
| A. Is each department and nursing station charged for the supplies used? | _____ | _____ |
| B. Do written procedures require that all patient-chargeable medical-surgical items be controlled and distributed by one department? | _____ | _____ |
| C. Is this department accountable for revenue earned and expenses incurred for patient-chargeable supplies? | _____ | _____ |
| D. Are charge slips reconciled with supplies used? If so: | _____ | _____ |
| 1. Are discrepancies investigated? | _____ | _____ |
| 2. Are departments accountable for lost charges? | _____ | _____ |
| E. Is there a consistent markup procedure for patient-chargeable medical-surgical supplies? | _____ | _____ |
| F. Does management periodically review the reasonableness of prices and markups? | _____ | _____ |

**Audit Steps for Charging Procedures**

This section is based on "Checklist and Guidelines for Evaluating Purchasing and Materials Management Functions in Private Hospitals: Opportunities for Improving Hospital Purchasing, Inventory Management and

Supply Distribution," part II, U.S. General Accounting Office, PSAD 79-58B, April 1979.

*Objective*: To determine if all materials are properly charged to the user department and/or to the patient where applicable.

*Audit Steps*:

1. If the institution has centralized distribution of medical-surgical supplies, determine what department is responsible for distribution and the type of system used. Observe the distribution of chargeable supplies and the processing of charge slips.
   a. If PAR-level or exchange-cart systems are in use, determine whether:
      i. Charge tickets are reconciled with usage at the time supplies are replenished.
      ii. Discrepancies are investigated and, if the patient owing charges cannot be identified, the using department is charged with the loss.
   b. If the supplies are obtained by requisition, observe the procedures. Determine whether a charge ticket is prepared by the requesting department before supplies are issued to patients.
   c. If it appears that patient charges are lost, estimate the amount for a representative period.
2. If central supply controls patient-chargeable medical-surgical supplies, select several departments for examination.
   a. Review each department's storeroom requisitions and determine whether patient-chargeable items were issued directly to the departments.
   b. If so, compare and reconcile patient charges with the department's receipts during the same period.
3. If it appears that patient charges are being lost, estimate the amount of charges lost for the period reviewed.
   a. Discuss your observations with the department managers and determine how they assure accountability for patient charges.
   b. Discuss your observations with the accounting department manager and determine how the department monitors control over patient-chargeable items.

# 3 Materials-Management Information Systems

## Information and Data

Materials-management information systems (MMIS) can be defined as *the combination of human and computer-based resources that results in the collection, storage, processing, retrieval, communication, and use of data for the purpose of cost-effective management of materials.* Because of the emphasis on cost effectiveness, each of the MMIS elements (collection, storage, processing, retrieval, communication, and use of data) must be considered at all times in terms of both their developmental and their operational costs. Such costs must be balanced against the value and the use of information, and finally against its potential effect on providing cost-effective care. Theoretically, it is possible to collect and store all data on every transaction taking place within an institution; to allow for its retrieval in any conceivable form; and to accomplish this within negligible or virtually zero time. Economics clearly do not justify such a system, as the vast majority of the data would have nominal or no information value for management.

Computer systems have been described as marriages of compromise. Clearly, data may be collected in a variety of ways, from written correspondence to an expensive teleprocessing network. The choice must depend on an analysis of the value of the information and its intended use. Moreover, a wide variety of data-storage media are available, ranging from filing cabinets through "Kardex"-type systems to high-speed computer-based random-access disks. The type of medium used to store the data involved must be related to the data's significance and their planned or potential use.

In the area of data retrieval, there are numerous choices. It may be most economical to use a clerk to search the files in the archives. In other cases the data may best be retrieved through reports. At higher levels of importance, urgency, or timeliness, retrieval through on-line inquiry terminals may be justified.

The communication and use of information may involve any one of several methodologies. A mailed report may suffice at one level. At higher levels, however, teleprocessed inquiry responses may be required. In addition, proper use of computer-based information may necessitate an educational effort orienting users and/or management to the capabilities of the system. Large institutions may facilitate communication of computer-provided reports, analyses, and exception messages through the use of weekly briefings for materials-management personnel.

The most difficult aspect of effective MMIS design involves determining what data to collect; how and at what organizational or institutional level to collect it; which medium to use; what retrieval method to adopt; what analyses to perform; and which control ratios to calculate. Information cannot be generated if the supporting data are absent, but the scope of the data base cannot be so broad that it prices the system out of range. Data are meaningless, and thus useless, unless interpreted, analyzed, and digested into information or operationally meaningful intelligence. At the same time, information does not exist without supporting data. These two issues deserve commensurate attention. What is needed is a way to tailor the information to the needs of the intended user in a cost-effective way. Beneath this phrase lies the framework of the entire MMIS structure.

Materials-management information systems should be capable of supporting various studies on an as-needed basis, as well as producing relevant periodic and exception reports. Consequently, in addition to the broad question of which data to collect, which data to store, and how, there are several fundamental questions in the area of exception processing. Historically and generally, computers have been used to process the volume- or "production"-paperwork tasks. This philosophy persists. In most installations, computer systems are not capable of cost-effectively addressing the unusual, irregular, and abnormal processing requirements.

Analysis must be performed to determine the extent of system design and processing requirements in order to provide the capability to satisfy requests for any unusual analyses or reports. Investment of several man-years to provide a capability for some special report that may be needed only once every two years should be given a second thought, unless, of course, that particular report carries a great deal of importance. Clearly the difficult questions do not arise in the extreme cases—the extremes are obvious. The difficult choices concern the borderline functions, items with a complexity of processing requirements and a sufficiently low frequency of occurrence to put into question the potential payback of computerization.

## Planning an MMIS Project

In a study of industrial applications of computers, J.T. Garrity [1] found that several characteristics were commonly present in organizations experiencing the greatest success with their computers. "First, . . . the quality of leadership that corporate executives provide. Next, . . . the planning and control tools that management has built into the computer-systems program.

Third, . . . the role operation management plays. Finally, . . . the caliber of the computer and systems staff.'' To increase the probability of a successful application and use of computers, management should set clear objectives to ensure that the computer program is focused on the major problems of the institution in general, and those concerned with materials management in particular. Adequate resources should be marshaled to get the job done, and the human and organizational barriers to progress should be brought down insofar as possible. Finally, top management should review and challenge the plans and programs of the computer group. They should monitor progress and insist on significant tangible benefits from the investment in computer systems.

There are several basic approaches to the planning and implementation of a materials-management information system. The *great-leap-forward* approach involves a complete ideological and organizational break with what now exists. Proponents of this approach argue that alternative approaches usually involve a continuation of the existing basic processing disciplines. Hence there is an absence of fresh, incisive institutional analysis of the real current and projected future needs.

Alternatively, the *building-block* approach calls for design and implementation of various logical MMIS sections as stepping stones to the total MMIS. Proponents of this approach argue that the great leap forward is too "blue sky," or too broad and general, ever to be implemented. A third alternative favors the complete design of the total MMIS to be followed by the systematic implementation of segments consistent with the overall plan [2].

An example of total failure in using the first type of approach, compared with the use of the third approach leading ultimately to a successful implementation, are documented in [3] for the case of a patient-management information system within a large health center.

Planning an effective MMIS requires a clear definition of the basic objectives of the system. The various milestones in achieving these objectives must also be delineated. Although this area may appear to be of nominal value, only a concise set of objectives can give the effort its direction. In addition, a review of the objectives and of the milestones provides a basis for evaluation of the success or failure of the effort.

After determining the basic objectives of the MMIS, the next step is the evaluation of the means by which these objectives are fulfilled. This effort requires an analysis of the organizational structure. A determination must be made of the patterns of information flow that exist among the various functional elements, departments, floors, divisions, and so on. Any decentralization trends must also be studied.

It is not enough to analyze the organizational form. The role, nature, extent of leadership, and degree of control exercised by each organizational entity must also be considered. Moreover, in introducing any new system into a health-provider institution, recognition must be given to the credibility of the administration in general and the systems-and-procedures function in particular in the eyes of the physicians, nurses, and other health providers. As shown in [3], the best conceived system will have difficulty in being implemented and properly used where such credibility does not exist. It is imperative to understand fully the decision-making process within the institution in order to service the health providers and administration with an accurate, timely, and effective materials-management information system.

Moreover, the analyst must be sensitive to the institutional plans for future growth and the means by which the projected growth is to be achieved. The effects of an expansion program in brick and mortar in the number of beds, physicians, research, teaching, and so on can be stated in quantitative terms. Growth along any or all of the above lines will result in the growth of materials usage within the institution. Hence the MMIS will be required to capture and process greater volumes and at times even different kinds of data. Clearly, the effects of diversification—for example, a community hospital branching out into research or teaching, or affiliating with a health-maintenance organization (HMO)—on the development of an MMIS are far more complex.

Management information systems in general and MMISs in particular should realistically be expected to be compatible with the present organizational direction and at best to be structurally consistent with any future institutional information needs.

The development of the MMIS should involve administration at levels where strategic decisions are made. The plan for an MMIS cannot otherwise be realistically expected to fulfill its potential for the institution. To state the matter more strongly, any effort to develop an MMIS without involving, at a strategic level, the ultimate users and managers of the materials-management system, is shortsighted.

A number of articles dealing with ways of structuring the process of designing new systems and procedures for organizations have recently appeared in the literature [4,5]. (Also see [6].) They generally agree on the need of using the task-force approach. They agree on the need for the task force to include systems professionals as well as line personnel from the user departments.

Thus an MMIS-design task force should include materials-management personnel and health-provider personnel from the client institution, in addition to systems personnel.

Moreover, there is agreement on the need to have such task forces periodically report to "watchdog" committees of top institutional management, such as administrators, physicians, and nurses. These review, evaluation, and planning sessions with top management should have as their objectives the sharing of information; the planning and direction of the project; and, most importantly, the *transferring* of *project ownership* from systems to the user and management personnel. Such approaches tend to maximize the probability of successful implementation of project results.

Whether or not the multidisciplinary approach to MMIS design is used, it is always a good idea to seek inputs from potential MMIS users regarding their perception of the kind of reporting they desire. The users should be queried as to the desired *content* and *frequency* of reports. The users should be informed that MMIS reports generally fall into the following categories:

*Periodic reports*: These are the reports that are provided on an ongoing basis at specified times throughout the year.

*Activity reports*: These reports summarize the activities performed over a specified time period (for example, requisitions by the department of medicine in May).

*Status reports*: These are snapshots taken of an entity at a particular time (for example, inventory levels of items in departments on Fridays).

*Exception reports*: These reports flag unusual developments. Therefore, threshold values are required so that situations falling above or below these performance levels are reported (for example, items with actual stock-out higher than the predetermined rate).

*Ad hoc or special-study reports*: These report the results of special studies involving analyses of some or all of the data. To accommodate such studies the data-retrieval and information system must be flexible and responsive to any number of possible study and report types. Often these studies require the ability to recall data for several years. This length of time is often required to determine trends or help identify usage-pattern changes.

Moreover, the users should be informed that the MMIS will contain timely information on the following basic data categories:

Status of:
    Inventory on hand

Transactions:
    Quantities ordered
    Dates of orders
    Quantities withdrawn
    Dates of withdrawal/shipment
    Dates of arrival
    Quantities received

These data will be known to the MMIS at the following organizational levels:

Warehouse/region

Central storerooms (CSRs)/facility

Departments

Modules (It is not always cost effective to capture materials-management data below the organizational level of a department.)

The following is an example of a questionnaire that may be used to solicit inputs from various materials managers, users, or general administrators regarding their perceptions of what is needed or desired.

## Information Requested for
## Materials-Management Reports

The following is a list of components for various materials-management reports. These can be generated for any single- or multifacility, multidepartmental hospital and/or HMO. Note that different types of reports are produced for different levels of management. First indicate the report that you will find useful and then circle the desired frequency of reporting for those informational items you will find useful, as follows: (1) monthly; (2) quarterly; (3) annually; or (4) on an exception basis (specify the threshold in the space provided).

*Top-Management Report*

|   |   |
|---|---|
|         | A. Facility name. |
|         | B. Facility number. |
| 1 2 3 4 | C. Dollar value of items used in the period. |
| 1 2 3 4 | D. Dollar value of items used to date. |
| 1 2 3 4 |    1. Last year. |
| 1 2 3 4 |    2. This year. |
| 1 2 3 4 | E. Percentage change of D (2) with regard to D (1). |
| 1 2 3 4 | F. Percentage of the dollar spent on supplies of a facility with regard to the total regional dollar spent on supplies for last year. |
|         | G. Dollar value of items used per work unit to date. Specify the facility and the work units appropriate to your function. For guidance, see Tables 2-3 and 2-4. |

1 2 3 4          1.  Last year.
1 2 3 4          2.  This year.
1 2 3 4     H.  Percentage change of G (2) with regard to G (1).
1 2 3 4      I.  Percentage of the work units of a facility with regard to the
                    total regional work units for last year.

*Middle-Management Reports*

These reports are produced for each facility. The information is reported on
a departmental basis. Each facility administrator receives the report pertinent to his or her own facility. These reports are available to top management in the form of backup or more detailed information. They contain the
following:

       I.  Heading: For the facility under consideration.
         A.  Facility name.
         B.  Facility number.
         C.  Number of departments in the facility.
      II.  Body: For each department in the above facility.
         A.  Department name.
         B.  Department number.
1 2 3 4          C.  Dollars spent on supplies in the period.
1 2 3 4          D.  Dollars spent on supplies to date.
1 2 3 4             1.  Last year.
1 2 3 4             2.  This year.
1 2 3 4          E.  Percentage change of D (2) with regard to D (1).
1 2 3 4          F.  Percentage of the dollar value spent on supplies of a
                        facility with regard to the total dollar spent for the
                        facility last year.
1 2 3 4          G.  Dollars spent per work unit to date. (Specify the facil-
                        ity and the work units appropriate to your function.)
1 2 3 4             1.  Last year.
1 2 3 4             2.  This year.
1 2 3 4          H.  Percentage change of G (2) with regard to G (1).
1 2 3 4           I.  Percentage of the work units of a department with
                        regard to the total-facility work units for last year.

*Departmental Report*

These reports are generated for each department in each of the facilities.
The person in charge of materials management receives the report pertaining

to his or her own department. These reports are available to the facility administrator as backup. These reports may contain the following:

    I.  Heading: For the department under consideration.
        A.  Facility name.
        B.  Facility number.
        C.  Department name.
        D.  Department number.
        E.  Number of items stocked at the department.
   II.  Body: For each item in the above department.
        A.  Item name.
        B.  Item number.

| | |
|---|---|
| 1 2 3 4 | C.  Item availability in the period (service level). |
| 1 2 3 4 | D.  Dollars spent on the item in the period. |
| 1 2 3 4 | E.  Dollars spent on the item to date. |
| 1 2 3 4 |     1.  Last year. |
| 1 2 3 4 |     2.  This year. |
| 1 2 3 4 | F.  Percentage change of E (2) with regard to E (1). |
| 1 2 3 4 | G.  Percentage of the dollar value spent on the item with regard to the total dollar spent on all the supplies for the department for last year. |
| 1 2 3 4 | H.  Dollars spent per work unit to date (the work unit used for the department in which the item is stocked). |
| 1 2 3 4 |     1.  Last year. |
| 1 2 3 4 |     2.  This year. |
| 1 2 3 4 | I.  Percentage change of H (2) with regard to H (1). |
| 1 2 3 4 | J.  Number of units used in the period. |
| | K.  Number of units of items used to date. |
| 1 2 3 4 |     1.  Last year. |
| 1 2 3 4 |     2.  This year. |
| 1 2 3 4 | L.  Percentage change of K (2) with regard to K (1). |
| | M.  Number of units used per work unit to date (the work unit used for the department in which the item is stocked). |
| 1 2 3 4 |     1.  Last year. |
| 1 2 3 4 |     2.  This year. |
| 1 2 3 4 | N.  Percentage change of M (2) with regard to M (1). |

*An Example of Specifications*
*for Requested MMIS Reports*

The following specifications of an MMIS were drawn up, based on input received from facility administrators and from the comptroller of a large HMO undergoing a study of its materials-management system.

The MMIS should generate reports providing management with concise, timely, accurate, and relevant information for decision making. The requested periodic activity reports were:

1. *Materials-usage standards report*

   This report registers measurements of actual usage against some standards (such as patient-day or doctor's-office visit) and will be issued monthly and/or quarterly.

2. *Allocation of CSR costs to user departments*

   This report:
   > Interfaces with the general ledger

   > Summarizes the allocation of CSR costs to the user departments for a period of one month.

3. *Department year-to-date volume and dollars*

   This report indicates year-to-date units and dollar usage of items listed by stock number and description.

   The information is broken down by department and shows prior year's volume as a basis for comparison.

   Results are presented as usage and costs per patient-day or doctor's office visit where appropriate.

4. *Report on turnover of items*

   This report:
   > Indicates items that are not turning over fast enough or items that are turning over much too rapidly.

   > The capability of looking at usage per workload unit makes it possible to differentiate trends caused by changes in usage patterns as opposed to changes in workload units and/or changes in replenishment decision rules used.

5. *Backorder and stockout report*

   This report:
   > To be issued daily.

   > It lists items backordered or stocked out.

   > It lists expected delivery dates on outstanding orders.

   > This information will be needed on a current basis in helping to determine the need to make special purchases at premium dollars.

The information system should capture data to analyze the activities of the following MMS functions:

1. Requisitioning

    Information on all requisitioning of standard-stock items and purchasing of nonstock items is to be obtained and classified into categories at least as detailed as the natural classes now used by the accounting system. It would be helpful to have the capability to break these down into subsections of "fixed" and "variable" expenditures and to indicate items that account for a large percentage of the natural-class expenditure. This can be done by using a different coding system for each department.

    Control of use and budgeting of these items, based on historical data, would be done. Based on a percentage increase in workload, it would be helpful to forecast the utilization of the various nonpayroll items and to price out that forecast. Also, a coding system should be used to group like items into subtotals (for example, all syringes).

2. Procurement.
3. Receiving.
4. Storage.
5. Shipping.
6. Distributions to facilities.
7. Distributions within a facility.

For the warehouse, facilities, and departments, the data base should contain timely information regarding

1. Quantity on hand and location.
2. Quantity on order and location (unfilled).
3. Usage:

    At each stocking locating, usage must be measured in terms of gross units, units per workload unit, gross price, and price per unit. Usage variances are to be separated from price variances. Comparisons of usage are to be made between the west-side and east-side facilities in order to compare readily differing purchasing, stocking, and other procedures.

4. Expected lead time:
    a. From vendors.
    b. From facility's central supplies.
    b. From warehouse.
5. Record of vendor's reliability.

The data base should contain inventory listings of items issued to a department with their dollar value in a given period:

1. Out-of-stock and/or backordered items (and items obtained from other sources).
2. Number of stockouts.
3. Unit prices, quantity discounts.
4. Oversupply items.
5. Returns to vendors (overload, damages, and so on).
6. Required cost information: Most specifically, inventory values should be recorded at net prices rather than gross prices to aid in reconciliation with the general ledger. Alternatively, discounts earned should be allocated into the issue system.

Actual service levels for each item:

1. Late deliveries by vendors.
2. Early deliveries by vendors.
3. Items to be shipped to facilities.
4. Alternative sources for urgent items.
5. Substitutable items (identified by a code).

Appendix 3A provides checklists for evaluating existing reports, for evaluating their distribution and control, and for evaluating the materials-management information system and its use in general.

## MMIS Characteristics

### Centralized and Decentralized Management Information Systems

Much like materials-management systems, the corresponding information-handling and -processing systems can be centralized or decentralized. Moreover, they need not be the same in this respect. Although it would be difficult to conceive of a centralized MMS with a decentralized MMIS, the reverse is indeed possible. Thus, radiology can buy and stock its own X-ray film and report all its transactions via standardized forms to a central MMIS which in turn provides radiology and high administrative councils with reports on usage, inventories, and so on. A centralized information system is one in which all function of the information system—data gathering, processing, storage, report generation, and transmission—are performed by the institution's information clearing house. All the reports and most of the forms and other documents that carry information to decision makers within the institution originate from this clearing house. Similarly, all the data collecting done by the organization is done by the centralized system, where the data are then stored and used to prepare the reports required.

A decentralized information system, on the other hand, is one that involves several rather autonomous information systems serving functional departments or suborganizations within the insitution. Each of these gathers its own data, produces reports as needed by the department it is serving, and stores data accordingly. Thus, in this case, radiology would keep and process its own X-ray-film transactions and generate its own reports. Good management information systems that are decentralized will have some form of centralized coordination (if the total information system is well designed), in order to achieve optimum institutional-level effectiveness.

### Distribution-Oriented and Storage-Oriented Information Systems

A distribution-oriented information system is one whose operations emphasize the transmission of information to decision-making stations throughout the organization. The storage-oriented system, on the other hand, is more concerned with efficient storage of data, as opposed to its transmission to information users. A medical-records library is a storage-oriented information system. Retrieving information from such a system requires some effort on the part of the information user. Airline-reservation systems, on the other hand, are devoted to the dissemination of information about aircraft-seat availability. These are distribution-oriented systems. Such systems provide reservation desks with information on seating availability on airline flights within a few seconds after an inquiry is made. Industry and many retailing organizations maintain materials-management information of this type. Some health centers have already installed such systems for entering and retrieving information concerned with appointment making and with fiscal and other matters. As computer-hardware and support technology becomes even less expensive and more accessible in the years to come, it is conceivable that health centers will enter some if not all of their MMIS onto the *interactive on-line* mode of operation. In this way health institutions will be able to shave the inventories of materials kept on hand even further while being able to serve users better.

### Data-Retrieval and Document-Retrieval Systems

Data-retrieval information systems have the ability to call out many different types of data kept in various kinds of storage devices and to manipulate the data in some predefined way.Such manipulations often involve complex statistical, arithmetic, and/or mathematical calculations. Materials-transactions data can thus be reported arrayed according to dollar or unit usage. Averages and variances can be calculated, as can various control ratios such as units consumed per patient day. Similarly, reorder points and quantities can be calculated based on sophisticated mathematical relationships between usage history, forecast of demand lead time, cost, and other information.

Document-retrieving systems, on the other hand, are able to reproduce a desired document, but with little or no manipulation of data. Such a system frequently makes use of microfilm and other recording techniques that utilize miniaturized reproduction in order to store documents and records. Upon inquiry, such a document can be reproduced on a television-screen-like device called a cathode ray tube (CRT). Alternately, a "hard" copy of the original document can be produced. The two types of systems are clearly not mutually exclusive. It is possible to have both capabilities and the same computer configuration if the costs justify the benefits.

## Manual and Automated Systems

Most information systems combine both manual and automated techniques in getting the work done. Institutions employing the most sophisticated computing equipment still find it necessary to buy pencils or ball-point pens. Some small hospitals or clinics still have information systems that are entirely manual, with all the gathering, storage, processing, and transmission of data accomplished without the use of automated devices of any kind. The degree to which an information system should be automated depends on the *speed* with which information must be processed, the *amount* of information to be *processed* and *stored*, and the *value* of the *information* to the *decision maker* compared with the *costs of automating* the system.

## Batch and Real-Time Systems

The most common data-processing systems use *batch*, or sequential, processing techniques. A batch technique is one that gathers and saves all transactions affecting a file of information and, after a specific time period has elapsed or after a given number of transactions have been accumulated, updates the file all at once using all transactions collected since the last processing cycle. For example, hotels typically accumulate all the transactions that affect charges against a room or a registered guest for a day and, the next day, record each transaction to the appropriate account. In this way the file of registered-guest accounts is always, at most, a day behind the actual transactions (telephone calls made or restaurant charges) that have taken place. Such a system is economical for a hotel to use because it permits considerable labor specialization and concentration of effort to do the updating job all at once. Updating each individual customer record as the transaction takes place is a much more costly practice.

*Real-time* systems, on the other hand, do not gather transactions for processing at some later time but process each transaction as it occurs. Perpetual inventories in the various locations, especially in the CSRs, can thus be instantaneously updated. Real-time systems promise to be the wave of the future in hospital and clinic information systems.

## Computers and MMIS

Earlier sections of this chapter addressed the broad issues dealing with what should be expected of an MMIS and how an MMIS might be organized. Some of the more detailed MMIS issues that should be considered in the design of a computer-aided MMIS will be discussed next.

### Computer Activity

Each distinguishable material that is stocked somewhere in the institution is typically assigned a "storeroom" *catalog* number. Each such catalog number in turn is assigned an *area* in the computer memory. The information contained in this memory segment remains constant (until changed) and acts as a source of reference. Whenever the computer needs to utilize this information, it searches, extracts the information, and replicates it for use in another area in the computer. This information stored in the computer memory is called a *file*. Changes in a file may be made either by people or by the computer.

A change made by a person might be, for example, the requirement to change the "current" purchase price to $12.50. Such a change might be accomplished via submission to the computer center of an Inventory-Control Setup/Change Form as shown in figure 3-1 [7].

The computer will make a change in the file when an item is issued. The computer will enter the file, find the current on-hand balance, and deduct the amount of the issue.

Files may be large or small, depending on what is required. In the case of the "Inventoried-Item File," many thousands of items are stored, each with its own memory. Many other activities occur in the computer, however. These are only two examples of computer activity.

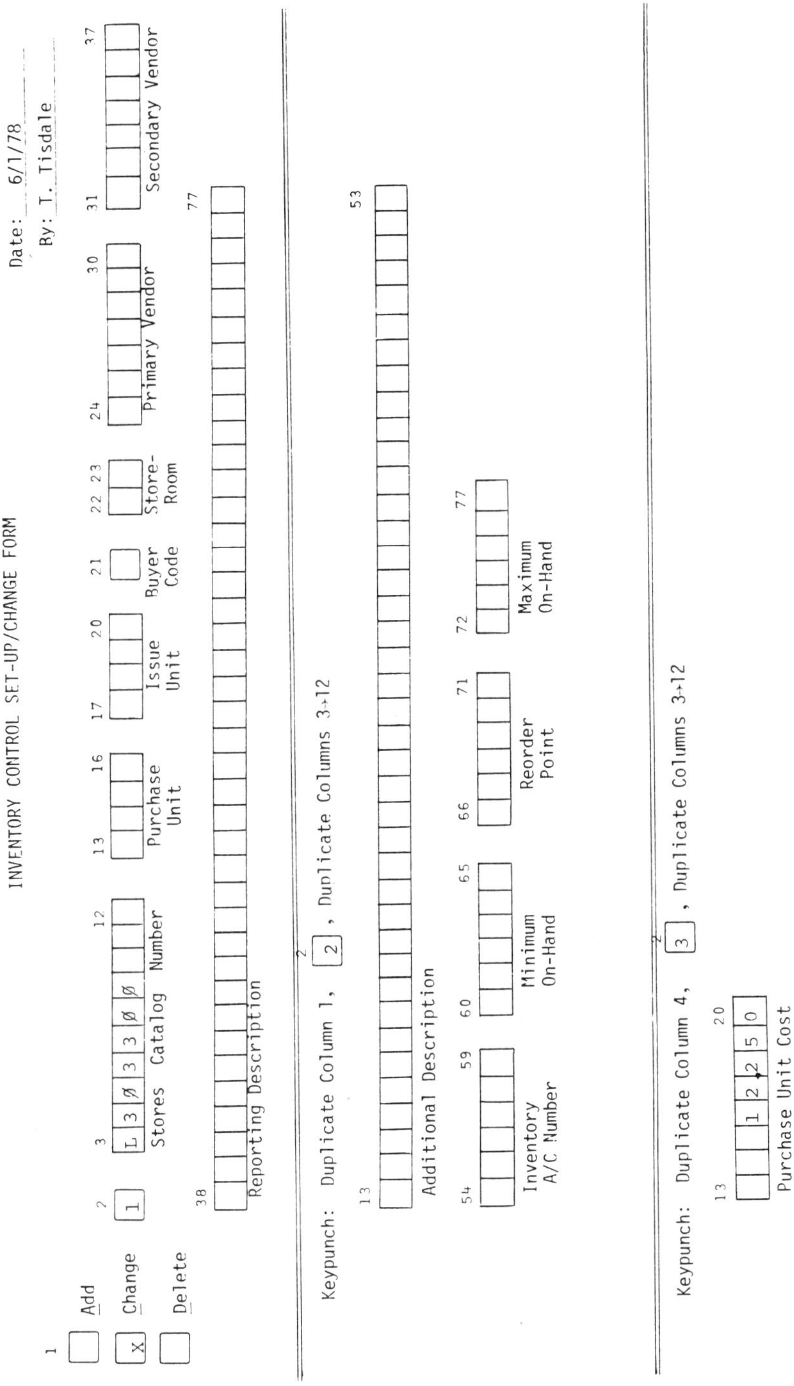

**Figure 3-1.** Inventory-Control Setup/Change

Source: Reproduced with permission from "Materiel Management Inventory Control Procedure" (Cleveland Clinic Foundation, 1979).

*Record Maintenance*

The inventory-control function typically establishes a master record for each item maintained within the "Inventory File." Clearly, a separate record is required for each item maintained within the inventory. As indicated earlier, this record is one of the primary sources of data used by the computer center in preparing reports for inventory control. The master record maintained in the computer files contains all the information required to process all daily transactions, along with general information required by the storeroom and the inventory-control function. Additions, changes, and deletions may be made to any data field of a master record. The change of a master record occurs by the submission of an "Inventory-Control Setup Change Form" to the computer center. The catalog number is the computer locating factor and therefore must appear on all change forms. For example, the change of the purchase-and-issue unit from boxes to cases is illustrated in figure 3-2.

*Quality Control*

Computers generally do not make mistakes—people do. Therefore, factors contributing to proper quality control of data entered include adequate supervision, proper management, and a thorough knowledge of the system. Although quality control must be practiced by all those associated with the maintenance of stock records, it is important that a single point of responsibility be established for the following activities:

> *Input*: Ensuring that the receipts, turn-ins, outshipments, credit to inventories, and so on are processed in an accurate and timely manner.

> *Output*: Source documents and computer reports are maintained in both the accounting and inventory-control sections for auditing purposes.

*Validating the Processing Cycle*

The input register and input audit register should provide for the correction of errors and should show and validate from listing to listing that corrections are being accomplished. It should be the responsibility of the inventory-control analyst to track the audit trail and make the corrections. Errors are to be corrected on a daily basis for reinput the following day. Figure 3-3 shows an Input Audit Register with Corrections and figure 3-4 shows a printout of an Input Register.

INVENTORY CONTROL SET-UP/CHANGE FORM

Date: 6/1/78

By: T. Tisdale

1

Add

Change [X]

Delete

2 [1]

3 [L 3 0 3 0]
Stores Catalog Number 12

13 [C S]
Purchase Unit 16

17 [C S]
Issue Unit 20

21
Buyer Code

22 23
Store-Room

24
Primary Vendor 30

31
Secondary Vendor 37

38
Reporting Description 77

Keypunch: Duplicate Column 1, [2], Duplicate Columns 3→12

13
Additional Description 53

54
Inventory A/C Number 59

60
Minimum On-Hand 65

66
Reorder Point 71

72
Maximum On-Hand 77

Keypunch: Duplicate Column 4, [3], Duplicate Columns 3→12

13
Purchase Unit Cost 20

Source: Reproduced with permission from "Materiel Management Inventory Control Procedure" (Cleveland Clinic Foundation, 1979).

**Figure 3-2.** Inventory-Control Setup/Change Form, B

```
CLEVELAND CLINIC FOUNDATION                   I N P U T   A U D I T   R E G I S T E R          RUN DATE  06-22-78
REPORT NO. HHK010 HHK011                                                                                 PAGE 1

COMPUTER  *  ***BATCH CONTROL***
USE ONLY  *  *                                                                  A/C 1  %1  A/C 2  %?  A/C 3  %3
1    4    *  DATE      NO  DOUC #  T/C  CATALOG #  QTY   DATE      A/C   55    61   63    ?? 71    77
             10        16  18      24   27         43    49
                                                                   49

C01 000003   06-20-78  11  030500  200  H137500   16    06-20-78  806500
C01 000005   06-20-78  15  030567  200  M033000   100   06-20-78  817100
```

**Figure 3-3.** Input Audit Register

Source: Reproduced with permission from "Materiel Management Inventory Control Procedure" (Cleveland Clinic Foundation, 1979).

CLEVELAND CLINIC FOUNDATION
REPORT NO. HH0010 HHX012

I N P U T   R E G I S T E R

RUN DATE 06-05-78
PAGE 3

| T/C | CATALOG # | P=QTY | I=QTY | TRAN DATE | P/O NO. | VENDOR | UNIT COST | C D | PUR COST | A/C 1 | % | A/C 2 | % | A/C 3 | % | DOUC # | BATCH DATE | BAT NO |
|---|---|---|---|---|---|---|---|---|---|---|---|---|---|---|---|---|---|---|
| 100 | P150000 | 36 | 432 | 06-01-78 | P70600G | | | | | | | | | | | 28059 | 06-01-78 | 1 |
| 100 | P155000 | 60 | 2080 | 06-01-78 | P70600G | | | | | | | | | | | 28059 | 06-01-78 | 1 |
| 100 | P156000 | 60 | 2880 | 06-01-78 | P70600G | | | | | | | | | | | 28059 | 06-01-78 | 1 |
| 100 | P159000 | 36 | 1728 | 06-01-78 | P70600G | | | | | | | | | | | 28059 | 06-01-78 | 1 |
| 100 | P169000 | 48 | 578 | 06-01-78 | P70600G | | | | | | | | | | | 28059 | 06-01-78 | 1 |
| 100 | P170000 | 80 | 760 | 06-01-78 | P70600G | | | | | | | | | | | 28059 | 06-01-78 | 1 |
| 100 | P171000 | 24 | 288 | 06-01-78 | P70600G | | | | | | | | | | | 28059 | 06-01-78 | 1 |
| 100 | P173000 | 24 | 288 | 06-01-78 | P70600G | | | | | | | | | | | 28060 | 06-01-78 | 1 |
| 100 | P175500 | 12 | 144 | 06-01-78 | P70600G | | | | | | | | | | | 28060 | 06-01-78 | 1 |
| 100 | P175900 | 60 | 720 | 06-01-78 | P70600G | | | | | | | | | | | 28060 | 06-01-78 | 1 |
| 100 | P176000 | 32 | 384 | 06-01-78 | P70600G | | | | | | | | | | | 28060 | 06-01-78 | 1 |
| 100 | P181000 | 144 | 1728 | 06-01-78 | P70600G | | | | | | | | | | | 28060 | 06-01-78 | 1 |
| 100 | P183000 | 60 | 720 | 06-01-78 | P70600G | | | | | | | | | | | 28060 | 06-01-78 | 1 |
| 100 | P183900 | 24 | 288 | 06-01-78 | P70600G | | | | | | | | | | | 28060 | 06-01-78 | 1 |
| 100 | P187500 | 12 | 144 | 06-01-78 | P70600G | | | | | | | | | | | 28060 | 06-01-78 | 1 |
| 100 | P190000 | 60 | 720 | 06-01-78 | P70600G | | | | | | | | | | | 28060 | 06-01-78 | 1 |
| 100 | P195000 | 48 | 576 | 06-01-78 | P70600G | | | | | | | | | | | 28060 | 06-01-78 | 1 |
| 100 | P196000 | 24 | 288 | 06-01-78 | P70600G | | | | | | | | | | | 28060 | 06-01-78 | 1 |
| 100 | P175750 | 12 | 144 | 06-01-78 | P70600G | | | | | | | | | | | 28060 | 06-01-78 | 1 |
| 100 | L226500 | 7 | 7 | 06-01-78 | P70720G | | | | | | | | | | | 28061 | 06-01-78 | 1 |
| 100 | M054100 | 30 | 30 | 06-01-78 | P70550G | | | | | | | | | | | 28061 | 06-01-78 | 1 |
| 100 | M064500 | 14 | 14 | 06-02-78 | P63620G | | | | | | | | | | | 28061 | 06-01-78 | 1 |
| 100 | M074900 | 6 | 6 | 06-01-78 | P57960G | | | | | | | | | | | 28061 | 06-01-78 | 1 |
| 100 | M075125 | 60 | 60 | 06-02-78 | P67870G | | | | | | | | | | | 28061 | 06-01-78 | 1 |
| 100 | M076900 | 75 | 225 | 06-01-78 | P68150G | | | | | | | | | | | 28061 | 06-01-78 | 1 |
| 100 | M107600 | 2 | 20 | 06-01-78 | P68040G | | | | | | | | | | | 28061 | 06-01-78 | 1 |
| 100 | M113600 | 48 | 48 | 06-01-78 | P68260G | | | | | | | | | | | 28061 | 06-01-78 | 1 |
| 100 | M113850 | 18 | 18 | 06-01-78 | P68260G | | | | | | | | | | | 28061 | 06-01-78 | 1 |
| 100 | M328700 | 12 | 12 | 06-01-78 | P63420G | | | | | | | | | | | 28061 | 06-01-78 | 1 |
| 100 | M631200 | 2 | 2 | 06-01-78 | P68120G | | | | | | | | | | | 28062 | 06-01-78 | 1 |
| 100 | M284950 | 360 | 18000 | 05-24-78 | 0523B0007G | | | | | | | | | | | 28062 | 06-01-78 | 1 |
| 400 | M286750 | 144 | 3600 | 06-02-78 | 0602B0010G | | | | | | | | | | | 28063 | 06-01-78 | 2 |
| 400 | M289530 | 68 | 2200 | 06-02-78 | 0602B0010G | | | | | | | | | | | 28063 | 06-01-78 | 2 |
| 400 | M350900 | 400 | 400 | 06-02-78 | 0602B0010G | | | | | | | | | | | 28063 | 06-01-78 | 2 |
| 400 | M408000 | 170 | 17000 | 06-02-78 | 0602B0010G | | | | | | | | | | | 28063 | 06-01-78 | 2 |
| 400 | M017920 | 12 | 12 | 06-02-78 | 0602B0010G | | | | | | | | | | | 28063 | 06-01-78 | 2 |
| 400 | M403000 | 48 | 48 | 06-02-78 | 0602B0010G | | | | | | | | | | | 28063 | 06-01-78 | 2 |
| 400 | H059000 | 4 | 40 | 06-02-78 | 0602B0010G | | | | | | | | | | | 28063 | 06-01-78 | 2 |
| 400 | M019000 | 360 | 360 | 06-02-78 | 0602B0010G | | | | | | | | | | | 28063 | 06-01-78 | 2 |
| 400 | M021000 | 12 | 12 | 06-02-78 | 0602B0010G | | | | | | | | | | | 28063 | 06-01-78 | 2 |
| 400 | M053000 | 2500 | 2500 | 06-02-78 | 0602B0010G | | | | | | | | | | | 28063 | 06-01-78 | 2 |
| 400 | M097150 | 18 | 18 | 05-03-78 | P57640G | | | | | | | | | | | 28064 | 06-01-78 | 2 |
| 400 | M028000 | 4 | 192 | 06-02-78 | P70840G | | | | | | | | | | | 28064 | 06-01-78 | 2 |
| 400 | M652000 | 12 | 12 | 06-02-78 | P70840G | | | | | | | | | | | 28064 | 06-01-78 | 2 |
| 400 | M691000 | 12 | 12 | 06-02-78 | P70860G | | | | | | | | | | | 28064 | 06-01-78 | 2 |
| 400 | D142000 | 300 | 1200 | 06-02-78 | P70870G | | | | | | | | | | | 28064 | 06-01-78 | 2 |
| 400 | M385000 | 36 | 36 | 06-02-78 | P70890G | | | | | | | | | | | 28064 | 06-01-78 | 2 |
| 400 | P037400 | 5 | 125 | 06-02-78 | P70890G | | | | | | | | | | | 28064 | 06-01-78 | 2 |
| 100 | P037800 | 5 | 5 | 06-02-78 | P70890G | | | | | | | | | | | 28064 | 06-01-78 | 2 |

Source: Reproduced with permission from "Materiel Management Inventory Control Procedure" (Cleveland Clinic Foundation, 1979).

**Figure 3-4. Input Register**

*Standard-Price Concept*

The standard-price concept is often used to maintain a current purchase price, and a standard issue price. This concept aids in controlling the dollar variance between price increases and shrinkage.

The accounting department receives a report, generally on a monthly basis, indicating the variance by line item with total dollar variance for proper book adjustment.

The inventory-control function receives a monthly purchase-price-variance report indicating:

1. The old price.
2. The new price.
3. The percentage difference by month.
4. A cumulative percentage of increase or decrease for a twelve-month period (figure 3-5).
5. A summary of the number of items unchanged, and the numbers of items decreased and increased respectively, is shown in figure 3-6.

This report can be used to identify:

1. The vendors or manufacturers with excessive price variances.
2. The calendar months in which most price changes occur.
3. Time buckets in which contracts should be negotiated.
4. Efficiency of contracts.

Upon determination that a *current* purchase price should be revised, the inventory-control section processes the price change in accordance with figure 3-6. This change will not normally affect the standard purchase and issue prices, which are set for a fixed period of time. Standard purchase and issue prices will not be changed without prior authorization of some authority such as the director of inventory control. When changes must occur to the standard prices, documentation will be initiated to support any variance that is not a true price change. This may occur because of corrective action, vendor and/or packaging changes, or establishment of a new data record.

*The Data Record*

This section is based on "Materiel Management Inventory Control Procedure" (Cleveland Clinic Foundation, 1979).

The data record is the heart of an MMIS data base [7]. Without it the

```
CLEVELAND CLINIC FOUNDATION                    PURCHASE   PRICE              RUN DATE 06-01-78
REPORT NO HHMOBO HHKOBO                         VARIANCE   REPORT                        PAGE 2

0000390   ABBOTT LABORATORIES
```

| CATALOG NO<br>DESCRIPTION OF ITEM | MAY-78<br>OLD<br>NEW<br>PCNT | APR-78<br>OLD<br>NEW<br>PCNT | MAR-78<br>OLD<br>NEW<br>PCNT | FEB-78<br>OLD<br>NEW<br>PCNT | JAN-78<br>OLD<br>NEW<br>PCNT | DEC-77<br>OLD<br>NEW<br>PCNT | NOV-77<br>OLD<br>NEW<br>PCNT | OCT-77<br>OLD<br>NEW<br>PCNT | SEP-77<br>OLD<br>NEW<br>PCNT | AUG-77<br>OLD<br>NEW<br>PCNT | JUL-77<br>OLD<br>NEW<br>PCNT | JUN-77<br>OLD<br>NEW<br>PCNT | ACCUM<br>PCNT |
|---|---|---|---|---|---|---|---|---|---|---|---|---|---|
| A000050 ABBOCATH-T, ABBOTT #4535-16, 16 GAX2", | 128.400<br>128.400 | | | | | | | | | | | | 0 |
| A000120 ABBOCATH, ABBOTT #4535-20, 20 GAX1-1/4", | 128.400<br>128.400 | | | | | | | | | | | | 0 |
| A005600 LT4-LARYNGOTRACH ANES KT, ABBOTT #4898-01 | 82.560<br>82.560 | | | | | | | | | | | | 0 |
| A007395 TRAY, SPINAL,25 GA, SPINAL, ABBOTT #4774-01 | 77.030<br>77.030 | | | | | | | | | | | | 0 |
| A007450 TRAY, SPINAL, WHITACRE, ADTT #4805-01 | 102.200<br>102.200 | | | | | | | | | | | | 0 |
| A007700 VENOTUBE, TWIN-SITE, ABBOTT22-48 | 49.440<br>49.440 | | | | | | | | | | | | 0 |
| M077710 LUMBAR PUNCTURE TRAY, 20 GA. X 3-1/2" | 61.120<br>61.120 | | | | | | | | | | | | 0 |
| M077761.120 LUMBAR PUNCTURE TRAY, 20 GA. X 2-1/2" | 61.120 | | | | | | | | | | | | 0 |
| P106000 BLOOD ADMINISTRATION SET, PLIAPAK, | 113.420<br>113.420 | | | | | | | | | | | | 0 |
| P121500 HEMOSETS, 20/CS, ABBOTT #8948-20 | 107.440<br>107.440 | | | | | | | | | | | | 0 |

Source: Reproduced with permission from "Materiel Management Inventory Control Procedure" (Cleveland Clinic Foundation, 1979).

**Figure 3-5.** Purchase-Price-Variance Report, A

```
CLEVELAND CLINIC FOUNDATION                    PURCHASE   PRICE           RUN DATE 06-01-78
REPORT NO. HHKOBO HHKOBO                       VARIANCE  REPORT                   PAGE 99


NO. ITEMS UNCHANGED: 1502    NO. ITEMS INCREASE:          NO. ITEMS DECREASE:
TOTAL ITEMS:  1502
```

Source: Reproduced with permission from "Materiel Management Inventory Control Procedure" (Cleveland Clinic Foundation, 1979).

**Figure 3-6.** Purchase-Price-Variance Report, B

computer can do nothing. Figure 3-7, an "Inventory-Control Setup Change Form," and figure 3-8, an "Issue Unit-Cost Change," represent forms used by one large health center to establish and maintain the data base (master or data record).

The nomenclaturé and specific instructions provided for filling in these forms are as follows:

1. *Catalog number*: A ten-digit alphanumeric code used to identify one specific item (seven digits are currently used).
2. *Purchase unit*: A four-digit alpha code used to identify the unit in which that item is bought from the procurement source (two digits are currently used). See table 3-1.
3. *Issue unit*: A four-digit alpha code used to identify the unit in which the item is accounted for, received, and issued (two digits are currently used). See table 3-1.
4. *Buyer code*: A one-digit alpha code denoting the buyer for that commodity.
5. *Storeroom number*: A two-digit alpha code denoting the physical locations of that line item.
   a. 01 = Main storeroom
   b. 02 = Gases
   c. 03 = Operating-room storeroom
   d. 04 = Carpeting (off-site)
6. *Primary vendor*: A seven-digit numeric code. This code always ends with "90," for computer location. The preceeding digits are obtained from the accounts-payable vendor master file.
7. *Secondary vendor*: Same as primary vendor except it will indicate a second source. Note: This is not a mandatory field.
8. *Reporting description*: Forty alphanumeric digits that appear on reports and picking tickets.
9. *Additional description*: An additional forty alphanumeric digits utilized to clarify and complete the total description.
10. *Inventory account number*: A six-digit numeric field containing the account number(s) assigned by the accounting department to the inventory(ies).
11. *Minimum level.*
12. *Reorder-point level.*
13. *Maximum level*: Six-digit numeric fields used by the computer to trigger:
    a. Replenishment orders
    b. Follow-up and *overstock* notifications.
14. *Purchase unit cost*: An eight-digit, third-position-decimal pricing structure.
15. *Issue unit cost*: An eight-digit, third-position-decimal based on latest information in figure 3-8.

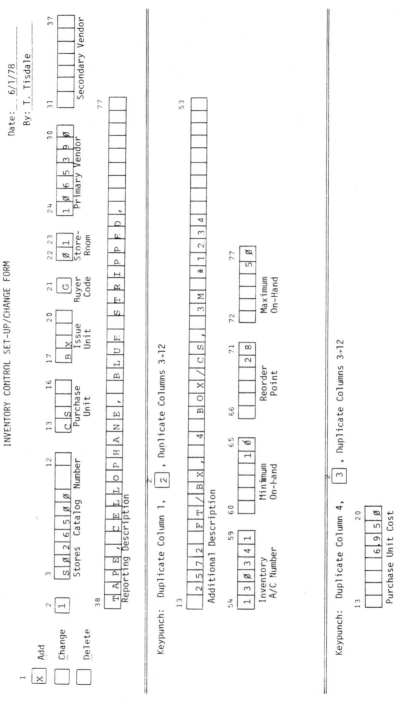

**Figure 3-7.** Inventory-Control Setup/Change Form, C

Source: Reproduced with permission from "Materiel Management Inventory Control Procedure" (Cleveland Clinic Foundation, 1979).

ISSUE UNIT COST CHANGE

DOCUMENT NO: 123456    DATE: 6/1/78    BY: THOMAS L. TISDALE

| T/C | CATALOG NUMBER | DATE CHNGD | 44 UNIT $ AMT. 52 |
|-----|----------------|------------|--------------------|
| 500 | SO26500        | 6/1/78     | 1.738              |
| 500 |                |            |                    |
| 500 |                |            |                    |
| 500 |                |            |                    |
| 500 |                |            |                    |
| 500 |                |            |                    |
| 500 |                |            |                    |
| 500 |                |            |                    |
| 500 |                |            |                    |
| 500 |                |            |                    |
| 500 |                |            |                    |
| 500 |                |            |                    |
| 500 |                |            |                    |

**Figure 3-8.** Procedure Flow Chart for Ordering Office Equipment

Source: Reproduced with permission from "Materiel Management Inventory Control Procedure" (Cleveland Clinic Foundation, 1979).

**Table 3-1**
**Issue-Unit Designation**

| Issue Unit | Abbreviation |
|------------|--------------|
| Pack | PK |
| Package | PG |
| Pad | PD |
| Pair | PR |
| Pound | LB |
| Roll | RL |
| Set | ST |
| Sheet | SH |
| Spool | SP |
| Square Yard | SY |
| Tank | TK |
| Tube | TU |
| Vial | VL |
| Yard | YD |

Reproduced with permission from "Materiel Management Inventory Control Procedure" (Cleveland Clinic Foundation, 1979).

## Computer-Selection Considerations

When health-care-delivery institutions consider purchasing or leasing computer capability, it is generally for purposes that include materials-management-information-systems needs, in addition to the information or data-processing needs of other functional units in the organization. Regardless of whether materials-management personnel are involved in the final computer-selection decisions, they should be knowledgeable in the various aspects of the selection process so that they can make intelligent contributions to the process. This section outlines the various economic and technical considerations that should affect a well-considered choice of hardware and software systems. The details can be found in [8].

*Costs* are exclusively tangible dollar cash flows, such as projections of payments to be made to the hardware manufacturer, the software supplier, and all those involved in the installation and continued use of the hardware-software system and the surrounding facilities wherever applicable. This also includes projections of any revenues attributable to the use of the system.

*Hardware characteristics* include a tremendous variety of factors, such as primary memory capacity, basic-instruction-cycle time, and possibly the required power supply.

*Expansion potential* typically consists of factors representing either the amount of slack time in the current system, expressed on a time scale; or an indication of maximum expansion in terms of numbers of certain physical units such as printers; or add-on memory expressed in K words or characters; and so on.

*Vendor support* involves such factors as programming assistance, training, and personnel loaned—probably best measured on a man-day scale. Maintenance and backup typically might be measured in terms of miles to the source, travel time, or some other measure of availability.

*Software rating* might occur in several dimensions, including execution time in seconds or minutes, or size in K words of primary memory required. Alternately, software may be rated subjectively on an arbitrary scale. If, for example, a specific software package provides 80 percent of the desired capabilities, then a rating of 80 percent would be given on, for example, a 0-100 scale.

### Changeovers from Manual to Computer-Aided Systems

Changeovers from manual to computer-aided materials-management information systems are never easy. Administrative and health-provider personnel must be led to recognize the ultimate advantages and the short-term dislocations. The philosophy and the optimum strategy for performing such changeovers are discussed in chapter 8 of a companion volume [6]. Basically, as indicated earlier in this chapter, the strategy calls for a meaningful involvement in its process of all those who will be affected by the changeover. They must be involved all the way from the inception of the study intended to identify the optimum system for their institution, through the implementation of that system. All concerned must recognize that, in general, the computer will handle the paperwork while people will handle the input and the material itself. Although the manner in which the computer works is fixed, the corrections and changes required can be made without conflicting with the computer activity.

The people involved must recognize that the objectives of the changeover are to establish a perpetual-inventory system that functions in an accurate and timely manner, controlling all aspects and requirements of inventory control; and to produce management reports necessary for that control.

They must recognize both the general and the specific advantages that occur when manual inventory records are computerized. The general advantages have been discussed earlier in this chapter. Some of the specific advantages are:

1. Reduction of posting time.
2. Perpetual-inventory calculations.
3. Purchase-order-requirement notification.

4. Notification of minimal inventory (followup required).
5. Overstock notification.
6. Control of unserviceable inventory.
7. Centralized control for all items.
8. Timely management and/or exception reports.
9. Easily accomplished storeroom-catalog-update procedures.
10. Physical-inventory facilitating procedures.
11. Daily update of all records.
12. Control of loaned and borrowed material.

After the changeover, the computer will process all transactions previously hand posted. The computer will process those transactions in a batch mode or post-post method, meaning the posting occurs after the action has been performed (for issues, receipts, and so on). The computer will process all transactions on a daily basis. Management reports will be produced on a daily, monthly, and/or annual basis to verify or correct the daily activity.

The computer will maintain all data records. The term *data record* in this context will apply to the method used in maintaining the perpetual inventory (also referred to as a *master record*). The computer will maintain all inventoried items on magnetic tape and disc. These items may have previously been maintained on manual Kardex-type systems. The inventory-control section will receive timely, if necessary daily, reports required to maintain the system within the established parameters from these tapes and discs.

Tom Scharf, a consultant in the area of computer-hardware-systems evaluation and installation lists nine errors commonly made in changing existing systems and designing new ones [9] (the statement is modified for health-care-service applicability).

1. Failure to consider the *motivation* (or lack of it) of the organization to use a new tool.
2. Failure to change the organizational structure in order to utilize the true potential of a new system. Failure also to recognize that this change process may require longer lead time than the machine installation.
3. Failure to attack and to give priority to the *real* problems of an organization. New soluions are often available but not even seriously considered in the rush to "improve" the old solutions to problems that were in fact solvable the last time around.
4. Failure to educate the organization's electronic-data-processing specialists and other personnel sufficiently well to avoid bad solutions, or to avoid good solutions to the wrong problems. The failure is in broad training and in updating knowledge to, and ahead of, current needs.

5. Failure to perceive the electronic-data-processing system and all associated costs as a capital investment and to compare such investment to alternative uses of capital.

6. Failure to place the electronic-data-processing organization in a sufficiently high organizational position so that it is responsible for serving the *whole* organization, not just a single department.

7. Failure of top management to:
   a. Explain their problems (their big problems).
   b. Clarify their goals and their policies.
   c. Demand (continual) economic and other justifications for the existence and installation of electronic-data-processing systems.

8. Failure to integrate technical and marketing problems into common-base solutions—for example, inventory control, production planning, and product design.

9. Failure to think in terms of *split solutions*. For example, hiring a smaller data-processing machine in house; using a larger one outside.

In the changeover process from manual to computer-aided systems, a discrepancy often exists between the basic information desired from an MMIS and the information available from the existing system. Such discrepancies can be depicted by an *incidence-type diagram*, as shown in figure 3-9. It depicts what the current system (CS) captured (✓) in a given institution, and what it did not (X). The figure also depicts what was required of the desired system (DS) (✓). The diagram also indicates what the "current" system with minor changes (m) and also with major changes (M) could have captured and hence provided. This diagram resulted from an MMS study for a multifacility health center using a multiechelon stocking system as depicted in figure 3-10.

A checklist for evaluating the kinds of reports needed and desired, and another one for evaluating the impact of information systems, are both provided in appendix 3A, as are audit procedures for the reporting functions.

**Documentation of Systems and Procedures**

In order that all concerned will understand a set of systems and procedures in the same way, such systems and procedures must be documented in an efficient and unambiguous manner. This is true both for systems and procedures in existence and for those contemplated.

Such a level of understanding is necessary prior to making meaningful changes, in order to teach users as well as systems personnel, and as a means of enforcement or control. It therefore behooves an integrated MMIS to maintain updated documentation on all systems and procedures concerned with the management of materials. Chapter 5 delineates various basic

| Level | Inventory On Hand | | Order Quantity | | Date of Order | | Quantity Withdrawn | | Date of Shipment | | Date of Arrival | | Quantity Received | |
|---|---|---|---|---|---|---|---|---|---|---|---|---|---|---|
| | CS | DS | CS | DS | CS | DS | CS | DS | CS | DS | CS | DS | CS | DS |
| Warehouse | ✓ | ✓ | ✓ | ✓ | ✓ | ✓ | ✓ | ✓ | X | ✓ | ✓ | ✓ | ✓ | ✓ |
| Facility CSR | X | ✓ | ✓ | ✓ | Xm | ✓ | XM | ✓ | ✓ | ✓ | Xm | ✓ | XmF | ✓ |
| Department | X | ✓ | WHSE. ✓ / CSR XM | ✓ | WHSE. Xm / CSR XM | ✓ | XG | ✓ | WHSE. ✓ / CSR XG | ✓ | WHSE. XmF / CSR XG | ✓ | WHSE. / CSR XM | |
| Module | X | X? | WHSE. X / CSR X | X? | WHSE. X / CSR X | X? | X | X? | WHSE. X / CSR X | X? | WHSE. XmF / CSR X | X? | WHSE. XMF / CSR Xm | |

*LEGEND:*

CS: Current system with *no* changes.
DS: Desired System.
✓: The information in this column *can* be easily obtained for the level of this row.
X: The information in this column *cannot* be easily obtained for the level of this row.
M: Major changes in current system can obtain the information.
m: Minor changes in current system can obtain this information.
F: Shipment arrives at facility but not necessarily the department.
?: It is questionable whether this information is needed at this row's level.

**Figure 3-9. Materials-Management System: Information Available and Desired**

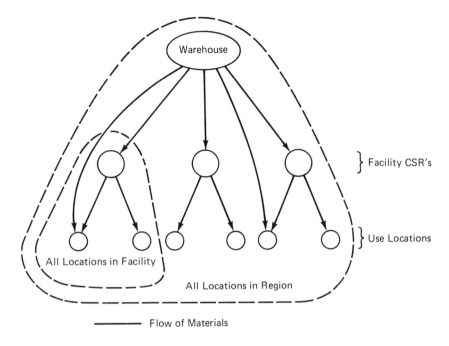

**Figure 3-10.** A Multiechelon Materials-Management System

techniques for describing systems involving personnel, products, and information flows. Figures 3-11 and 3-12 depict a documentation developed for an existing system of procuring nonstandard-stock items in a large HMO.

**References**

1. Garritty, J.T. *Getting the Most Out of Your Computer.* New York: McKinsey and Company, 1964.
2. Gallagher, James D. "Management Information Systems and the Computer." *AMA Research Study,* no. 51. New York: American Management Association, 1961.
3. Reisman, A.; Silva, J.; and Mantell, J. "Systems and Procedures of Patients and Information Flow in the Outpatient Clinic of a Large Health Center." *Hospital and Health Services Administration* 23 (Winter 1978).
4. Schultz, R.L. and Slevin, D.P., eds. *Implementing Operations Research/Management Science.* New York: Elsevier, North Holland, 1975.

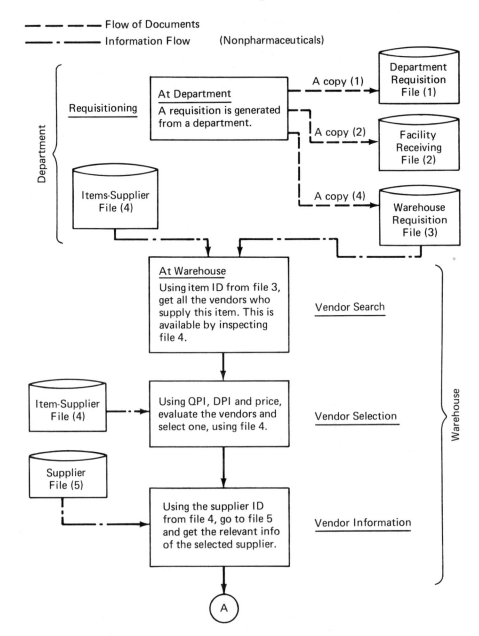

— — — — — Flow of Documents
———— · ———— Information Flow        (Nonpharmaceuticals)

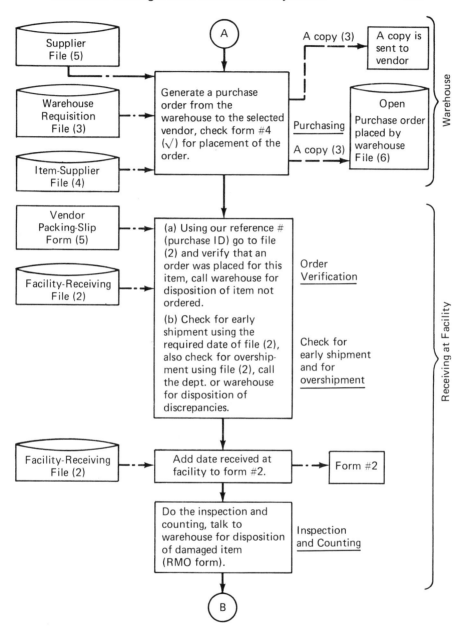

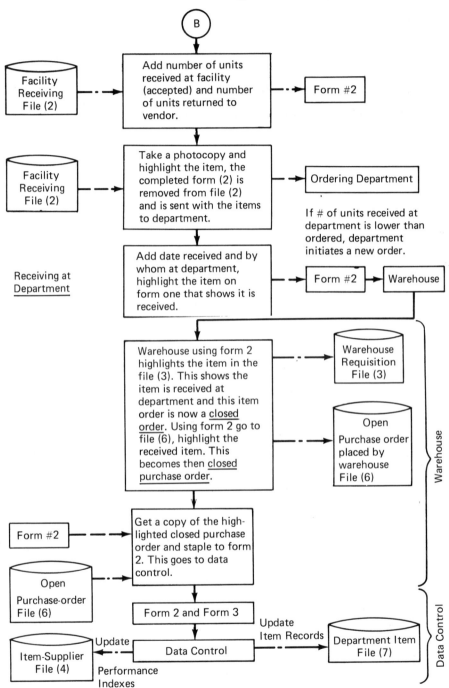

**Figure 3-11.** Example of Procurement Procedures for Nonstandard-Stock Items

*FILES OF NON STANDARD STOCK*

FILE # :              1

FILE NAME:            DEPARTMENT REQUISITION FILE

PRIMARY KEY:          REQUISITION ID AND LINE #

KEPT AT:              ORIGINATING DEPARTMENT

CONTENT:              DEPARTMENT REQUISITION FORM (FORM #1)

FUNCTION:             WHAT ITEMS ARE PLACED ON ORDER, WHEN, AND HOW MUCH.

FILE # :              2

FILE NAME:            FACILITY RECEIVING FILE

PRIMARY KEY:          REQUISITION ID AND LINE # (WHICH IS PURCHASE ORDER ID)

KEPT AT:              FACILITY RECEIVING DOCK

CONTENT:              A COPY OF DEPARTMENT REQUISITION FORM (FORM #2)

FUNCTION:             TO VERIFY THE PLACEMENT OF AN ORDER WHEN A
                      SHIPMENT ARRIVES.

                      TO CHECK THE ARRIVAL DATE OF THE ITEM.

                      TO CHECK THE NUMBER OF UNITS ORDERED.

                      TO RECORD THE ARRIVAL DATE.

                      TO RECORD THE NUMBER OF UNITS ACCEPTED.

FILE # :              3

FILE NAME:            WAREHOUSE REQUISITION FILE

PRIMARY KEY:          REQUISITION ID AND LINE #

KEPT AT:              WAREHOUSE

CONTENT:              A COPY OF DEPARTMENT REQUISITION FORM
                      (WAREHOUSE COPY) (FORM #4)

FUNCTION:     WHICH DEPARTMENTS HAVE REQUISITIONED WHAT ITEMS IN WHAT QUANTITY, TO USE THE ITEM ID TO FIND THE VENDORS

FILE # :     4

FILE NAME:     ITEM, SUPPLIER FILE

PRIMARY KEY:     ITEM ID

KEPT AT:     WAREHOUSE, THIS IS A FILE KEPT IN A COMPUTER STORAGE AND IS UPDATED FOR ITS CONTENT. A HARD COPY (PRINT OUT) OF IT IS KEPT AT WAREHOUSE

CONTENT:

| ITEM ID | SUPPLIED ID | DATE UNTIL WHICH QUOTATION IS VALID | PRICE BREAKS | | QUOTED LEAD TIME |
|---|---|---|---|---|---|
| | | | MIN QTY | PRICE | |

| EMERGENCY DELIVERY | | | QUALITY [1] PERFORMANCE INDEX | DELIVERY PERFORMANCE INDEX |
|---|---|---|---|---|
| PRICE BREAKS | | | | |
| MIN QTY | PRICE | LEAD TIME | | |

[1] NEW QPI = $\alpha$ OLD$_{QPI}$ + (1 − $\alpha$) CALCULATED QPI FROM A RECEIPT

NEW DPI = $\alpha$ OLD$_{DPI}$ + (1 − $\alpha$) CALCULATED DPI FROM A RECEIPT

$0 < \alpha < 1$, i.e., $\alpha$ = .10, GIVES APPROPRIATE WEIGHT TO PREVIOUS PERFORMANCE

$1 - \alpha$ GIVES APPROPRIATE WEIGHT TO THE LATEST PERFORMANCE

FILE # :     6

FILE NAME:     SUPPLIER FILE

PRIMARY KEY:     SUPPLIER ID

KEPT AT:     THIS IS KEPT IN A COMPUTER STORAGE AND IS UPDATED. A HARD COPY (PRINT OUT) IS KEPT AT WAREHOUSE FOR REFERENCE.

CONTENT:

| SUPPLIER ID | SUPPLIER NAME | SUPPLIER ADDRESS | CONTACT PERSON | PHONE # |
|---|---|---|---|---|

FUNCTION:     TO GET THE SELECTED SUPPLIER INFORMATION USING SUPPLIER ID

FILE # :          6

FILE NAME:        OPEN PURCHASE ORDER FILE

PRIMARY KEY:      PURCHASE ORDER ID (DEP. REQUISITION ID – LINE #)

KEPT AT:          WAREHOUSE

CONTENT:          PURCHASE ORDER FORM (FORM #3)

FUNCTION:         TO FACILITATE ANSWERING THE QUERIES OF DEPT.
                  ABOUT THEIR REQUISITION

FILE # :          7

FILE NAME:        DEPARTMENT, ITEM FILE

PRIMARY KEY:      DEP ID AND ITEM ID

KEPT AT:          COMPUTER STORAGE DATA BASE

| DEP ID, ITEM ID | $ UP TO DATE | $ UP TO DATE LAST YEAR | UNIT UP TO DATE |
|---|---|---|---|

| UNIT UP TO DATE LAST YEAR | TOTAL $ LAST YEAR | TOTAL UNITS LAST YEAR |
|---|---|---|

FUNCTION:         PROVIDE COMPARATIVE COST INFORMATION FOR AN
                  ITEM IN A DEP. SOURCE FOR ANY TYPE OF REPORTING OF
                  COSTS AND NUMBER OF UNITS ACROSS DEPARTMENTS
                  AND FACILITIES.

*FORMS OF NON STANDARD STOCK*

FORM #1:          DEPARTMENT REQUISITION FORM

CONTENT OF THE FORM:

| REQUISITION ID[1] | DEPT ID[2] | DEPT. NAME | FACILITY NAME | ITEM ID[3] | ITEM DESCRIPTION UNIT OF ISSUE INCLUDED |
|---|---|---|---|---|---|

| QUANTITY REQUIRED | REQUESTED BY | TODAY'S DATE | DATE REQUIRED | APPROVED BY | DATE APPROVED | DEA[4] ITEM |
|---|---|---|---|---|---|---|
| | | | | | | |

1) THIS IS A PREPRINTED NUMBER AND IS UNIQUE.

2) THIS IS A NUMBER WHICH HAS THE ENTITY (FACILITY) # AND ALSO THE DEPARTMENT #, THIS NUMBER IS ALREADY IN USE.

3) NUMBER BY WHICH AN ITEM IS UNIQUELY IDENTIFIED. THE WAREHOUSE SHOULD BE ABLE TO COME UP WITH THESE FOR NON-STOCK ITEM.

4) IT IS A CHECK FOR CONTROLLED ITEMS.

NOTE: ALL THE FIELDS APPEARING ARE FILLED WHEN A REQUISITION IS PLACED BY A DEPARTMENT.

FORM #2:        A COPY OF DEPARTMENT REQUISITION FORM

CONTENT OF THE FORM:

| FORM #1 | DATE RECEIVED AT DOCK OF FACILITY | NUMBER OF UNITS ACCEPTED | NUMBER OF UNITS REJECTED (OR RETURNED) | RECEIVED BY AT FACILITY DOCK |
|---|---|---|---|---|
| | | | | |

THIS PART IS FILLED IN WHEN THE REQUISITION IS GENERATED FROM A DEPARTMENT

THIS PART IS FILLED IN WHEN THE ITEM IS RECEIVED AT THE RECEIVING DOCK OF THE FACILITY

| DATE RECEIVED AT DEPARTMENT | RECEIVED AT DEPT. AT |
|---|---|
| | |

THESE WILL BE FILLED OUT WHEN ITEM IS RECEIVED IN THE DEPARTMENT

FORM #3:        PURCHASE ORDER FORM

CONTENT OF THE FORM:

| PURCHASE ORDER ID[1,2] | ITEM ID[2] | ITEM DESCRIPTION[2] | ORDER PLACED[3] AT DATE BY WAREHOUSE | DATE REQUIRED[2] |
|---|---|---|---|---|
| | | | | |

| QUANTITY[2] REQUIRED | UNIT PRICE[4] | TOTAL $ AMOUNT | SUPPLIER ID[5] | SUPPLIER NAME[5] | LEAD TIME[5] | TAX INDICATOR[6] | SHIP TO ADDRESS[7] |
|---|---|---|---|---|---|---|---|
| | | | | | | | |

1) THIS IS SAME AS REQUISITION ID — LINE #, USING DEPT. REQUISITION FORM.

2) USE DEPARTMENT REQUISITION FORM KEPT IN FILE (3).

3) THIS IS FILLED OUT BY WAREHOUSE AT THE TIME PURCHASE ORDER IS BEING FILLED OUT.

4) USE FILE (4) TO GET THIS.

5) USE FILE (5) TO GET THESE.

6) WHETHER THE ITEM IS TAXABLE OR NOT (1 FOR TAXABLE, 0 FOR NON-TAXABLE).

7) THE ADDRESS TO WHERE ITEM IS SUPPOSED TO BE SHIPPED (FACILITY ADDRESS).

NOTE: THIS FORM IS FILLED OUT BY WAREHOUSE.


FORM #4:             DEPARTMENT REQUISITION FORM (WAREHOUSE COPY)

CONTENT OF THE FORM:

| FORM #1 | ORDER PLACED[1] INDICATOR |
|---|---|
| | |

1) A √ SHOWS THAT WAREHOUSE HAS PLACED ORDER FOR THIS ITEM.


FORM #5:             VENDOR PACKING SLIP

CONTENT OF THE FORM (AMONG OTHER THINGS):

| PURCHASE ORDER ID[1] | QUANTITY |
|---|---|
| | |

1) THE FIRST PART OF THIS SHOWS THE REQUISITION # AND THE REST LINE #.

**Figure 3-12.** Files of Nonstandard Stock

5. Schultz, R.L.; Slevin, D.P.; and Henry, M.D. "A Bibliography on the Implementation of Operations Research/Management Science." *Report*. West Lafayette, Ind.: Graduate School of Management, Purdue University, August 1978.
6. Reisman, A. *Systems Analysis in Health-Care Delivery*. Lexington, Mass.: Lexington Books, D.C. Heath and Company, 1979.
7. "Materiel Management Inventory Control Procedure." Cleveland, Ohio: Cleveland Clinic Foundation, 1979.
8. Clark, J.D., and Reisman, A. *Computer Systems Selection: An Integrated Approach*. New York: Praeger, 1981.
9. Scharf, Tom G. "How Not to Choose an EDP System." *Datamation* (April 1969).

# Appendix 3A:
# Checklists and
# Audit Procedures for
# Materials-Management
# Information Systems

**Checklist for Evaluating Existing Reports**

| Questions | *Comments (Provide data on "yes" answers. Explain "no answers.)* | |
|---|---|---|
| | *Yes* | *No* |
| A. Are the principal items in the report emphasized? | _____ | _____ |
| B. Are the reports timely, that is, current and up-to-date? | _____ | _____ |
| C. Are the reports promptly available? | _____ | _____ |
| D. Are the reports understandable? | _____ | _____ |
| E. Are the reports accurate and reliable? | _____ | _____ |
| F. Are the reports valid? | _____ | _____ |
| G. Are the reports clearly and simply designed? | _____ | _____ |
| H. Are the reports expressed in language and terms familiar to the reader? | _____ | _____ |
| I. Is it possible adequately to judge current performance and identify trends from the report? | _____ | _____ |
| J. Are actual performances compared to reasonable standards? | _____ | _____ |
| K. Are explanatory comments included to direct the users' attention to important |

|  | *Comments (Provide data on "yes" answers. Explain "no" answers.)* | |
|---|---|---|
| *Questions* | *Yes* | *No* |

items and to interpret the significance and
meaning of those items? _____  _____

L.  Does the report provide meaningful and
needed information? _____  _____

**Checklist for Evaluating Distribution
and Control of Existing Reports**

A.  Is a report catalog of the existing reports
available that will indicate what information is now being supplied and to whom? _____  _____

B.  Does a report-request form exist that can
be used by operating managers to request
information they may need in carrying
out their responsibilities? _____  _____

C.  Does a policy exist to determine who will
receive reports and how and when they
will receive them? _____  _____

D.  Are the reports designed for the ultimate
users' needs? _____  _____
    1.  Is the policy covering the distribution
        of information and reports made
        available to those charged with
        designing and preparing reports? _____  _____

E.  Are the internal management reports
secure, that is, not made available to persons outside the institution unless
specifically authorized by higher management? _____  _____

F.  Is there a system of reviewing the
usefulness of reports on a periodic basis? _____  _____

|  | Comments |
|---|---|
|  | *(Provide data on "yes" answers. Explain "no" answers.)* |

| *Questions* | *Yes* | *No* |
|---|---|---|

G. Does there exist a system of authorizing new reports?  _____  _____

H. Are the generated reports properly reviewed and evaluated?  _____  _____

I. Does the records-management program contain a retention schedule for reports?  _____  _____

J. Who are the ultimate users of the reports:
  1. Is the report to be used by a doctor?  _____  _____
  2. Is the report for departmental use?  _____  _____
  3. Is the report to be used by a chief-executive officer or controller or both?  _____  _____

**Checklist for Evaluating the Kinds of Reports Needed and Desired**

A. Do control reports exist for the detection of errors occurring during the processing of transactions?  _____  _____

B. Are monitoring reports available for monitoring necessary activities and expenses required for the conduct of business?  _____  _____

C. Do the regularly scheduled reports provide the necessary information to support managerial decision-making efforts?  _____  _____
  1. Are these schedules prepared at definite intervals and in a fixed format?  _____  _____
  2. Are these schedules automatically generated?  _____  _____

|  | *Comments (Provide data on "yes" answers. Explain "no" answers.)* | |
| --- | --- | --- |
| *Questions* | *Yes* | *No* |

D. Are exception reports available, which signal out-of-bounds conditions?   _____   _____

E. Can unscheduled reports be prepared when requested by managers?   _____   _____

F. Can special-analysis reports be prepared when requested by managers?   _____   _____

G. Are inquiry-processing reports needed, which would generate information through terminals directly to the user upon request?   _____   _____

**Checklist for an MMIS and Its Use**

This section is based on "Checklist and Guidelines for Evaluating Purchasing and Materials Management Functions in Private Hospitals: Opportunities for Improving Hospital Purchasing, Inventory Management and Supply Distribution," part II, U.S. General Accounting Office, PSAD 79-58B, April 1979.

A. Do perpetual-inventory records show receipts, issues, and inventory balances for each stock item?   _____   _____
   1. Are these records kept by people other than those with access to the inventory?   _____   _____
   2. Are the perpetual-inventory balances periodically compared to the actual stock; and are discrepancies investigated, corrected, and documented?   _____   _____

B. Are the medical-surgical supplies stored in nursing stations and other departments carried as inventory?   _____   _____

| *Questions* | *Yes* | *No* |
|---|---|---|

C.  Are records kept of:
   1. High-dollar-value items?
   2. Major supply sources?
   3. Emergency-supply sources?
   4. Order frequencies?
   5. Vendor performance?
   6. Product performance?

D.  If pharmaceutical purchases are made by
   the purchasing department, does the
   pharmacy:
   1. Maintain a list of drug manufacturers
      and wholesalers and their local
      representatives?
   2. Maintain a list of emergency sources
      with special attention to critical items
      not widely available?
   3. Prepare detailed specifications?
   4. Prepare requisitions?
   5. Prepare receiving reports?
   6. Prepare return-goods memos for any
      items returned for credit?

E.  Does the pharmacy's written instructions
   require it to:
   1. Forecast future needs?
   2. Record past usage?
   3. Rank its pharmaceutical items accord-
      ing to annual dollar volume?

F.  Does the pharmacy maintain the data
   needed to effectively manage its purchasing function, such as:
   1. Major high-dollar-value items?
   2. Major supply sources?
   3. Emergency-supply sources?
   4. Quantities purchased and prices for
      each item?

|  | *Comments (Provide data on "yes" answers. Explain "no" answers.)* | |
| :--- | :---: | :---: |
| *Questions* | *Yes* | *No* |
| 5. Usage histories? | _____ | _____ |
| 6. Order frequencies? | _____ | _____ |
| 7. Vendor performance? | _____ | _____ |
| 8. Product performance? | _____ | _____ |
| G. Are perpetual-inventory records kept for high-dollar-volume and critical pharmaceutical items? | _____ | _____ |
|    1. Are the records kept by people other than those with access to the inventory? | _____ | _____ |
|    2. Are they used to obtain usage histories for each item? | _____ | _____ |
|    3. Are the perpetual-inventory balances periodically compared to the actual stock; and are discrepancies investigated, corrected, and documented? | _____ | _____ |
| H. Are annual physical inventories reconciled with accounting department control accounts? | _____ | _____ |
|    1. Is the physical inventory taken or supervised by a member of another department (such as the accounting department)? | _____ | _____ |
|    2. Is the physical inventory verified by the hospital's external auditors? | _____ | _____ |
| I. If food purchases are made by the purchasing department does the dietary department: | | |
|    1. Maintain a list of food suppliers, including wholesalers and local vendors? | _____ | _____ |
|    2. Prepare requisitions? | _____ | _____ |
|    3. Prepare receiving reports? | _____ | _____ |

|  | *Comments (Provide data on "yes" answers. Explain "no" answers.)* | |
|---|---|---|
| *Questions* | *Yes* | *No* |

4. Prepare return-goods memos for any items returned for credit? _____ _____

J. Does the dietary department maintain the data needed to effectively manage its purchasing functions, such as:
  1. Major high-dollar-value items? _____ _____
  2. Major supply sources? _____ _____
  3. Emergency-supply sources? _____ _____
  4. Quantities purchased and prices for each item? _____ _____

K. If the dietary department purchases food, does it have written instructions? _____ _____

L. If so, are they specific instructions that:
  1. Cannot be changed without review by the purchasing chief or central manager and approval by top management? _____ _____
  2. Restrict dietary department purchases to food supplies and require it to requisition capital items and other supplies through the purchasing department? _____ _____
  3. Promote maximum use of competition? _____ _____
  4. Encourage the dietary department to purchase other than brand-name foods? _____ _____

M. Do the written instructions require the dietary department to:
  1. Forecast future needs? _____ _____
  2. Record past usage? _____ _____
  3. Record usage history? _____ _____
  4. Record order frequency? _____ _____

|  | *Comments (Provide data on "yes" answers. Explain "no" answers.)* | |
|---|---|---|
| *Questions* | *Yes* | *No* |

5. Record vendor performance?      _____      _____

6. Record product performance?      _____      _____

N. Are perpetual dietary-department-inventory records kept for high-dollar-value and critical items?      _____      _____

     1. Are the records kept by people other than those with access to the inventory?      _____      _____

     2. Are they used to obtain usage histories for each item?      _____      _____

     3. Are the perpetual-inventory balances periodically compared to the actual stock and are discrepancies investigated, corrected, and documented?      _____      _____

O. Are annual dietary-department inventories reconciled with the accounting department control accounts?      _____      _____

     1. Is the physical inventory taken or supervised by a member of another department (such as the accounting department)?      _____      _____

     2. Is the physical inventory verified by the hospital's external auditors?      _____      _____

**Checklist for Evaluating Impact of Information Systems**

A. Have information systems changed the cost of operation?      _____      _____

B. Have information systems changed the way in which operations are performed?      _____      _____

|  | *Comments (Provide data on "yes" answers. Explain "no" answers.)* | |
|---|---|---|
| *Questions* | *Yes* | *No* |

C.  Have information systems changed the accuracy of information that users receive? _____ _____

D.  Have information systems changed the timeliness of information and reports that users receive? _____ _____

E.  Have information systems brought about organizational changes? Are these changes for the better or for the worse? _____ _____

F.  Have information systems changed the completeness of the information? _____ _____

G.  Have information systems changed control or centralization? What is the effect of such changes? _____ _____

H.  Have information systems changed the attitudes of systems users or persons affected by the systems? _____ _____

I.  Have information systems changed the number of users? _____ _____

J.  Have information systems changed the interactions between members of the organization? _____ _____

K.  Have information systems changed productivity? _____ _____

L.  Have information systems changed the effort that must be expanded to receive information for decision making? _____ _____

**Checklist for Appraising Forms**

A.  Is the form necessary? _____ _____

| Questions | *Comments (Provide data on "yes" answers. Explain "no" answers.)* | |
| --- | --- | --- |
| | *Yes* | *No* |
| 1. Is a new form necessary, or is there some existing form that could be adopted as is or with some revisions? | _____ | _____ |
| 2. Has the entire system been checked? Would a written procedure for the use of this form help to put it into more efficient operation? | _____ | _____ |
| 3. Can the information furnished by this form be combined with some other form, or can some other form be eliminated by or consolidated with this form? | _____ | _____ |
| 4. Could the period covered be lengthened from daily to weekly or from weekly to monthly? | _____ | _____ |
| 5. Are all copies necessary? Could a copy be routed from one department to another, thereby cost-effectively eliminating one or more copies? | _____ | _____ |
| 6. Have persons who will use the form been consulted for suggested improvements? Have those responsible for the form approved it? | _____ | _____ |
| B. Is it well designed? | _____ | _____ |
| 1. If this is a revised form, can it be distinguished from the previous form? | _____ | _____ |
| 2. Does the form clearly indicate its purpose by its title and arrangement? | _____ | _____ |
| 3. If this form is to take information from or pass information to another form, do both have the same sequence of items? | _____ | _____ |

*Comments
(Provide data on
"yes" answers.
Explain "no"
answers.)*

| *Questions* | *Yes* | *No* |
|---|---|---|
| 4. Is the size standard and no larger than necessary? Is the form convenient for filing, mailing, and handling? | _____ | _____ |
| 5. If the form is to be filled in with a typewriter, is it suited for straight typing, that is, for a minimum number of tab stops, rollbacks, and carriage returns? | _____ | _____ |
| 6. Will routing or handling instructions printed on each copy facilitate use? | _____ | _____ |
| 7. Have sufficient margins been allowed for printing, office machine, fill-in, duplicating, binding, and filing? | _____ | _____ |
| 8. If it is an external form, should it be designed for use in a window envelope? | _____ | _____ |
| 9. Could the form be designed as a self-mailer? | _____ | _____ |
| 10. Should the copies of this form be numbered consecutively or have a place for inserting a number? | _____ | _____ |
| 11. Is the spacing, both horizontal and vertical, correct for fill-in? | _____ | _____ |
| 12. Is there space for date of issue, and is it properly located? | _____ | _____ |
| 13. Is all fixed information to be printed, so that only variable items need to be filled in? | _____ | _____ |
| 14. Are the important items, which should be seen first, properly placed (near the top, if practicable)? | _____ | _____ |
| 15. Are items properly grouped for other departments to fill in or refer to? | _____ | _____ |

|  | *Comments (Provide data on "yes" answers. Explain "no" answers.)* | |
| *Questions* | *Yes* | *No* |

16. Are items properly located to make reference easy when the copies are filed or bound? _____ _____

17. Are spaces provided for signatures and approvals with date spaces for each? _____ _____

18. Has the number of digits or the typical fill-in been indicated? _____ _____

19. If the form is to be sent from one person to another, are proper spaces for "to" and "from" provided? _____ _____

20. Is the form identified by the name of the hospital or by a code number to aid in reordering? _____ _____

C. Are specifications and volume right? _____ _____

  1. Is the duplication process contemplated consistent with the number required and the desired character of the form? _____ _____

  2. If a nonpermanent duplication process is involved, has consideration been given to deterioration? _____ _____

  3. Are detailed printing specifications complete (paper, type, rules, punch, perforate, score, fold, gather, pad, carbon sheet, stitch, and so on)? _____ _____

  4. Should the form be on colored paper to speed writing, distribution, sorting, and filing; to designate departments; to indicate days, months, or years; to distinguish manifold copies; or to identify rush orders? _____ _____

  5. Have requirements been estimated correctly and is the quantity to be ordered the most economical? (Con-

|  | Comments *(Provide data on "yes" answers. Explain "no" answers.)* |  |
| :--- | :---: | :---: |
| *Questions* | *Yes* | *No* |

sider the probability of revision and the rate of use.)  \_\_\_\_\_  \_\_\_\_\_

6. Has an order point been properly established with due regard for the time required to secure a new supply? (Consider the type of form and the source of supply.)  \_\_\_\_\_  \_\_\_\_\_

7. Has the disposition of old or superceded forms been decided?  \_\_\_\_\_  \_\_\_\_\_

8. Will sample or proofs be needed for distribution? How many?  \_\_\_\_\_  \_\_\_\_\_

9. Has consideration been given to the number of forms that will be used in a given time, the possibility of changes, and the length of time that the form will remain in use?  \_\_\_\_\_  \_\_\_\_\_

## Audit Procedures for the Reporting Functions

*Objective*: To determine whether the report is tailored specifically to the purpose it serves, the use to which it will be put, and the person who will receive it.

*Audit steps*:

1. Determine whether the management of the purchasing department and others in the hierarchical structure are kept informed for decision and control purposes through reports including the following:
   a. Market conditions, including current and anticipated future price and supply developments.
   b. Inventory position, including stock on hand, turnover, and anticipated demand.
   c. Purchase commitments, by inventory category, showing orders placed and delivery schedules.

    d.  Open-to-buy, the amount of additional inventory that can be ordered without exceeding anticipated usage and inventory positions.

    e.  Open requisitions, awaiting processing into purchase orders.

    f.  Survey of vendor performance, showing inspection information, lapsed time between order and receipt, and percentage of items backordered.

    g.  Summary of purchase by vendor and by expense, to identify the major suppliers of particular items.

    h.  Expense and activity analysis, detailing the activities of the department in dollars and other quantitative measures.

2.  Determine whether the inventory reports are providing the information necessary in order to evaluate the effectiveness of day-to-day inventory operations and controls. The present reports should provide the following information:

    a.  Inventory analysis by item class, age, value, or department.

    b.  Purchase commitments and open-to-buy amounts.

    c.  Analysis of obsolete, damaged, stolen, slow-moving, or frequently restocked items.

    d.  Material price-and-quantity-variance analysis, to reveal market-price trends, purchasing efficiency, and efficiency in use of inventory items.

    e.  Analysis of scrapped and reworked items.

    f.  Analysis of turnover and investment in particular classes or items.

    g.  Analysis of differences between physical count and book amounts of inventory, to reveal accuracy in accounting for and handling of items.

3.  Determine whether there are formal procedures for authorizing, reproducing, and distributing information in the form of reports.

    a.  Review the report catalogue of existing reports (if one is available), establish what information is now being supplied and to whom, and identify areas where there is duplication of information and reports.

    b.  Determine whether requests for a regular continuing report are handled according to an established review procedure.

    c.  Review the report-authorization process when a report is requested.

        1.  Is determination made of whether the requested information is already available in an existing report?

        2.  If the information is not available in an existing report, is the relevant data being recorded at present, and in what form?

        3.  Determine whether the information can be made available within the time restraints, and calculate the cost.

d. Review the reports and observe whether they indicate trends by including past figures and budgeted figures and whether the latter are compared against actual amounts.

e. Examine the reports to see if they are complete, accurate, and easily read.

f. Interview some of the receivers of these reports to determine whether the reports are timely.

g. Identify who will receive the reports and how and when they will receive them.

   1. Ascertain and evaluate whether these individuals should receive reports; that is, do they need the information in order to carry out their responsibilities?

h. Check to see whether procedures are established to deliver reports to the user as soon as they are produced.

   1. Determine whether there are procedures for reviewing and editing the reports after they are produced.

# 4 Decision Rules

## Materials Inventory Control: An Analogy

A simple, liquid flow and storage system can serve as a useful *analogy* in discussions of materials-inventory systems. Figure 4-1 illustrates a tank being filled with a liquid substance through a valve-controlled nozzle. The tank is provided with an outflow nozzle, which can be used to draw the liquid out of the bottom of the tank. For purposes of this analogy, both the liquid inflow and the outflow are considered to take place intermittently. If the liquid is assumed to have a fairly high unit cost, then the inventory problem in this case might be to have enough material available when and if it is needed, but not much more than that. To do otherwise would tie up material, and therefore money, unnecessarily. This problem may be solved in one of two ways. The materials manager can periodically check the level of the tank and fill it to the top whenever the liquid level is clearly at less than full tank capacity. At times this may require a replenishment of only a fraction of a gallon or a liter; at other times the entire tank may have to be refilled. Alternatively, the materials manager may wish to do nothing in terms of replenishment until the liquid falls below a certain predefined level. This might be accomplished by having a reserve tank that is drawn on when and if the first tank has been emptied.

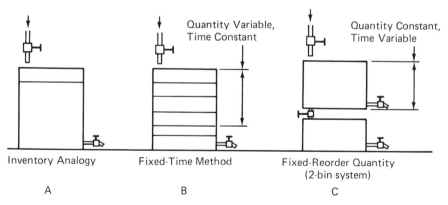

**Figure 4-1.** Inventory Concepts

Checking the tank at equal time intervals is considered a fixed-review-time method of replenishment, frequently referred to as the *ordering-cycle method*. On the other hand, a replenishment policy that is triggered only when the tank reaches a certain level is a *fixed-reorder-point method*, frequently referred to as the *two-bin method*. The reason for the two-bin terminology is evident from the analogy just stated. The liquid system includes one tank or bin holding the regular supply, and another tank or bin holding a reserve supply. The second tank is drawn on only after the first tank has been emptied. Figure 4-2 can be used to indicate the difference between these two approaches. It is a typical sawtooth diagram, very often used to illustrate inventory-control problems. The horizontal axis corresponds to time; the vertical axis corresponds to the quantity in storage. Withdrawals of different-sized lots at different time intervals is illustrated by the dashed "staircase"-shaped lines. When both the quantities withdrawn each time and the time durations between such withdrawals are fairly equal or uniform, then the solid, straight line is clearly a good approximation to the actual situation. The quantity represented by $Q_0$ is the initial amount of inventory in storage, and this is reduced over time as a result of the various withdrawals. The quantity in storage approaches a zero level at a certain time interval, $t$. The slope of the line, $Q_0 t$, is indicative of the amount of inventory withdrawn per unit of time.

Figure 2(B) shows the case in which the time intervals between replenishments are equal, but the replenishment quantity varies from order to order. This, then, is the fixed-review-time, or cyclic, ordering method. As indicated earlier, the inventory items under this schema, or policy, are kept under periodic surveillance so that once a month, or once a week, or once a day, a replenishment order is placed, bringing the inventory levels up to the a priori established maximum.

On the other hand, figure 4-2(C) depicts the case of a *constant-replenishment*-quantity policy with varying time intervals between reorders. This is referred to as the *fixed-order-point method*. Under this policy, the on-hand inventory is theoretically checked every time any material is withdrawn from inventory. When the inventory of the amount stocked reaches a certain point, a quantity of a fixed size is reordered. In summary:

In the fixed-review-time method:

The quantity is reviewed periodically at fixed intervals of time.

The order is placed for a quantity sufficient to replenish the inventory to a predefined maximum level, which was calculated to optimize the costs of holding and management of inventories.

In the fixed-quantity method:

The inventory is withdrawn to a point where there is just sufficient material to cover the demand during the replenishment lead time. The

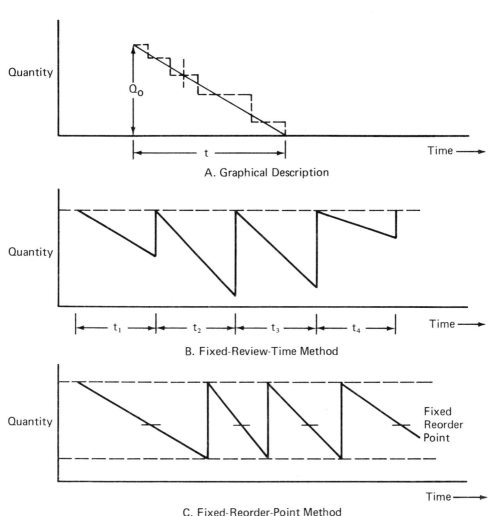

A. Graphical Description

B. Fixed-Review-Time Method

C. Fixed-Reorder-Point Method

**Figure 4-2.** Graphical Inventory Concepts

concept of replenishment lead time will be discussed in a subsequent section.

The order is placed for a quantity that optimizes the cost factors. This quantity is fixed regardless of the period under consideration, hence the name.

This discussion addresses the questions of *when* and *how much* to order. The above two notions will be further explored next.

As shown in figure 4-3, the shorter the review period and/or the less the maximum amount of inventory carried, the less will be the amount of average inventory carried, and hence the lower are the various costs associated with holding inventory. As indicated in chapter 1 and further discussed in this chapter, these amount to approximately 30 percent of the dollar purchase value of the inventory carried (when the cost of money tied up is approximately 10 percent). On the other hand, more frequent reordering increases both the monetary and the "nuisance" costs of maintaining inventories. As shown in figure 4-4, tradeoffs between holding and reorder costs must be made in an enlightened manner.

**Materials-Inventory Decision Guidelines**

*Fixed-Review-Time Methods*

With the introduction of modern digital computers, and their expanding use in materials-management systems in industry as well as in health-care institutions, there is an increasing interest in the fixed-review-time method. Clearly, a computer can very quickly and at relatively low cost check a large number of inventory items on a periodic basis. This is not to say that fixed-review-time methods cannot be used without computers. Whenever the

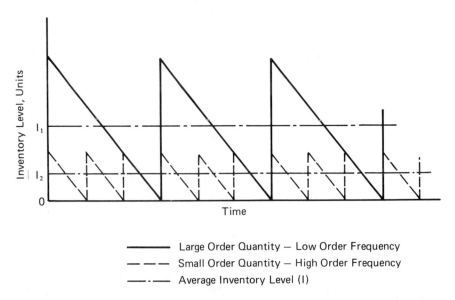

Large Order Quantity — Low Order Frequency
Small Order Quantity — High Order Frequency
Average Inventory Level (I)

**Figure 4-3.** Effect of Extreme Inventory Policies on Inventory Level under Constant-Demand and Constant-Lead-Time Conditions

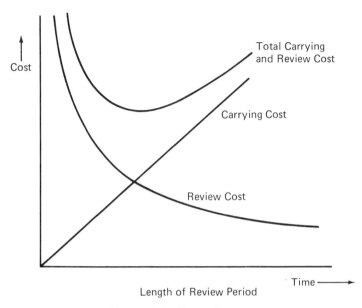

**Figure 4-4.** Cost of Review

number of items inventoried is relatively low, or where and when records are displayed graphically on some form of bar charts for quick review and evaluation, fixed-review-time methods can be used with relative ease. The length of the review period clearly depends on tradeoffs between costs and benefits, as is true of everything else in materials management. The clerical and/or computer costs decrease as the length of the review period increases. To compensate for this, larger reserve stocks are needed in order to maintain cerain service levels. This, in turn, increases the carrying costs of the materials inventoried. More specifically, the longer the review period, the greater must be the average inventory carried in order to maintain the same level of service. Figure 4-4 depicts the total costs, that is, the sum of the carrying and the review or reordering costs, as the length of the period increases. The total costs are shown to go down to some minimum level and then to start climbing again. Thus there is generally an optimum review and reorder period in any given organization.

*Fixed-Order-Quantity Methods*

To keep the discussion simple, it will be assumed initially that all parameters and all variables in the inventory-replenishment situation are known with certainty. That is, there are no random variations or fluctuations in the withdrawal quantity, in its timing, or in the replenishment lead-time. Expanding on figure 4-3, the slope of the line again represents the average material rate of usage or withdrawals. The basic economic-lot-size or economic-ordering-quantity equations assume that the replenishment of stock is accomplished instantaneously after zero level is reached. Clearly in this case the replenishment order could have been placed at some time prior to the no-stock condition for delivery when the stock reaches the zero level. The difference in the timing of these two events should reflect the delivery *lead time*, the elapsed time between order placement and materials delivery, as discussed in a subsequent section and as shown in figure 4-5. In other words, this assumption requires that the materials delivery not be spread over time, as might be the case where materials are produced in house and delivered as they come off the production line or work center.

To set up a system based on these assumptions is clearly far too risky. The risk of running out of stock because of the human element in the system is significant under such assumptions, even if the probabilistic nature of demand or withdrawals is overlooked as is the case in this initial development of the theory. Inventory-control methods, especially as they apply to the health-care-delivery arena, must recognize that even the most mechanized or computerized inventory systems do include the possibility of human oversight. Humans form the numerous links between the health providers and service departments on the one hand, and the inventory record-keeping functions—the storage and distribution of material functions—on the other. Human errors or oversights may take place on the health-provider side; the nurse, medical assistant, or clerk may overlook the need to reorder. On the other hand, oversights may take place at the purchasing department or vendor levels. The channels of communication between these two extremes in any one institution may vary in length. Each stage may involve a human link and hence the possibility for an oversight. In order to cover the needs for materials in light of such potential oversight, a reserve or safety stock is required. The question is what the size of this reserve or safety stock should be.

*Application of the Two-Bin or Min-Max System*

The "two-bin" approach to the control of inventories clearly implies two separate groups of inventory items. One group (the "first bin") includes all the items above the reorder point, and the other group (the "second bin") includes all items below the reorder point. However, this does not imply that the two groups of material need to be physically separated from each other or stored in different bins or areas. The two-bin system is simply a concept or a theoretical construct. The materials may be stored together; in

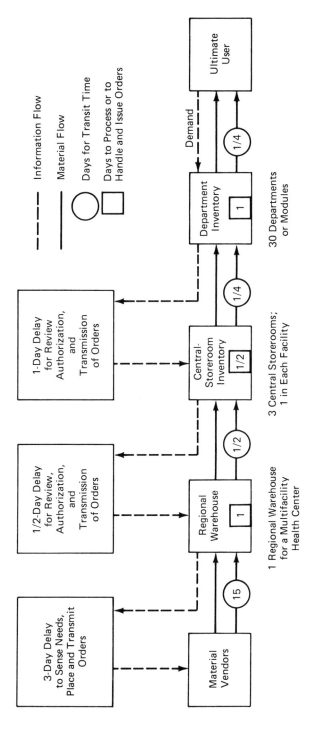

**Figure 4-5.** Example of Materials-Management-System Lead Times

fact, one group may be indistinguishable from the other. The distinction will be made only on the inventory record or, in many instances, specifically on the inventory card.

In institutions or in specific areas of institutions where a *perpetual inventory* is not in fact kept on record (that is, the files are not updated with every transaction) the two groups of inventories may indeed, be physically separated. It is not uncommon to box up a reserve quantity and set it aside in the stocking area. Whenever the first "bin" is depleted and the reserve box is opened, an order is placed. Some institutions include a preprinted materials requisition with the reserve-material requirements. When the package is opened, the requisition is routinely sent to the purchasing department. Since the boxed material could be, and indeed historically has been, placed in a reserve bin, we call this a two-bin system.

The two-bin system is sometimes referred to as the *Min-Max* replenishment policy. For a given good and at a given organizational level, the minimum (Min) quantity kept on shelves represents the reserve quantity typically expressed in terms of days', weeks', or months' supply. The orders placed under this policy are such that the preset maximum (Max) is not exceeded. Both the Min and the Max quantities must reflect projected usage rates and replenishment lead times.

Inasmuch as the projections of usage for these purposes are typically short-term (days or weeks), the most recent experience, adjusted for any seasonalities, generally suffices as a basis of forecasting. The process of translating historical data into forecasts of future demands can clearly take on a number of formats depending on the level or organizational sophistication in this respect and the cost/benefit of using mathematical-statistical methods of tracking, analyzing, and projecting a time series of data.

The technology of forecasting is beyond the scope of this book. A number of articles [1,2,3] and of books [4,5] dealing with this subject and written for the layman or the user are recommended.

*Safety-Reserve Quantity*

The safety-reserve quantity or buffer stock is, as the name implies, the additional inventory that is carried to cover for unusual demands, that is, those that exceed the level forecasted and planned for. It must take into account the time needed to obtain a certain stocked-out item under emergency or great-urgency conditions. Typically, the purchasing personnel in an institution know what delay can be expected in obtaining a given item in the normal course of events. Moreover, these people also know how much time can be shaved off the usual time under emergency or special-priority conditions. This may necessitate revising schedules, shipping by air express, "robbing" standing orders, or, alternatively, borrowing from other institutions. Clearly, this will be more expensive than standard operating procedures and should not be relied on nor permitted to occur too frequently. The emergency safety reserve or buffer stock should be automatically signaled by the existing inventory record-keeping system. Moreover, inventory personnel should be aware of the danger point and should act and react almost instinctively.

Figure 4-6 depicts the notion of the safety-reserve quantity or buffer stock superimposed on the basic economic order quantity (EOQ) concept. Whereas the basic sawtooth-shaped inventory-variation graph is based on the average demand or withdrawal rate, the buffer stock is set for the maximum demand or rate of withdrawals during the replenishment lead time—the time between order placement and fulfillment. Clearly, having a safety reserve increases the inventory carying costs which will be discussed later in this chapter. These additional costs must be offset or justified by the costs and ramifications of being out of stock temporarily, that is, shortage costs. Obviously, in the case of items for which the costs of shortage are lower than the carrying costs and the ramifications are inconsequential, it is cost-beneficial to allow temporary stockouts.

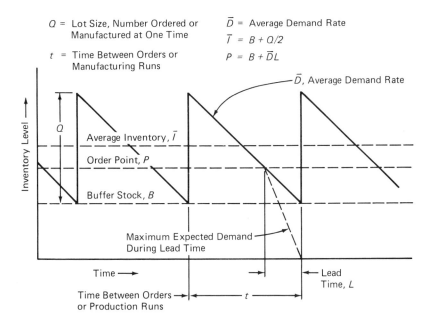

Idealized structure of inventory levels in relation to time shows relationships between lot size ($Q$), buffer stock ($B$), order point ($P$), average inventory ($\overline{I}$), time between orders ($t$), demand rate ($\overline{D}$), and lead time ($L$).

**Figure 4-6.** Idealized Structure of Inventory Levels in Relation to Time

*Replenishment Lead Times*

As indicated earlier in this chapter, materials-replenishment decision rules must take into account the fact that a certain amount of time will elapse between the instant at which someone is aware of a need for additional stock and the actual replenishment of that stock. It takes time to place and transmit an order. Depending on the materials-management system and on the organizational level of the unit seeking replenishment, the order may have to be reviewed and authorized. This too takes time, especially in a multilevel MMS where approval must be sought at several tiers of hierarchy, as shown in figure 4-5.

A certain amount of time also elapses after the authorized order reaches the appropriate inventory backup level such as the central store room, the warehouse, or the vendor. It takes time to process and fill the order, to ship or deliver the materials; to receive and inspect the materials received (for quantity if not for quality). Finally, it takes time to place the materials on the appropriate shelves. All this must be taken into consideration in the timing and in the quantity of replenishment decision rules.

Figure 4-5 depicts an example of a multilevel MMS in a multifacility health-maintenance organization (HMO). The various delays in the information-flow channels are fairly typical, as are the transit and processing times for the goods within the HMO. The response time of vendors, however, varies widely from vendor to vendor and, moreover, sometimes varies for different kinds of goods even if they are supplied by the same vendor. Finally, these delays may change over time for any one item obtained from any one vendor.

*Reorder Point*

The reorder-point quantity generally does appear on the inventory records and is a "flag" or signal for inventory personnel, the computer, or the purchasing agents that an order must be placed. If, as was initially assumed in this discussion, the demand for a particular item is constant, the reorder point is then the *safety-reserve quantity plus the usage anticipated during the time the order is being placed, processed, and acted on.* Viewed another way and shown in figure 4-6, it is the *lead time multiplied by the maximum usage rate* on a per-day or per-week basis. The "normal" reorder time will clearly vary from vendor to vendor. Although a trend among American hospitals toward the use of the *prime*-vendor concept is beginning to gain some momentum, most institutions still prefer or are required by law to use several vendors and thereby avoid dependence on any one. As indicated earlier, this has the advantage of making vendors more competitive. The names of the respective vendors can be listed on the inventory record, along with delivery lead times experienced with the respective vendors by the institution in the recent past. These lead times, however, must not be fixed for all time, but should be reviewed and revised periodically. Alternatively, as it is recognized that the lead times have changed significantly, a revision must be made on a by-exception basis. Needless to say, delivery-lead-time performance may vary greatly between vendors.

Under these conditions, the safest policy is to establish the reorder point assuming the *highest* or maximum reorder time. An alternative approach, when and where feasible, is to allow the purchasing personnel to choose a vendor, taking into account the rate of withdrawal and any foreseeable or unplanned exigencies. When and if the demand is great, then the order can be placed with the vendor who can deliver the materials in the shortest time.

*The Order Quantity*

The previous discussion focused on the question of *when* to place a replenishment order. The next question is that of *how much* to reorder for replenishment purposes. The fixed-order-quantity method described earlier requires the knowledge of the *economic order quantity* (EOQ) in order to make the discussion complete. The EOQ, to be discussed later, is normally posted visibly on the inventory record along with the reorder-point quantity for the convenience of the inventory-control clerk or the purchasing agent.

The quantity ordered within a certain time interval can involve one or more *lots*. The lot is a group or batch of materials that normally have the same identity and therefore serve the same function. *Economic lot size* is the quantity of material that can be purchased or produced on the one hand, and stored or kept on the other, so that the total cost is kept at a minimum. The generic "prescription" or formula for the economic lot size is the same for purchased lots as for manufactured lots. The factors entering the prescription and hence the decision are, however, somewhat different. For purchased items, quantity discounts in the unit price, as well as in the transportation and order processing, are traded off against the costs of holding a larger amount of inventory in the stores and on the shelves all the time.

Clearly, the smaller the reorder lot size, the more often are the lots produced or purchased. The reverse is also true. The larger lots need to be produced or requisitioned less frequently. Figure 4-3 shows the relationship between lot size and number of lots in a given time frame. In the one case, the original order included three times the replenishment. The second case, in turn, required placement of three replenishment orders. It can be seen from this figure that in the first case the average amount of inventory carried is much greater than in the second. Indeed, the *average* is one and one-half times the *maximum* ever carried in the second case. This does not imply, however, that smaller order quantities are always beneficial. As will be shown in the sections that follow, the optimal order quantities allow for optimum tradeoffs between the various inventory-related costs, yet take account of other considerations.

### The Basic Economic-Lot-Size Equation

In attacking this problem, it is usually assumed that a planning period of length $T$ is used, and that the average amount of product required at a uniform (constant) rate over this period is known to be $\bar{D}$ units. If the lot size is given by $Q$, then $\bar{D}/Q$ equals the number of lots required during the planning period $T$, and $TQ/\bar{D} = $ time between lots. For example, if 12 months represents a planning horizon ($T$) during which the forecasted average demand ($\bar{D}$) for sutures is 12,000 units and the lot size ($Q$) is 2,000 units, then 6 lots (12,000/2,000 = $\bar{D}/Q$) will need to be purchased during this planning period in order to satisfy the demand. The time between orders will be 12(2,000/12,000) or 2 months.

The costs that depend on the choice of $Q$ (the lot size) are generally taken to be of two kinds: those that depend on the lot size (variable costs) and those that are independent of the lot size (fixed costs). Costs of setups are usually assumed to be independent of the lot size and are defined to include all costs of getting the production or procurement of a lot underway and terminating production when the lot requirements are fulfilled. Costs of storage are considered to vary with the size of the lot, since they are generally computed on the basis of the maximum or average amount of product in storage. If the following costs are given or can be established

$C_1 = $ setup and/or reorder cost per lot

$C_2 = $ holding or storage cost per piece per unit time, based on average number of units in storage

and

$C(Q) = $ total cost, for example, setup and/or reorder cost and holding or storage cost for a planning period $T$, using a lot size of $Q$.

then the cost may be computed as follows:

$C_1 \dfrac{\bar{D}}{Q} = $ total setup and/or reorder cost = setup or reorder cost × number of lots during the planning period

$\dfrac{Q}{2}$ = average number of units in storage

$C_2 \dfrac{Q}{2} T$ = total holding or storage cost = unit holding cost × average inventory held × planning period

then the total cost = setup and/or reorder cost + holding or storage cost.

$$C_1 \frac{D}{2} + C_2 \frac{Q}{2} T \qquad (4.1)$$

The next step is to find the value of $Q$ that will yield the *minimum* total cost of a lot. This occurs where the marginal holding cost is equal to the marginal setup or reorder cost. Alternatively, it can be found graphically, as shown in figure 4-7 at the point where the total cost is a minimum. Mathematically, this is accomplished by finding the first derivative of the total cost with respect to $Q$, equating it to zero, and solving it for $Q$. This lowest point in the total-cost curve is given by the formula

$$Q^\circ = \sqrt{\frac{2C_1 D}{C_2 T}} = \text{square root of} \left\{ \frac{2 \times \text{setup and/or reorder cost per lot} \times \text{usage or demand}}{\text{holding cost} \times \text{planning period}} \right\}$$

$$(4.2)$$

Figure 4-7 provides an almost classic form for many decision problems. As the choice is moved from one extre e to another along the range of alternatives, some costs increase and others decrease. The best policy is

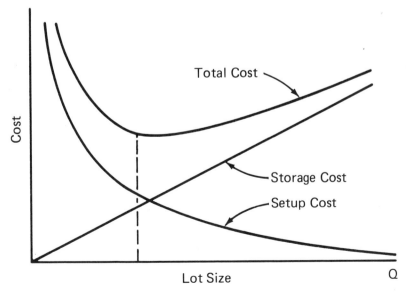

**Figure 4-7.** The Relationship between Costs and Lot Sizes

to select not an extreme alternative but an *optimum*, one that brings about a compromise between the increasing and decreasing costs. As indicated earlier, at the point where the total cost is minimum, the marginal storage cost is just equal to the negative or the marginal setup cost. Industry has developed various charts, monographs, and even slide rules that make it possible to solve the resulting basic EOQ equation [6]. However, the worksheets of a subsequent section of this chapter circumvent the need for relying on such devices.

Equation 4.2 is the basic lot-size equation, which has been widely reprinted and even more widely used by industry, including the health-services sector. This equation minimizes the sum of setup or reorder costs and storage costs. Once $Q$ is determined, the time between lots is also determined, since $\bar{D}$ and $T$ are assumed to be known. The following example will demonstrate the use of this equation:

What quantity of widgets should a hospital materials manager order each time if it costs \$14 to make up or process an order and if the widgets are worth \$7 each? The manager estimates his overall carrying charges for insurance, storage, interest on capital, and so on to be 36 percent of product value. All his other costs are fixed, that is, not dependent on the inventory carried. The demand for the widgets is 360,000 per year.

The total annual cost pertinent to this problem is made up of the reorder costs, the storage costs, and the fixed costs. The total reorder costs are

$$C_1 \frac{\bar{D}}{Q} = \frac{14 \times 360,000}{Q}$$

This is the *annual* cost of placing $\bar{D}/Q = 360,000/Q$ orders. The total storage or carrying cost in this particular case is $0.36 \times 7.00 \times (Q/2) \times 1 = C_2(Q/2)T$. The planning period $T$ in this case is one year.

Thus the total cost per annum is the sum of these costs plus any fixed costs. The fixed costs, however, drop out in arriving at equation 4.2 since they are the same no matter what the value of $Q$, within reason. Therefore, the economic ordering quantity is

$$\sqrt{\frac{2C_1\bar{D}}{C_2T}} = \sqrt{\frac{2 \times 14 \times 360,000}{0.36 \times 7.00 \times 1}} = \sqrt{4,000,000}$$

From figure 4-24, from square-root tables, or from any other source, this is seen to be equal to 2,000 widgets per order, and the optimum number of orders is

$$N = \frac{D}{Q} = \frac{360,000}{2,000} = 60 \text{ orders/year}$$

*Volume Discounts*

Suppliers often offer price discounts in order to encourage larger orders. The purchaser's benefits from bigger orders include lower unit prices, lower shipping and handling costs, and a reduction in costs of ordering owing to fewer orders placed. However, these benefits must be traded off against the incremental increase in carrying costs. With increasing order sizes more space is required for storage, and the costs of holding the larger inventories correspondingly increase. The risk of obsolescence or functional depreciation is also pertinent (although difficult to quantify) unless the supplier offers to take back any stock rendered obsolete at any time for any reason. Larger inventories magnify losses resulting from design or usage changes.

Basically, there are two types of quantity discounts. As seen from figure 4-8 one type of discount allows for different unit costs (slopes of the line) in each discount range. Specifically, the greater the quantity bought, the lower the unit price within each range. A supplier might thus offer the following price schedule:

| Number of Items | Price per Unit |
|---|---|
| 0-100 | $50 |
| 100-500 | $45 |
| 500-1000 | $40 |

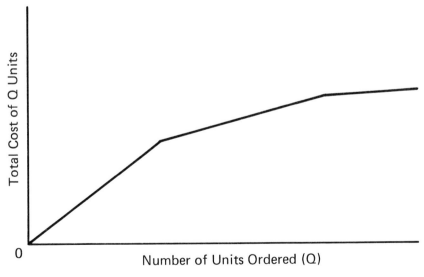

**Figure 4-8.** Graduated Quantity Discounts, Total Cost of *Q* Units

An order of 600 units under this schema would cost

$$
\begin{array}{lr}
\text{First } 100 \ @ \ \$50 & \$ \ 5,000 \\
\text{Next } 400 \ @ \ \$45 & \$18,000 \\
\text{Next } 100 \ @ \ \$40 & \underline{\$ \ 4,000} \\
& \$27,000
\end{array}
$$

$$
\text{or } \frac{27,000}{600} = \$45/\text{unit}
$$

The other form of quantity discount is shown in figure 4-9. Under this schema, the supplier gives a cash discount (a discount related to the timing of payment) of some fixed percentage of total purchase price if the quantity purchased falls within such a prescribed range. An example of such a discount policy follows:

| Number of Items | Discount (%) |
|:---:|:---:|
| 0-100 | 0 |
| 100-500 | 10 |
| 500-1000 | 20 |

If the base price per unit is again $50, then 600 units would qualify for the 20-percent discount, and the total value of the contract is

$$
50 \times 600 \times 0.80 = 24,000
$$

$$
\text{or } \frac{24,000}{600} = \$40 \text{ per unit}
$$

The discount scheme depicted in figure 4-8 results in an average-total-cost relationship depicted in figure 4-10. Clearly, the points of discontinuity on the solid curve represent the price break or discontinuity of slope in the line segments of figure 4-8.

The total stocking cost of the cash-discount policy depicted in figure 4-9 results in the relationship shown in figure 4-11. Again the discontinuities represent the price-break points.

The lowest-unit-cost ordering policy when price breaks of the cash discount variety are in effect is determined by calculating the total annual stocking cost for each *feasible* economic order quantity and the minimum quantity at which the quantity discount is allowed. A feasible order quantity is found when the calculated $Q^0$ is within the price break range of the $C_1$ utilized in the calculation.

When the following procedures are used, fewer computations for the minimum-cost solution are required for most of the common quantity-discount patterns. However, all feasible order quantities should be checked whenever an unusual discount pattern is encountered.

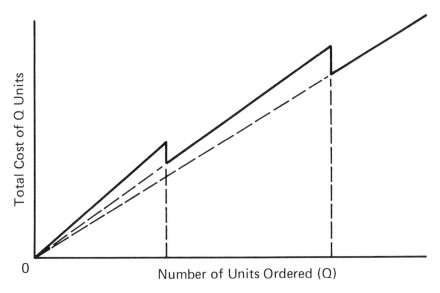

**Figure 4-9.** Cash Discounts, Total Cost of $Q$ Units

1.  Compute the EOQ using the lowest unit price. If the EOQ thus obtained is feasible ($Q^o$ is large enough to qualify for the lowest price), it is the optimal order quantity. Stop.

2.  If the EOQ obtained is not feasible, calculate the total annual stocking cost for the minimum order quantity allowed at that price.

3.  Compute the EOQ using the next lowest unit price.

    a.  If the EOQ is feasible, calculate the total annual stocking cost using the EOQ and compare it with the cost obtained in step 2; the lot size producing the lower total cost is the optimal order quantity. Stop.

    b.  If $Q$ is not feasible, repeat steps 2 and 3a until the minimum-cost solution is identified.

Any savings resulting from ordering larger quantities should be evaluated against the risks incurred from maintaining higher inventories. Risks are gauged by the stability of past usage, resale value of stock, and projections of future demand for health services within the institution. Prepaid plans and/or HMOs should be especially sensitive to the latter consideration as new groups of members are projected to enroll. Alternatively, groups have been known to disenroll.

The following example shows the calculation performed to find the optimum order quantity when volume discounts are offered. A supplier offers the following quantity discount schedule:

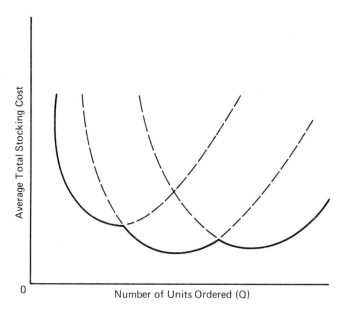

**Figure 4-10.** Graduated Quantity Discounts, Stocking Cost

| Price | Quantity |
|-------|----------|
| $0.40/unit | < 10,000 |
| $0.36/unit | 10,000-19,999 |
| $0.35/unit | 20,000 + |

A hospital buys 80,000 units of some consumable item each year. The order cost (cost of processing an order) $C_1$ = $80.00 per order and the storage component of the holding cost in this case is $0.20 per unit per year. Moreover, the insurance as well as the interest component of the holding cost is 15 percent of the average value of inventory.

**Step 1.** Using the steps shown in figure 4-12, the lowest price per unit obtained is $0.35. The EOQ is computed as follows:

$$EOQ = \sqrt{\frac{2 \times 80 \times 80,000}{(0.20 + 0.15 \times 0.35) \times 1}} = \sqrt{50,694,400}$$

From figure 4-25, square-root tables, or any other calculation aid, this is seen to equal 7,120 units.

**Step 2.** Since the order quantity is below the number needed to qualify for the $0.35-per-unit price, the annual stocking cost from ordering the minimum lot size (20,000 containers) that qualifies for the lowest price break is computed to be

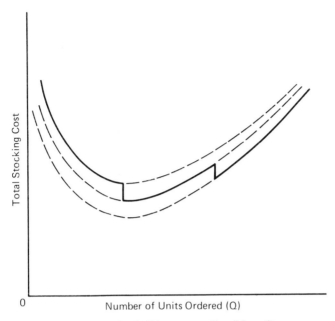

**Figure 4-11.** Cash Discounts, Stocking Cost

$$\text{Total annual stocking cost} = \frac{(\$80)\,(80{,}000)}{20{,}000} + \frac{(\$0.20 + 0.15 \times \$0.35)\,20{,}000}{2}$$
$$+ \,\$0.35 \times 80{,}000$$
$$= \$320 + \$2525 + \$28{,}000 = \$30{,}845$$

**Step 3.** Using the next-highest price break, $0.36 per unit, the EOQ is now shown to be

$$\sqrt{\frac{2 \times 80 \times 80{,}000}{(0.02 + 0.15 \times 0.36) \times 1}} = \sqrt{50{,}395{,}801} = 7{,}099$$

**Step 4.** The EOQ does not again fit within the range of the quantities required for the price used in its computation. Therefore, the total annual stocking cost for the minimum lot size (10,000 units) required to take advantage of the $0.36 price is calculated:

$$\frac{(\$80)(80{,}000)}{10{,}000} + \frac{(\$0.20 + 0.15 \times \$0.36)\,10{,}000}{2} + \$0.36 \times 80{,}000$$

or

$$\$640 + \$1270 + \$28{,}000 = \$30{,}710$$

Note that the reduction on carrying costs for the EOQ of 10,000 units compared to the EOQ of 20,000 units outweighs the added costs for purchasing and procurement.

The total cost for using a lot size of 10,000 versus one of 20,000 units is calculated, disclosing a savings of $30,845 − $30,710 = $135.

Finally, the highest-purchase-price alternative must be checked because a feasible EOQ was not calculated previously. This is calculated next:

$$\sqrt{\frac{2 \times 80 \times 80,000}{(0.20 + 0.15 \times 0.40) \times 1}} = \sqrt{49,230,769} = 7,016$$

The total annual stocking cost for shipping containers in this case is

$$\frac{(\$80)(80,000)}{7,016} + \frac{(2 \times \$0.10 + 0.15 \times \$0.40)\,7,016}{2} + \$0.40 \times 80,000$$

or

$$\$912 + \$912 + 32,000 = \$33,824$$

Note the equality between procurement and carrying costs. Thus the total annual stocking cost in this case is $33,824 for an order quantity of 7,016 when $0.40 is the price assigned per unit. The policy of ordering 10,000 units at a time is considerably less expensive, with $33,824 − $30,710 = $3114 savings. However, the preference for an order size of 10,000 units should receive a final check to ascertain whether any changes are anticipated in usage rates, and with the stores manager to be sure storage facilities can handle the larger inventories with no increase in per-unit carrying charges. The logic used in calculating the optimum EOQ with volume discounts is diagrammed in figure 4-12.

### Economic-Lot-Size-Equation Modifications and Aids to Computation

Having introduced the *basic* EOQ equation, as well as that with volume discounts, in earlier sections, this section will introduce a number of extensions of the basic theory. The basic EOQ equation, which does not allow for backlogging or planned shortages, will be modified to do so. A further modification will allow for deliveries to be distributed over time, as is the case when items are produced within the facility where they are used. Next, these two modifications will be combined into a single EOQ model.

A modification of the basic EOQ model is dictated when a number of different products must be produced in the same work center, and the center can produce only one product at a time. Similarly, modifications are needed whenever space or budgetary considerations place a constraint on

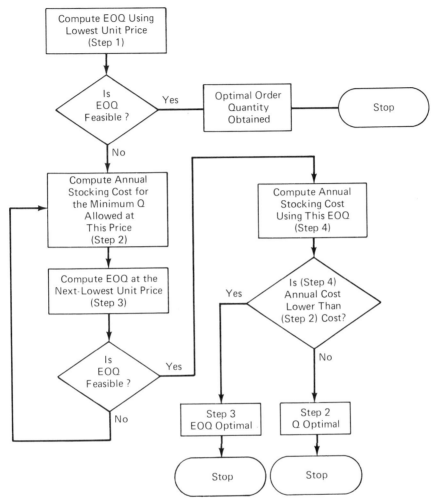

**Figure 4-12.** Computation Process for Finding Minimum EOQ in a Volume-Discount Environment

the total inventory, involving a number of different products, that can be carried. These modifications will also be shown.

Straightforward worksheets for calculating the respective EOQs in each of these cases will be provided in this section. For those with access to a computer with interactive capability, this section will provide a printout of a program showing the questions asked by the computer, the problem solver's responses, and the EOQ solutions that correspond to the responses (the program listing is available from the author). Clearly, the computer program can handle each of the modified EOQ models mentioned earlier in this section.

Appendix 4A provide checklists for materials-management-system decision rules and their use, as well as audit procedures for the inventory-control policies in place. Audit steps for materials-management-system decision rules, and their use, are also provided.

**Worksheets for Various Economic-Lot-Size Equations**

*Case I: Basic Economic-Lot-Size Equation*

The basic EOQ equation is founded on the following assumptions:

1.  Demand rate is constant, continuous, and known.
2.  Items are ordered in equal numbers, $Q$ at a time.
3.  Production or replenishment is instantaneous.
4.  There is no limit on production capacity.
5.  No shortage is allowed.

These assumptions in an inventory-replenishment policy result in the stock pattern depicted in figure 4-13. As seen earlier, this rather simple pattern requires a calculation involving the solution of a square-root equation. To facilitate calculations involving the basic EOQ equation, as well as some more complex extensions thereof, a series of worksheets are presented next (figures 4-14, 4-16, 4-18, 4-20, and 4-21).

*Case II: Basic Economic Lot Size with Shortages Allowed*

The policy represented by case II differs from the case-I set of assumptions only in the fact that some shortages can be tolerated, albeit at a cost. Stockouts, when and if they occur, could be handled by asking the client to return at some future date, as may be the case with some pharmaceuticals. Alternatively, delivery may be expedited or a more expensive item used as a

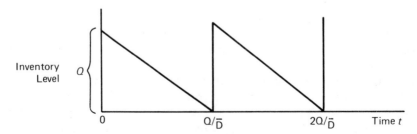

**Figure 4-13.** Basic EOQ Concept

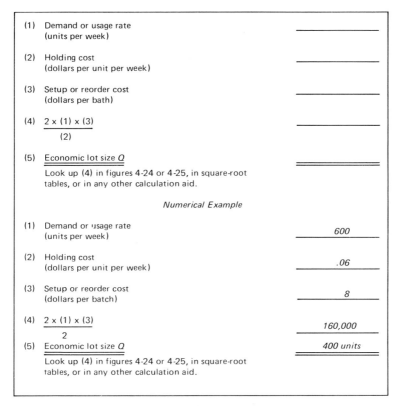

(1)  Demand or usage rate
     (units per week)                                    _____

(2)  Holding cost
     (dollars per unit per week)                         _____

(3)  Setup or reorder cost
     (dollars per bath)                                  _____

(4)  $\dfrac{2 \times (1) \times (3)}{(2)}$             _____

(5)  Economic lot size $Q$                              _____
     Look up (4) in figures 4-24 or 4-25, in square-root
     tables, or in any other calculation aid.

                        *Numerical Example*

(1)  Demand or usage rate
     (units per week)                                       600

(2)  Holding cost
     (dollars per unit per week)                            .06

(3)  Setup or reorder cost
     (dollars per batch)                                     8

(4)  $\dfrac{2 \times (1) \times (3)}{2}$                 160,000

(5)  Economic lot size $Q$                              400 units
     Look up (4) in figures 4-24 or 4-25, in square-root
     tables, or in any other calculation aid.

**Figure 4-14.** Worksheet for Case I: Calculation of Basic Economic Lot Size

substitute, for example, a larger X-ray film substituting for the one required. Thus this case is based on the following assumptions:

1. Demand rate is constant, continuous, and known.
2. Items are ordered in equal number, $Q$ at a time.
3. Production or replenishment is instantaneous.
4. There is no limit on production or procurement capacity.
5. *Shortages are allowed.*

This case is depicted in figure 4-15.

*Case III: Economic Lot Size with Delivery
Spread over Time*

The policy represented by case III differs from the case-I set of assumptions only in the fact that the delivery of items ordered takes place over some time

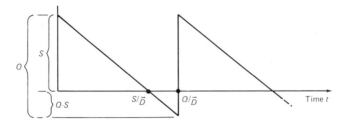

**Figure 4-15.** EOQ with Shortages Permitted

period, that is, it is not instantaneous. This is often the case when items are manufactured and inventoried in house, as may be the case in the preprocessing of some foods by the dietary department or the making up of unit doses from pharmaceuticals purchased in bulk. Thus this case is based on the following assumptions:

1. Demand rate is constant, continuous, and known.
2. Items are ordered in equal numbers, $Q$ at a time.
3. Delivery is *not* instantaneous, *but over a period of time.*
4. *No shortages* are allowed.

This case is depicted in figure 4-17.


*Case IV: Economic Lot Size with Production Spread
over Time and Shortages Allowed*

This case represents a combination of case-II and case-III policies. That is, it represents a situation involving in house production, such as preprocessing of foods or pharmaceuticals, at a rate that is clearly faster than the rate of demand or withdrawals. Any shortages are made up through expediting the preprocessing on a less-than-efficient basis, hence the shortage cost. Thus this case is based on the following assumptions:

1. Demand rate is constant, continuous, and known.
2. Delivery is made *over a period of time* at a constant rate greater than the demand rate.
3. Items are ordered in equal numbers, $Q$ at a time.
4. *Shortages are allowed.*

This case is depicted in figure 4-19.

(1) Demand or usage rate
(units per week)                          _____

(2) Holding cost
(dollars per unit per week)               _____

(3) Setup or reorder cost
(dollars per batch)                       _____

(4) Shortage cost
(dollars per unit per week)               _____

(5) (2) + (4)                             _____

(6) $\dfrac{2 \times (1) \times (3) \times (5)}{(2) \times (4)}$      _____

(7) Economic lot size $Q$                 ═══════════

Look up (6) in figures 4-24 or 4-25, in square-root
tables, or in any other calculation aid.

(8) $\dfrac{2(1) \times (3) \times (4)}{(2) \times (5)}$      _____

(9) For $S$, look up (8) in figures 4-24 or 4-25, in square-root
tables, or in any other calculation aid.    _____

(10) Optimal highest shortage level to be permitted $Q$ - $S$
(9) - (7)                                 _____

*Numerical Example*

(1) Demand or usage rate
(units per week)                          200

(2) Holding cost
(dollars per unit per week)               5

(3) Setup or reorder cost
(dollars per batch)                       5

(4) Shortage cost
(dollars per unit per week)               10

(5) (2) + (4)                             15

(6) $\dfrac{2 \times (1) \times (3) \times (5)}{(2) \times (4)}$      600

(7) Economic lot size                     24.5

Look up (6) in figures 4-24 or 4-25 in square-root
tables, or in any other calculation aid.

(8) $\dfrac{2(1) \times (3) \times (5)}{(2) \times (5)}$      266.66

(9) For $S$, look up (8) in figures 4-24 or 4-25, in square-root
tables, or in any other calculation aid.    16.33

(10) Optimal highest shortage level to be permitted $Q$ - $S$
(9) - (7)                                 8.2

**Figure 4-16.** Worksheet for Case II: Calculation of Economic Lot Size
with Shortages Allowed

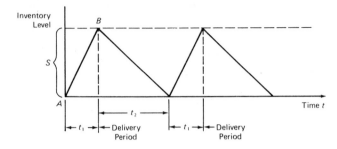

**Figure 4-17.** EOQ with Deliveries over a Period of Time

*Case V: Calculation of Multiproduct Economic Lot Size
with Production Spread over Time*

If a number of products must be manufactured on a single unit of equipment, case III may be inadequate when applied to the various products independently. These may be inconsistent with each other or with the availability of the machine.

In many situations it is desirable to make a sequence of products, with each product manufactured once in each cycle. The only open question is the total length of the cycle across all products. In most cases, the sequence of products will be established by analysis of changeover costs from one product to another. This case is based on the following assumptions:

1. Demand rate for each product is constant and known.
2. There is no limit on production capacity.
3. Items are manufactured in equal quantities for a given product in all the cycles.
4. The number of orders for each product are the same.
5. *No shortages* or backorders are allowed.
6. Delivery is not instantaneous but takes place over a period of time.

*Cases VI and VII: Multiple Items with Space or
Budgetary Constraints*

Most, if not all, real-world inventory systems stock many items. It is permissible to study and set stocking policies for individual items only as long as there are no significant interactions among them. However, when the warehouse capacity is limited and the items may be competing for floor space, or when there is an upper limit on the maximum investment in inventory and the respective items are competing for investment dollars, the traditional approach to EOQ development and use fails if it is only partial. The approaches delineated in cases VI and VII, on the other hand,

| | |
|---|---|
| (1) | Demand or usage rate (units per week) | _____ |
| (2) | Holding cost (dollars per unit per week) | _____ |
| (3) | Setup or reorder cost (dollars per batch) | _____ |
| (4) | Delivery or production rate (units per week) | _____ |
| (5) | (4) - (1) | _____ |
| (6) | $\dfrac{2 \times (1) \times (4) \times (3)}{(2) \times (5)}$ | _____ |
| (7) | Economic lot size $Q$ Look up (6) in figures 4-24 or 4-25 in square-root tables, or in any other calculation aid. | ══════════════ |

*Numerical Example*

| | | |
|---|---|---|
| (1) | Demand or usage rate (units per week) | 2,500 |
| (2) | Holding cost (dollars per unit per week) | 0.6 |
| (3) | Setup or reorder cost (dollars per batch) | 50 |
| (4) | Delivery or production rate (units per week) | 10,000 |
| (5) | (4) - (1) | 7,500 |
| (6) | $\dfrac{2 \times (1) \times (4) \times (3)}{(2) \times (5)}$ | 555,555 |
| (7) | Economic lot size Look up (6) in figures 4-24 and 4-25 in square-root tables, or in any other calculation aid. | 745.4 |

**Figure 4-18.** Worksheet for Case III: Calculation of Economic Lot Size with Production Spread over Time

recognize interactions due to floor space or budgetary constraints, respectively. (The problem becomes somewhat complex when it has financial and space constraints.)

Case VI is based on the following assumptions:

1. Demand rate for each product is continuous, known, and constant.
2. *No shortages* or backorders are allowed.
3. The number of orders for each of the products is the same.
4. Production or replenishment is instantaneous.
5. There exists a floor-space constraint on the sum of all items carried.

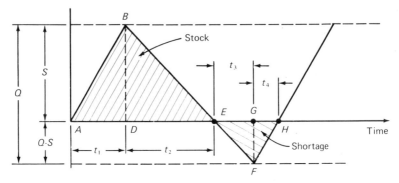

**Figure 4-19.** EOQ with Shortages Permitted and Deliveries over a Period of Time

The assumptions in case VII are identical to those just listed except that item 5 should read: "There exists a budgetary constraint on the sum of all items carried." These assumptions result in the stock pattern depicted in figure 4-13 for each of the products. Worksheets for cases VI and VII are found in figures 4-22 and 4-23.

### An Interactive Computer Program for Various Economic-Lot-Size Equations

Solutions of the basic EOQ equation require very little mathematical sophistication, especially when worksheets such as those in the previous section are available. But even in a simple case involving a number of stocking points and/or a number of different products, the solution can become tedious; and as the EOQ model used becomes more complex, the calculations become more and more demanding. In such instances, programmable calculators or computers can help expedite calculation, especially if these must be made on a repetitive basis. There is no unique or best way to use such devices in this context. Since the programs required to solve any of the cases shown in the previous section are not very complex, they should be tailored to each situation depending on user requirements, available computer capability, and so on.

One way to solve problems expeditiously that involve any of the EOQ cases discussed earlier is to use a computer in an *interactive* mode. In this mode, the problem solver interacts with the computer via a teletype terminal. Once the computer has been instructed to provide this program capability and the user has been properly identified, the terminal will print out certain

(1) Demand or usage rate
(units per week) _____

(2) Holding cost
(dollars per unit per week) _____

(3) Setup or reorder cost
(dollars per batch) _____

(4) Shortage cost
(dollars per unit per week) _____

(5) Delivery or production rate
(units per week) _____

(6) (2) + (4) _____

(7) $\dfrac{(1)}{(5)}$ _____

(8) 1 - (7) _____

(9) $\dfrac{2 \times (1) \times (3) \times (6)}{(2) \times (4) \times (8)}$ _____

(10) Economic lot size $Q$ ===============

Look up (9) in figures 4-24 or 4-25 in square-root
tables, or in any other calculation aid.

(11) $\dfrac{2 \times (1) \times (2) \times (3) \times (8)}{(6) \times (4)}$ _____

(12) For $S$, look up (11) in figures 4-24 or 4-25, in
square-root tables, or in any other calculation aid. _____

(13) Optimal highest shortage level to be permitted $Q$ - $S$
(10) - (12) _____

*Numerical Example*

(1) Demand or usage rate
(units per week) *5,000*

(2) Holding cost
(dollars per unit per week) *5*

(3) Setup or reorder cost
(dollars per batch) *75*

(4) Shortage cost
(dollars per unit per week) *15*

(5) Delivery or production rate
(units per week) *10,000*

(6) (2) + (4) *20*

(7) $\dfrac{(1)}{(5)}$ *0.5*

(8) 1 - (7) *0.5*

(9) $\dfrac{2 \times (1) \times (3) \times (6)}{(2) \times (4) \times (8)}$     *400,000*

(10) Economic lot size $Q$
Look up (9) in figures 4-24 or 4-25 in square-root
tables, or in any other calculation aid.     *632.5*

(11) $\dfrac{2 \times (1) \times (2) \times (3) \times (8)}{(6) \times (4)}$     *.6250*

(12) For $S$, look up (11) in figures 4-24 or 4-25, in
square-root tables, or in any other calculation aid.     *79.1*

(13) Optimal highest shortage level to be permitted $Q - S$
(10) - (12)     *553.4*

**Figure 4-20.** Worksheet for Case IV: Calculation of Economic Lot Size
with Production Spread over Time and Shortages Allowed

messages. Some of these messages are informational in nature, and others
request a response. Once all the questions have been raised by the computer
and the responses given in the proper format, the terminal prints out a solution.

Specifically, figure 4-26 shows a computer printout of a message spelling out the assumptions underlying the various EOQ cases that the computer has been programmed to handle. These cases clearly correspond to those in the previous section. Figure 4-27 depicts the printout for sample numerical solutions involving each of the cases.

## The History of Inventory-Control Theory

Inventory-control theory is one of the best-explored fields of study in operations research, industrial engineering, management science, and the other related professions. The roots of inventory theory can be traced to the H.H. Franklin Manufacturing Company, which was known to use the concept of economic order quantities as early as 1912. In 1915 Ford W. Harris of the Westinghouse Electric Company developed a simple lot-size formula [7]. R.H. Wilson published a classic work in the field of inventory-control theory in 1926 [8]. This was followed in 1931 by Fairfield E. Raymond's *Quantity and Economy in Manufacture* [9]. *Optimal Inventory Policy*, published in 1951 and jointly written by K. Arrow, T. Harris, and J. Marshak [10], gave inventory theory a rigorous mathemathical underpinning. In 1953 T.M. Whitin [11] showed that the theory must recognize the fact that at times withdrawals from inventories cannot be known with any precision.

Product

| | 1 | 2 | 3 | . . . | n |
|---|---|---|---|---|---|
| (1) Demand or usage rate for each product (units per week) | | | | | |
| (2) Holding cost for each product (dollars per unit per week) | | | | | |
| (3) Setup or reorder cost for each product (dollars per batch) | | | | | |
| (4) Production rate for each product (units per week) | | | | | |
| (5) (1) × (2) for each product | | | | | |
| (6) (1) ÷ (4) for each product | | | | | |
| (7) 1 - (6) for each product | | | | | |
| (8) (5) × (7) for each product | | | | | |

(9) Add all entries in (3) and multiply by 2.  _____

(10) Add all entries in (8).  _____

(11) (10) ÷ (9)  _____

(12) <u>Number of cycles</u>
Look up (11) in figures 4-24 and 4-25 in square-root tables, or in any other calculation aid.  _____

Product

| | 1 | 2 | 3 | . . . | n |
|---|---|---|---|---|---|
| (13) <u>Lot size</u> for each product (1) ÷ (12) | | | | | |

*Numerical Examples*

Product

| | 1 | 2 | 3 | . . . | n |
|---|---|---|---|---|---|
| (1) Demand or usage rate for each product (units per week) | 1,000 | 1,000 | 2,000 | | |
| (2) Holding cost for each product (dollars per unit per week) | 5 | 5 | 5 | | |
| (3) Setup or reorder cost for each product (dollars per batch) | 25 | 25 | 25 | | |
| (4) Production rate for each product (units per week) | 1,500 | 1,500 | 2,500 | | |
| (5) (1) × (2) for each product | 5,000 | 5,000 | 10,000 | | |
| (6) (1) ÷ (4) for each product | 0.66 | 0.66 | 0.8 | | |
| (7) 1 - (6) for each product | 0.34 | 0.34 | 0.2 | | |
| (8) (5) × (7) for each product | 1,700 | 1,700 | 2,000 | | |

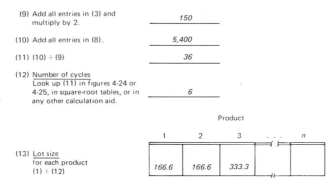

**Figure 4-21.** Worksheet for Case V: Calculation of Lot Size and Number of Cycles

Specifically, such withdrawals may follow more or less random patterns. Thus the *probabilistic*, or what are otherwise known as *stochastic*, components of inventory-control theory were first treated in Whitin's book.

Many publications pertaining to inventory-control theory appeared in the 1920s. There appears to have been a lull in activity in the 1930s and early 1940s, followed by a great resurgence of interest in the 1950s, 1960s and 1970s. The advent and expanding use of computer technology can be credited with much, if not all, of the upsurge of interest within academia, in industry, and more recently in the health-care-services sector for the general field of management science and particularly in inventory-control theory.

A complete coverage of the entire body of inventory-theory knowledge is clearly beyond the scope of this book. This section will, however, present a more detailed overview of the field through a classification or taxonomic format.

**Classification of Characteristics of Inventory-Control Problems**

In the previous sections the basic EOQ equation was derived and discussed. It was indicated that the basic EOQ equation has imbedded within it a large number of simplifying assumptions regarding demand, lead time, shortages, and so on. In later sections some of these assumptions were relaxed, one or more at a time. In each case the specific inventory problem was depicted both verbally and graphically, and the resulting economic ordering-lot-size calculations have been indicated on the worksheets. Their derivations shown in [8] are considered outside the scope of this book. The reader should note that as one or more of the simplifying assumptions in the

Wilson EOQ equation are relaxed, the resulting equations are more complex, as is their derivation. The scope of this book clearly does not permit an exhaustive review of all possible combinations and permutations of inventory-control-problem characteristics, and hence the resulting equations. As indicated earlier, the theory of inventory control is rather extensive and is perhaps one of the most explored areas of management science. In order to provide students and practitioners with a feeling for the breadth of possibilities, S. Javad [12] proposed a taxonomic plan for identification of inventory systems. The scheme is modeled on similar developments elsewhere [6] and is based on the idea that each inventory model has twelve elemental constituents. These are:

1. *Demand*—The demand for an item may be known with certainty, and its rate may or may not be constant over time.
2. *Ordering cycle*—The review and replenishment of inventory can be continuous or periodic, depending on the constraints of the system and/or management preference.
3. *Lead time*—The period of time that elapses before the order is on the shelves. It can be zero in cases where the system can acquire instantaneous delivery. The degree of certainty in its behavior is yet another consideration.
4. *Stock replenishment*—It is often considered instantaneous if the items are not manufactured by the system. It is considered to take place at a uniform rate if the items are produced on site.
5. *Number of items*—A system may carry more than one item; however, until these item interact (by means of space and/or budgetary constraints) inventory-control models consider them on an individual basis. The items are considered dependent on each other if, for example, they are substitutable.
6. *Time period*—This can be a single period if the system behaves like in the "newsboy's inventory" problem, or it can be a multiperiod model.
7. *Number of supply echelons*—The most general model is similar to a multilevel supply network with inventories maintained at all levels.
8. *Item characterization*—The items can be consumable, perishable, and reusable.
9. *Treatment of excess demand*—The excess demand may be backordered or may be lost forever.
10. *Objective of the model*—This addresses the question of whether it is a cost- or a service-oriented model.
11. *Modeling*—This deals with specification of the approach to formulating the problem and whether it is an exact or approximate model.
12. *Solution method*—This deals with identification of the approach to

problem solving and whether it is an optimization, suboptimization, or heuristic procedure.

The details of the taxonomy—which is called DOLRIPECTOMS—are addressed in table 4-1. Any model can be characterized by simply taking its appropriate identifier (for example, $d_3$, $o_2$, $l_3$, and so on) from each of the primary constituents (demand, ordering cycle, and so on) of table 4-1 and constructing some special case of DOLRIPECTOMS (for example, $d_1o_1l_2$-$r_1i_1p_3e_2c_2t_1o_2m_1s_3$). In this way both the student of inventory theory and the practitioner can categorize any proposed or existing model and easily specify its form, objectives, and built-in assumptions.

## Measures of Materials Service Performance

In the preceding sections of this chapter, various methods for optimizing the costs of inventory were presented under various combinations of assumptions and real-life constraints. The focus, however, was on inventory management from the cost-minimization point of view. Inasmuch as materials management in the health setting is a service function, it is necessary to look at the performance of each of these decision rules from the user's or service point of view. This section will address the *service-oriented* measures of performance.

### Inventory Efficiency

In general, efficiency is expressed as follows:

$$\text{Efficiency} = \frac{\text{Output}}{\text{Input}}$$

In real life, output rarely exceeds input. Therefore, efficiency, as defined here, is always one or less and is frequently stated as a percentage.

Inventory-efficiency measures, however, are not expressed in terms of output/input but nevertheless indicate how efficiently the inventory is being managed. They are a measure of the probability of stockouts.

Often the interest is not in the percentage delivered but in the percentage not delivered yet requested and/or needed in a period of time.

$$\text{Percentage of shortages} = \frac{\text{Number of units short} \times 100}{\text{Number of units demanded}}$$

**Table 4-1**
**A Taxonomic Scheme for Classification of Inventory-Control Systems**

| | | | |
|---|---|---|---|
| Demand | Deterministic | Static | ($d_1$) |
| | | Dynamic | ($d_2$) |
| | Stochastic | Stationary | ($d_3$) |
| | | Nonstationary | ($d_4$) |
| Ordering cycle | Continuous | | ($o_1$) |
| | Periodic | | ($o_2$) |
| Lead-time | Zero | | ($l_1$) |
| | Deterministic | | ($l_2$) |
| | Stochastic | | ($l_3$) |
| Stock replenishment | Instantaneous | | ($r_1$) |
| | Uniform | | ($r_2$) |
| Number of items | Single | | ($i_1$) |
| | Multi | Dependent | ($i_2$) |
| | | Independent | ($i_3$) |
| Time period | Single | | ($p_1$) |
| | Multi | Finite horizon | ($p_2$) |
| | | Infinite horizon | ($p_3$) |
| Number of supply echelons | Single | | ($e_1$) |
| | Multi | General | ($e_2$) |
| | | Arborescence   General | ($e_3$) |
| | | Parallel | ($e_4$) |
| | | Series | ($e_5$) |
| Item characterization | Consumable | | ($c_1$) |
| | Perishable | | ($c_2$) |
| | Reusable | | ($c_3$) |
| Treatment of excess demand | Backorder | | ($t_1$) |
| | Lost sale | | ($t_2$) |
| Objective of the model | Cost oriented | | ($o_1$) |
| | Service oriented | | ($o_2$) |
| Modeling | Exact | | ($m_1$) |
| | Approximate | | ($m_2$) |
| Solution method | Optimization | | ($s_1$) |
| | Suboptimization | | ($s_2$) |
| | Heuristics | | ($s_3$) |

See appendix A, "Glossary of Terms."

Iteration _____

Product

| | 1 | 2 | 3 | . . . | n |
|---|---|---|---|---|---|
| (1) Demand or usage rates (units per year) | | | | | |
| (2) Holding cost/year $/unit/year | | | | | |
| (3) Setup or reorder cost (dollars per batch) | | | | | |
| (4) Space required in square feet per item | | | | | |
| (5) Item unit cost | | | | | |
| (6) Set $\theta = 0$ For each item $j=1, \ldots n$ on first iteration and increment in steps of 0.01 or greater until line (18) is zero or less. | | | | | |
| (7) Multiply (4) by (6). (4) x (6) | | | | | |
| (8) Multiply (7) by 2. 2 x (7) | | | | | |
| (9) Add (2) and (8). (2) + (8) | | | | | |
| (10) Multiply (1) by (3). (1) x (3) | | | | | |
| (11) Multiply (10) by 2. 2 x (10) | | | | | |
| (12) Divide (11) by (9). | | | | | |

Entries (1) to (5) are the same for all iterations.

Product

| | 1 | 2 | 3 | . . . | n |
|---|---|---|---|---|---|
| (13) Look up (12) in figures 4-24 and 4-25, in square-root tables, or in any other calculation aid. | | | | | |

(14) Total floor space available in square feet.

(15) Multiply (4) by (13) for each item (4) × (13)

(16) Sum (15) for all items.

(17) Subtract (16) from (14).
$(14) - (16)$

(18) If (17) is less than or equal to zero, go to (20).

(19) Increment previous $\theta$ by 0.01 or more and go to (8).

|  | Product | | | | |
|---|---|---|---|---|---|
|  | 1 | 2 | 3 | . . . | n |

(20) Optimal solution found
Write $Q_j$ $j$=1,2, . . . $n$ from (13).

*Numerical Examples*

Iteration ___1___

| | Product | | | | |
|---|---|---|---|---|---|
| | 1 | 2 | 3 | . . . | n |
| (1) Demand or usage rates (units per year) | 5,000 | 2,000 | 10,000 | | |
| (2) Holding cost/year $/unit/year | 2 | 3 | 1 | | |
| (3) Setup or reorder cost (dollars per batch) | 100 | 200 | 75 | | |
| (4) Space required in square feet per item | 0.7 | 0.8 | 0.4 | | |
| (5) Item unit cost | 10 | 15 | 5 | | |
| (6) Set $\theta = 0$ For each item $j$=1, . . . $n$ on first iteration and increment in steps of 0.01 or greater until line (18) is zero or less | 0 | 0 | 0 | | |

| | 1 | 2 | 3 | | |
|---|---|---|---|---|---|
| (7) Multiply (4) by (6)<br>(4) x (6) | 0 | 0 | 0 | | |
| (8) Multiply (7) by 2<br>2 x (7) | 0 | 0 | 0 | | |
| (9) Add (2) and (8)<br>(2) + (8) | 2 | 3 | 1 | | |
| (10) Multiply (1) by (3)<br>(1) x (3) | 500,000 | 400,000 | 750,000 | | |
| (11) Multiply (10) by 2<br>2 x (10) | 1,000,000 | 800,000 | 1,500,000 | | |
| (12) Divide (11) by (9) | 500,000 | 266,667 | 1,500,000 | | |

Entries (1) to (5) are the same
for all iterations.

Product

| | 1 | 2 | 3 | . . . | n |
|---|---|---|---|---|---|
| (13) Look up (12) in figures 4-24 and 4-25, in square-root tables, or in any other calculation aid. | 707.1 | 516.4 | 1224.7 | | |

(14) Total floor space available in
square feet.      700

| | 1 | 2 | 3 | | |
|---|---|---|---|---|---|
| (15) Multiply (4) by (13) for each item<br>(4) x (13) | 494.97 | 413.12 | 489.88 | | |

(16) Sum (15) for all items      1397.97

(17) Subtract (16) from (14)<br>(14) − (16)      697.97

(18) If (17) is less than or equal to
zero, go to (20)      greater than zero

(19) Increment previous $\theta$ by 0.01 or
more and go to (8)      $\theta = 0.01$

Product

| | 1 | 2 | 3 | . . . | n |
|---|---|---|---|---|---|
| (20) Optimal solution found<br>Write $Q_j$ $j$=1,2, . . . $n$ from (13). | | | | | |

Iteration ___2___

Product

| | 1 | 2 | 3 | . . | n |
|---|---|---|---|---|---|
| (1) Demand or usage rates (units per year) | 5,000 | 2,000 | 10,000 | | |
| (2) Holding cost/year $/unit/year | 2 | 3 | 1 | | |
| (3) Setup or reorder cost (dollars per batch) | 100 | 200 | 75 | | |
| (4) Space required in square feet per item | 0.7 | 0.8 | 0.4 | | |
| (5) Item unit cost | 10 | 15 | 5 | | |
| (6) Set $\theta = 0$ For each item $j=1, \ldots n$ on first iteration and increment in steps of 0.01 or greater until line (18) is zero or less | 0.01 | 0.01 | 0.01 | | |
| (7) Multiply (4) by (6) (4) × (6) | 0.007 | 0.008 | 0.004 | | |
| (8) Multiply (7) by 2 2 × (7) | 0.014 | 0.016 | 0.008 | | |
| (9) Add (2) and (8) (2) + (8) | 2.014 | 3.016 | 1.008 | | |
| (10) Multiply (1) by (3) (1) × (3) | 500,000 | 400,000 | 750,000 | | |
| (11) Multiply (10) by 2 2 × (10) | 1,000,000 | 800,000 | 1,500,000 | | |
| (12) Divide (11) by (9) | 496,524.33 | 265,252 | 1,488,095 | | |

Entries (1) to (5) are the same for all iterations.

Product

| | 1 | 2 | 3 | . . . | n |
|---|---|---|---|---|---|
| (13) Look up (12) in figures 4-24 and 4-25, in square-root tables, or in any other calculation aid. | 704.6 | 515.0 | 1,219.9 | | |

(14) Total floor space available in square feet.

| | 700 | | | |
|---|---|---|---|---|

(15) Multiply (4) by (13) for each item (4) × (13)

| 493.3 | 412.0 | 488 | | |
|---|---|---|---|---|

(16) Sum (15) for all items

1393.3

(17) Subtract (16) from (14) (14) − (16)

693

(18) If (17) is less than or equal to zero, go to (20)

*greater than zero and much like first iteration*

(19) Increment previous $\theta$ by 0.01 or more and go to (8)

$\theta = .11$

Product

| 1 | 2 | 3 | . . . | n |
|---|---|---|---|---|

(20) Optimal solution found Write $Q_j$ $j$=1,2, . . . $n$ from (13).

| | | | | |
|---|---|---|---|---|

*Numerical Examples*

Iteration   $\theta = 4.43$

Product

| | 1 | 2 | 3 | . . . | n |
|---|---|---|---|---|---|
| (1) Demand or usage rates (units per year) | 5,000 | 2,000 | 10,000 | | |
| (2) Holding cost/year $/unit/year | 2 | 3 | 1 | | |
| (3) Setup or reorder cost (dollars per batch) | 100 | 200 | 75 | | |
| (4) Space required in square feet per item | 0.7 | 0.8 | 0.4 | | |
| (5) Item unit cost | 10 | 15 | 5 | | |
| (6) Set $\theta = 0$ For each item $j$=1, . . . $n$ on first iteration and increment in steps of 0.01 or greater until line (18) is zero or less | 4.43 | 4.43 | 4.43 | | |
| (7) Multiply (4) by (6) (4) × (6) | 3.101 | 3.544 | 1.772 | | |

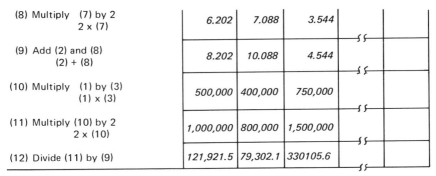

| (8) Multiply (7) by 2<br>2 × (7) | 6.202 | 7.088 | 3.544 | | |
|---|---|---|---|---|---|
| (9) Add (2) and (8)<br>(2) + (8) | 8.202 | 10.088 | 4.544 | | |
| (10) Multiply (1) by (3)<br>(1) × (3) | 500,000 | 400,000 | 750,000 | | |
| (11) Multiply (10) by 2<br>2 × (10) | 1,000,000 | 800,000 | 1,500,000 | | |
| (12) Divide (11) by (9) | 121,921.5 | 79,302.1 | 330105.6 | | |

Entries (1) to (5) are the same
for all iterations.

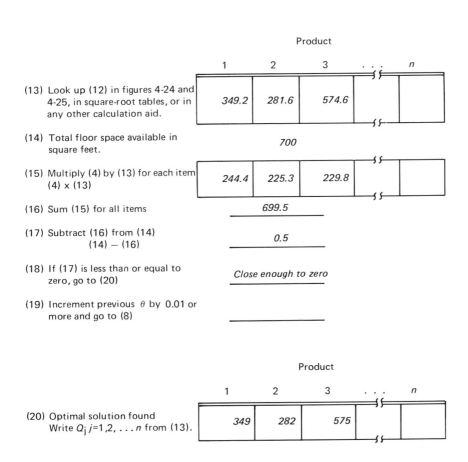

Product

| | 1 | 2 | 3 | . . . | n |
|---|---|---|---|---|---|
| (13) Look up (12) in figures 4-24 and 4-25, in square-root tables, or in any other calculation aid. | 349.2 | 281.6 | 574.6 | | |

(14) Total floor space available in square feet.                    700

| (15) Multiply (4) by (13) for each item<br>(4) × (13) | 244.4 | 225.3 | 229.8 | | |
|---|---|---|---|---|---|

(16) Sum (15) for all items                    699.5

(17) Subtract (16) from (14)
(14) − (16)                    0.5

(18) If (17) is less than or equal to zero, go to (20)        *Close enough to zero*

(19) Increment previous $\theta$ by 0.01 or more and go to (8)

Product

| | 1 | 2 | 3 | . . . | n |
|---|---|---|---|---|---|
| (20) Optimal solution found<br>Write $Q_j$ j=1,2, . . . n from (13). | 349 | 282 | 575 | | |

**Figure 4-22.** Worksheet for Case VI: Multiple Items with Space Constraint

Iteration _____

Product

|  | 1 | 2 | 3 | . . . | n |
|---|---|---|---|---|---|
| (1) Demand or usage rate (units per year) |  |  |  |  |  |
| (2) Holding cost ($/unit/year) |  |  |  |  |  |
| (3) Setup cost or reorder cost (dollars per batch) |  |  |  |  |  |
| (4) Item unit cost |  |  |  |  |  |
| (5) Set $\theta = 0$. For each item $j=1, \ldots n$ on first iteration and increment in steps of 0.01 or greater until line (18) is zero or less |  |  |  |  |  |
| (6) Multiply (3) by (1) (3) x (1) |  |  |  |  |  |
| (7) Multiply (6) by (2) (6) x (2) |  |  |  |  |  |
| (8) Multiply (4) by $\theta$ (4) x (5) |  |  |  |  |  |
| (9) Multiply (8) by (2) (2) x (8) |  |  |  |  |  |
| (10) Add (2) to (9) (2) + (9) |  |  |  |  |  |
| (11) Divide (7) by (10) (7) ÷ (10) |  |  |  |  |  |
| (12) Look up (12) in figures 4-24 and 4-25, in square-root tables, or in any other calculation aid. |  |  |  |  |  |

(13) Total dollars available for inventory investment. _____

Product

|  | 1 | 2 | 3 | . . . | n |
|---|---|---|---|---|---|
| (14) Multiply (12) by (4) for each item. (4) x (12) |  |  |  |  |  |

(15) Sum (14) for all items. _____

(16) Subtract (13) from (15). (15) - (13) _____

(17) If (16) is less than or equal to zero, go to (19); otherwise go to (18).

(18) Increment $\theta$ by 0.01 or more and go to 7.

|  | | | Product | | |
|---|---|---|---|---|---|
| 1 | 2 | 3 | . . . | n |

(19) Optimal solution found. Write $Q_j, j$ - 1, 2 . . . $n$; from (12).

*Numerical Examples*      Iteration      1

| | | Product | | | |
|---|---|---|---|---|---|
| | 1 | 2 | 3 | . . . | n |
| (1) Demand or usage rate (units per year) | 1,000 | 500 | 2,000 | | |
| (2) Holding cost ($/unit/year) | 4 | 20 | 10 | | |
| (3) Setup cost or reorder cost (dollars per batch) | 50 | 75 | 100 | | |
| (4) Item unit cost | 20 | 100 | 50 | | |
| (5) Set $\theta$ = 0. For each item $j$=1, . . . $n$ on first iteration and increment in steps of 0.01 or greater until line (18) is zero or less. | 0 | 0 | 0 | | |
| (6) Multiply (3) by (1). (3) x (1) | 50,000 | 37,500 | 200,000 | | |
| (7) Multiply (6) by (2). (6) x (2) | 100,000 | 75,000 | 400,000 | | |
| (8) Multiply (4) by $\theta$. (4) x (5) | 0 | 0 | 0 | | |
| (9) Multiply (8) by (2). (2) x (8) | 0 | 0 | 0 | | |
| (10) Add (2) to (9). (2) + (9) | 4 | 20 | 10 | | |
| (11) Divide (7) by (10). (7) ÷ (10) | 25,000 | 3,750 | 40,000 | | |
| (12) Look up (12) in figures 4-24 and 4-25, in square-root tables, or in any other calculation aid. | 158.1 | 61.2 | 200 | | |

(13) Total dollars available for inventory investment.          14,000

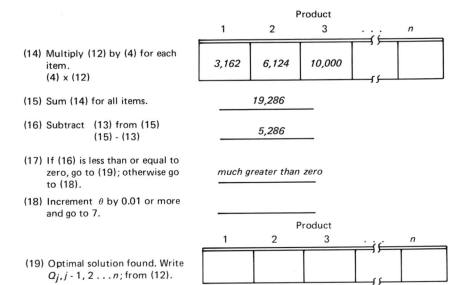

| | Product | | | . . . | |
|---|---|---|---|---|---|
| | 1 | 2 | 3 | | n |
| (14) Multiply (12) by (4) for each item. (4) x (12) | 3,162 | 6,124 | 10,000 | | |

(15) Sum (14) for all items.     19,286

(16) Subtract (13) from (15)   (15) - (13)     5,286

(17) If (16) is less than or equal to zero, go to (19); otherwise go to (18).     *much greater than zero*

(18) Increment $\theta$ by 0.01 or more and go to 7.

(19) Optimal solution found. Write $Q_j, j - 1, 2 \ldots n$; from (12).

| Product | | | . . . | |
|---|---|---|---|---|
| 1 | 2 | 3 | | n |
| | | | | |

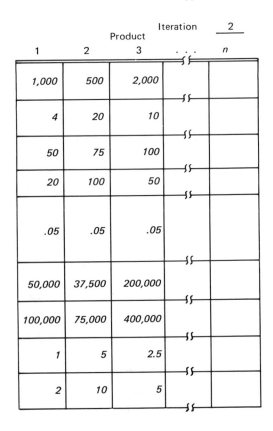

Iteration    2

| | Product | | | . . . | |
|---|---|---|---|---|---|
| | 1 | 2 | 3 | | n |
| (1) Demand or usage rate (units per year) | 1,000 | 500 | 2,000 | | |
| (2) Holding cost ($/unit/year) | 4 | 20 | 10 | | |
| (3) Setup cost or reorder cost (dollars per batch) | 50 | 75 | 100 | | |
| (4) Item unit cost | 20 | 100 | 50 | | |
| (5) Set $\theta = 0$. For each item $j=1$, ...$n$ on first iteration and increment in steps of 0.01 or greater until line (18) is zero or less. | .05 | .05 | .05 | | |
| (6) Multiply (3) by (1). (3) x (1) | 50,000 | 37,500 | 200,000 | | |
| (7) Multiply (6) by (2). (6) x (2) | 100,000 | 75,000 | 400,000 | | |
| (8) Multiply (4) by $\theta$ (4) x (5) | 1 | 5 | 2.5 | | |
| (9) Multiply (8) by (2). (2) x (8) | 2 | 10 | 5 | | |

(10) Add (2) to (9).
     (2) + (9)

| | | | | |
|---|---|---|---|---|
| 6 | 30 | 15 | | |

(11) Divide (7) by (10).
     (7) ÷ (10)

| | | | | |
|---|---|---|---|---|
| 16,666 | 2,500 | 26,666 | | |

(12) Look up (12) in figures 4-24 and 4-25, in square-root tables, or in any other calculation aid.

| | | | | |
|---|---|---|---|---|
| 129.1 | 50 | 163 | | |

(13) Total dollars available for inventory investment.

_14,000_

Product

| 1 | 2 | 3 | . . . | n |
|---|---|---|---|---|

(14) Multiply (12) by (4) for each item.
     (4) x (12)

| | | | | |
|---|---|---|---|---|
| 2,581 | 5,000 | 8,164 | | |

(15) Sum (14) for all items.

_15,746_

(16) Subtract (13) from (15)
     (15) - (13)

_1747_

(17) If (16) is less than or equal to zero, go to (19); otherwise go to (18).

_greater than zero_

(18) Increment $\theta$ by 0.01 or more and go to 7.

Product

| 1 | 2 | 3 | . . . | n |
|---|---|---|---|---|

(19) Optimal solution found. Write $Q_j, j$ - 1, 2 . . . n; from (12).

| | | | | |
|---|---|---|---|---|

Iteration    _3_

Product

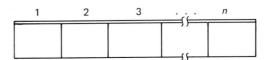

| | 1 | 2 | 3 | . . . | n |
|---|---|---|---|---|---|
| (1) Demand or usage rate (units per year) | 1,000 | 500 | 2,000 | | |
| (2) Holding cost ($/unit/year) | 4 | 20 | 10 | | |
| (3) Setup cost or reorder cost (dollars per batch) | 50 | 75 | 100 | | |
| (4) Item unit cost | 20 | 100 | 50 | | |

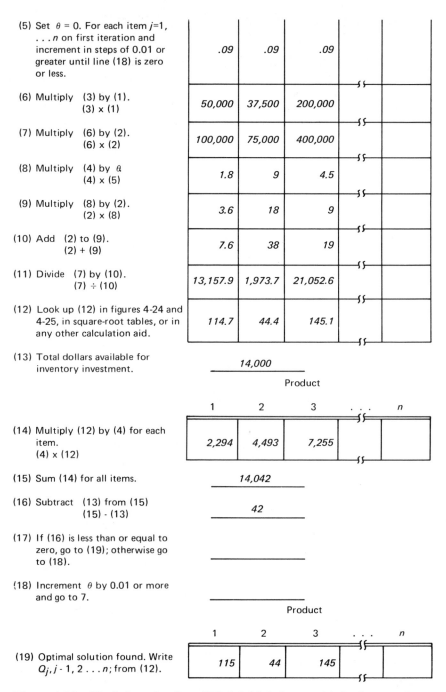

| | | | | | |
|---|---|---|---|---|---|
| (5) Set $\theta = 0$. For each item $j=1$, ...$n$ on first iteration and increment in steps of 0.01 or greater until line (18) is zero or less. | .09 | .09 | .09 | | |
| (6) Multiply (3) by (1).<br>(3) x (1) | 50,000 | 37,500 | 200,000 | | |
| (7) Multiply (6) by (2).<br>(6) x (2) | 100,000 | 75,000 | 400,000 | | |
| (8) Multiply (4) by $\theta$<br>(4) x (5) | 1.8 | 9 | 4.5 | | |
| (9) Multiply (8) by (2).<br>(2) x (8) | 3.6 | 18 | 9 | | |
| (10) Add (2) to (9).<br>(2) + (9) | 7.6 | 38 | 19 | | |
| (11) Divide (7) by (10).<br>(7) ÷ (10) | 13,157.9 | 1,973.7 | 21,052.6 | | |
| (12) Look up (12) in figures 4-24 and 4-25, in square-root tables, or in any other calculation aid. | 114.7 | 44.4 | 145.1 | | |

(13) Total dollars available for inventory investment.   <u>14,000</u>

Product

| 1 | 2 | 3 | . . . | n |
|---|---|---|---|---|
| 2,294 | 4,493 | 7,255 | | |

(14) Multiply (12) by (4) for each item.
(4) x (12)

(15) Sum (14) for all items.   <u>14,042</u>

(16) Subtract (13) from (15)
(15) - (13)   <u>42</u>

(17) If (16) is less than or equal to zero, go to (19); otherwise go to (18).   _____

(18) Increment $\theta$ by 0.01 or more and go to 7.   _____

Product

| 1 | 2 | 3 | . . . | n |
|---|---|---|---|---|
| 115 | 44 | 145 | | |

(19) Optimal solution found. Write $Q_j$, $j$ - 1, 2 ...$n$; from (12).

**Figure 4-23.** Worksheet for Case VII: Multiple Items with Budgetary Constraint

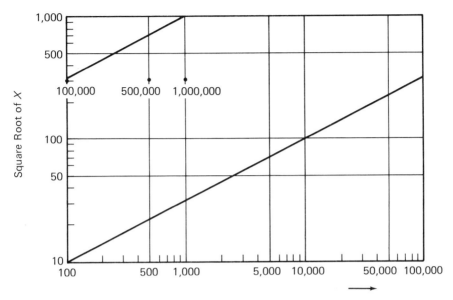

**Figure 4-24.** Plot of Square Roots of $X$, 100-100,000

Some inventory-management decisions may be made on the basis of stockouts, expressed in days.

$$\text{Stockout days} = \frac{(\text{Number of days inventory goes to zero}) \times 100}{\text{Total number of working days}}$$

There are other measures that can be used to determine inventory efficiency.

*Service level* is of concern to the manager because, in spite of methods used to prevent stockouts, there will probably always be some. Service level for some time period is defined as:

$$\text{Service level} = \frac{\text{Units supplied without delay} \times 100}{\text{Units demanded}}$$

For example:

$$\text{Service level} = \frac{398 \text{ units supplied} \times 100}{502 \text{ units demanded}}$$

$$\text{Service level} = 69.3 \text{ percent}$$

A more useful form of the equation is:

$$\text{Service level} = \frac{(\text{Units demanded} - \text{Units short}) \times 100}{\text{Units demanded}}$$

Stockouts in periods are also of concern to a manager.

$$\text{Percentage of stockouts} = \frac{(\text{Number of order periods inventory goes to zero}) \times 100}{\text{Total number of order periods}}$$

*The Average Scrap-loss* ratio is a measure of performance closely related to the service level in settings where items are "produced," as in a hospital pharmacy, a dietary department, or even a laundry. When production creates faulty units that must be scrapped, the question is how many units should be started into the production process so that just the right number is produced—not too many and not too few.

The proper quantity to start into production can be calculated by the following equation:

$$\text{Quantity started} = \frac{\text{Quantity desired}}{1 - \text{Average percentage defective}}$$

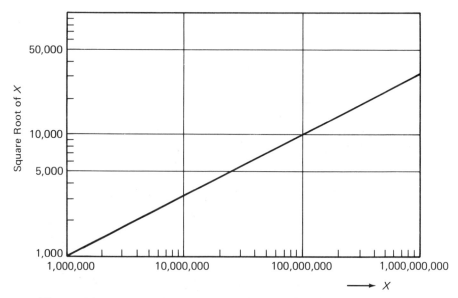

**Figure 4-25.** Plot of Square Roots of $X$, 1,000,000-1,000,000,000

For example, a lot of 2,000 finished units is desired from a process that has produced an average of 10 percent defective units in the past.

$$\text{Quantity started} = \frac{2,000}{1 - 0.10} = 2,220$$

Frequently, this problem is incorrectly calculated by the following equation, which will obviously give the wrong results.

Quantity started = Quantity desired (100% + Average percentage defective)

Quantity started = 2,000 (1 + 0.10) = 2,200

Notice that if the process has 10 percent defectives, 2,200 − (2,200 × 0.10), or 1,980 good units will be produced. This is not very helpful since a quantity of 2,000 was needed. This policy would result in a shortage of 20 units.

The scrap loss calculated previously is accurate but is considered the *average* scrap loss only. In reality there may be considerable variation. Frequently one runs into a situation in which a product has very high setup costs. To start a few products through again in order to make up for defective items can be excessively expensive. Yet this may be a product for which there is no other user department, and it might be extremely expensive to store the excess production while waiting for the user to place another order. In this situation, one can have the user bill enough to absorb the risk of either over- or underproducing.

Measures of efficiency and of effectiveness in any endeavor often are expressed as ratios or as ratios of ratios. Performance of automobiles is typically stated in terms of miles per gallon or miles per tire. Performance of an investment or savings account is given in dollars per dollar. Materials managers also need to use some yardstick for performance in these days of cost-containment pressures. Reference [13] provides a glossary of ratios for all kinds of endeavors. However, caution must be exercised in picking a measure of performance to make sure that care for the ill, the main function of a health-provider institution, is not put in significant jeopardy as a result.

In connection with this, it is necessary to point out once again that management must make enlightened tradeoffs between the service level and the total inventory-related costs associated with any given stocking policy. As further discussed later in this chapter, the tradeoffs must be made for each category of items or in some cases for each line item in consideration of the item's urgency level and possible substitutability with other, perhaps more-costly, items.

INVENTORY MODELS

CASE 1

ASSUMPTIONS IN CASE 1

1. DEMAND RATE IS CONSTANT, CONTINIOUS AND KNOWN.

2. ITEMS ARE ORDERED IN EQUAL NUMBERS, Q AT A TIME.

3. PRODUCTION OR DELIVERY IS INSTANTANEOUS.

4. NO LIMIT ON PRODUCTION CAPACITY.

5. NO SHORTAGES AND NO BACKORDERS ALLOWED.

CASE 2

ASSUMPTIONS IN CASE 2

1. DEMAND RATE IS CONSTANT.

2. ITEMS ARE ORDERED IN EQUAL NUMBERS, Q AT A TIME.

3. PRODUCTION OR DELIVERY IS INSTANTANEOUS.

4. NO LIMIT ON PRODUCTION CAPACITY.

5. SHORTAGES ARE ALLOWED.

CASE 3

ASSUMPTIONS IN CASE 3

1. DEMAND RATE IS CONSTANT, CONTINIOUS AND KNOWN.

2. ITEMS ARE ORDERED IN EQUAL NUMBERS, Q AT A TIME.

3. DELIVERY IS MADE OVER A PERIOD OF TIME AT A CONSTANT RATE GREATER THAN THE DEMAND RATE.

4. NO SHORTAGES ARE ALLOWED.

CASE 4

ASSUMPTIONS IN CASE 4

1. DEMAND RATE IS CONSTANT, CONTINIOUS AND KNOWN.

2. DELIVERY IS MADE OVER A PERIOD OF TIME AT A CONSTANT RATE GREATER THAN DEMAND RATE.

3. ITEMS ARE ORDERED IN EQUAL NUMBERS, Q AT A TIME.

**4.** SHORTAGES ARE ALLOWED.
---------- --- -------


CASE 5

ASSUMPTIONS IN CASE 5

1. DEMAND RATES FOR ALL ITEMS ARE CONSTANT, CONTINIOUS, KNOWN
   AND INDEPENDENT.

2. DELIVERIES ARE MADE OVER A PERIOD OF TIME AT CONSTANT RATES
   EACH GREATER THAN THE RESPECTIVE DEMAND RATE, THEY ARE
   CONTINIOUS, KNOWN AND INDEPENDENT OF ONE ANOTHER.

3. TIME BETWEEN ORDERS FOR ALL THE ITEMS IS SAME.

4. NO SHORTAGES ARE ALLOWED.
   -- ---------


CASE 6

ASSUMPTIONS IN CASE 6

1. DEMAND RATES FOR ALL ITEMS ARE CONSTANT, CONTINIOUS, KNOWN
   AND INDEPENDENT.

2. PRODUCTION IS INSTANTANEOUS FOR ALL THE ITEMS.

3. NO LIMIT ON PRODUCTION CAPACITY.

4. NO SHORTAGES ARE ALLOWED.
   -- --------- --- -------

5. TOTAL FLOOR SPACE AVAILABLE IS THE ONLY CONSTRAINT.


CASE 7

ASSUMPTIONS IN CASE 7

1. DEMAND RATES FOR ALL ITEMS ARE CONSTANT, CONTINIOUS, KNOWN
   AND INDEPENDENT.

2. PRODUCTION IS INSTANTANEOUS FOR ALL THE ITEMS.

3. NO LIMIT ON PRODUCTION CAPACITY.

4. NO SHORTAGES ARE ALLOWED.
   -- --------- --- -------

5. TOTAL CAPITAL AVAILABLE FOR INVENTORY INVESTMENT IS LIMITED.

**Figure 4-26.** Inventory Models

```
CASE NUMBER
1

DEMAND OR USAGE RATE?
600

HOLDING COST?
.06

SET UP COST?
8

OPTIMAL ORDER QUANTITY    =           400.00
TIME PERIOD OF ONE CYCLE   =        0.6666667   YEARS'    OR    34.666667   WEEKS
ARE THERE ANY MORE MODELS TO BE ANALYZED?
ANSWER YES OR NO, IF YES GIVE A VALUE EQUAL TO 1 OTHERWISE GIVE A VALUE EQUAL TO
 0
1

CASE NUMBER
2

DEMAND RATE OR USAGE RATE?
200

HOLDING COST?
5

SETUP OR REORDER COST?
5

SHORTAGE COST?
10

OPTIMAL ORDER QUANTITY    =          24.49
OPTIMAL INVENTORY LEVEL TO START   =          16.33
OPTIMAL NUMBER OF SHORTAGES   =            8.16
TIME PERIOD FOR ONE CYCLE   =      .1224745   YEARS     OR     6.36867   WEEKS
ARE THERE ANY MORE MODELS TO BE ANALYZED?
ANSWER YES OR NO, IF YES GIVE A VALUE EQUAL TO 1 OTHERWISE GIVE A VALUE EQUAL TO
 0
1

CASE NUMBER
3

DEMAND RATE OR USAGE RATE?
2500

DELIVERY RATE OR PRODUCTION RATE?
10000

HOLDING COST?
0.6

SETUP COST OR ORDERING COST?
50

OPTIMAL ORDERING QUANTITY   =        745.36
TIME PERIOD OF ONE CYCLE =      .2981424   YEARS   OR    15.50340   WEEKS
ARE THERE ANY MORE MODELS TO BE ANALYZED?
ANSWER YES OR NO, IF YES GIVE A VALUE EQUAL TO 1 OTHERWISE GIVE A VALUE EQUAL TO
 0
1

CASE NUMBER
4

DEMAND RATE OR USAGE RATE?
5000

DELIVERY RATE OR PRODUCTION RATE?
10000

HOLDING COST?
5

SET UP COST OR ORDERING COST?
75

SHORTAGE COST?
15

OPTIMAL ORDER QUANTITY   =        632.46
ORDER WHEN THE LEVEL OF SHORTAGES   =         79.06
TIME PERIOD FOR ONE CYCLE   =     0.1264911   YEARS  OR   6.577538   WEEKS
ARE THERE ANY MORE MODELS TO BE ANALYZED?
ANSWER YES OR NO, IF YES GIVE A VALUE EQUAL TO 1 OTHERWISE GIVE A VALUE EQUAL TO
 0
1
```

```
CASE NUMBER
5

TOTAL NUMBER OF DIFFERENT ITEMS ?
3

READ THE DEMAND OR USAGE RATE r1 r2 ....... rN ONE BY ONE
1000
1000
2000

READ THE PRODUCTION RATE k1 k2 ............ kN ONE BY ONE
1500
1500
2500

READ THE HOLDING COST C11 C21 ............ CN1 ONE BY ONE
5
5
5

READ THE SETUP COST C12 C22 .............. CN2 ONE BY ONE
25
25
25

TOTAL NUMBER OF CYCLES FOR EACH PRODUCT =   5.96285    CYCLES/YEAR       0.114670
 CYCLES/WEEK
OPTIMAL ORDER QUANTITIES Q1 Q2 ........QN ARE ONE BY ONE
     167.71
     167.71
     335.41
ARE THERE ANY MORE MODELS TO BE ANALYZED?
ANSWER YES OR NO, IF YES GIVE A VALUE EQUAL TO 1 OTHERWISE GIVE A VALUE EQUAL TO
 0
1

CASE NUMBER
6

TOTAL NUMBER OF DIFFERENT ITEMS ?
3

READ THE DEMAND OR USAGE RATE R1 R2 ....... RN ONE BY ONE
5000
2000
10000

READ THE HOLDING COST C11 C12 ............ CN1 ONE BY ONE
2
3
1

READ THE SETUP COST C12 C22 .............. CN2 ONE BY ONE
100
200
75

READ THE FLOOR SPACE REQUIRED IN SQUARE FEET F1 F2 .......FN ONE BY ONE
0.7
0.8
0.4

TOTAL FLOOR SPACE AVAILABLE IN SQUARE FEET EQUAL TO ?
700

OPTIMAL ORDER QUANTITIES Q1 Q2 ....... QN ARE ONE BY ONE
   349.3218    ,
   281.7182    ,
   574.8014    ,
VALUE OF THETA  =      4.42500
IF THE VALUE OF THETA EQUALS TO ZERO SPACE IS NOT A CONSTRAINT
ARE THERE ANY MORE MODELS TO BE ANALYZED?
ANSWER YES OR NO, IF YES GIVE A VALUE EQUAL TO 1 OTHERWISE GIVE A VALUE EQUAL TO
 0
1

CASE NUMBER
7

TOTAL NUMBER OF DIFFERENT ITEMS ?
3

READ THE DEMAND OR USAGE RATE R1 R2 ....... RN ONE BY ONE
1000
500
2000

READ  THE PRODUCTION COST ONE BY ONE
20
```

```
100
50

READ THE HOLDING COST C11 C12 ............ CN1 ONE BY ONE
4
20
10


READ THE SETUP COST C12 C22 .............. CN2 ONE BY ONE
50
75
100

TOTAL CAPITAL AVAILABLE FOR INVENTORY INVESTMENT ?
14000

OPTIMAL ORDER QUANTITIES Q1 Q2 ....... QN ARE ONE BY ONE
   114.7079      ,
   44.42616      ,
   145.0952      ,
VALUE OF THETA  =      0.09000
IF THE VALUE OF THETA EQUALS TO ZERO BUDGET FOR INVENTORY IS NOT A CONSTRAINT
ARE THERE ANY MORE MODELS TO BE ANALYZED?
ANSWER YES OR NO, IF YES GIVE A VALUE EQUAL TO 1 OTHERWISE GIVE A VALUE EQUAL TO
   0
1

CASE NUMBER
7

TOTAL NUMBER OF DIFFERENT ITEMS ?
3

READ THE DEMAND OR USAGE RATE R1 R2 ....... RN ONE BY ONE
1000
1000
2000


READ   THE PRODUCTION COST ONE BY ONE
50
20
80

READ THE HOLDING COST C11 C12 ............ CN1 ONE BY ONE
10
4
16


READ THE SETUP COST C12 C22 .............. CN2 ONE BY ONE
50
50
50

TOTAL CAPITAL AVAILABLE FOR INVENTORY INVESTMENT ?
15000

OPTIMAL ORDER QUANTITIES Q1 Q2 ....... QN ARE ONE BY ONE
   87.37041      ,
   138.1447      ,
   97.68308      ,
VALUE OF THETA  =      0.03100
IF THE VALUE OF THETA EQUALS TO ZERO BUDGET FOR INVENTORY IS NOT A CONSTRAINT
ARE THERE ANY MORE MODELS TO BE ANALYZED?
ANSWER YES OR NO, IF YES GIVE A VALUE EQUAL TO 1 OTHERWISE GIVE A VALUE EQUAL TO
   0
0

STOP

END OF EXECUTION
CPU TIME: 4.87  ELAPSED TIME: 9:23.97
EXIT
```

**Figure 4-27.** Sample Computer Solutions of the Various EOQ Cases

**Break-Even Analysis**

*Introduction*

Break-even analysis is one of the most widely used methodologies in materials-management practice. It is an integral part of the practice of such professions as accounting, business and engineering economics, finance, industrial engineering, marketing, and production management.

Break-even analysis is used to answer such questions as: What is the quantity of item $X$ that must be produced and sold or billed at price $Y$ in order for the income to equal the costs of production?

As it is commonly used, this methodology does not address itself to the time value of money in the sense of discounting future cash flows [6]. It is commonly applied to decisions regarding actions taking place at a given instant of time or regarding actions having a rather short time horizon. Hence it can be argued that compounding effects of interest or of the cost of capital are negligible.

In its common usage break-even analysis is essentially a graphic device for combining costs, revenues, and the production level so as to illustrate the probable effects of alternative courses of action on net revenues. The technique contains many variations and applications. In this section a few of its essential characteristics are highlighted in order to provide a basic understanding of its nature.

The economic basis of break-even analysis stems from the cost-output and revenue-output functions of price theory illustrated in figure 4-28. The diagram shows the total-revenue curve *TR*, the total-cost curve *TC*, and the corresponding net-revenue curve *NR*, as these relationships are commonly expressed in the literature of economics. They represent the short-run cost and revenue data for a single institution under static conditions, that is, a fixed plant, no change in technology—in general, a given "state of the art." The total-revenue line, determined by price/unit times number of units sold, is curved concave to the base, indicating that the institution can sell additional units only by charging a lower price per unit on all units sold. However, if the institution could sell additional units at the same price, as in pure competition, the *TR* curve would be a straight line. Total revenue starts at zero output, indicating that when there is no output there is no revenue. Inventories are assumed not to exist, so that the institution sells and/or bills for all it produces.

The total-cost curve represents the sum of both fixed costs, *FC*, and variable costs. Fixed costs are those that do not vary with (are not a function of) output. They include what is commonly considered overhead, pro-

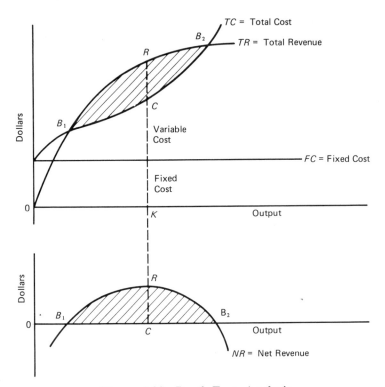

**Figure 4-28.** Break-Even Analysis

rated building or space costs, administrative salaries, insurance, and all other constant costs associated with fixed resources during the production period regardless of the level of output.

Variable costs are those that vary with or are a function of output. They include all payments associated with production that vary according to the level of production. Examples of variable costs are direct labor, raw materials, energy, and so on. In figure 4-28 the variable-cost area lies between the *TC* and *FC* curves. In short, total cost equals fixed cost plus variable cost. The total-cost curve or cost function thus represents the dependent relationship between cost and output.

The difference between *total revenue* and *total cost* represents net revenue, *NR*, and is shown by the shaded area in figure 4-28. When the net-revenue (and -loss) data are plotted, the result is the *NR* curve. The segments of the *NR* curve below the horizontal axis represent losses or negative revenue. Net revenue is a maximum where $TR - TC$ = maximum, as at the output *K* in the upper panel ($= C$ in lower panel).

Another way of looking at this is to note that the net revenue is at a maximum when the marginal revenue equals the marginal cost.

The chart reveals two break-even points—two levels of output at which the institution's revenues associated with this item just cover its costs, so that net revenue is zero. These break-even levels occur at points $B_1$ and $B_2$ in figure 4-28.

This is essentially the way in which the cost, revenue, and profit functions, as well as the break-even points, are portrayed in economics. The break-even chart, considered next, is a more typical formulation of this construction.

### The Break-Even Chart

With a few modifications, the upper panel of figure 4-28 forms a basis for the construction of the break-even chart shown in figure 4-29. The nature of these modifications rests mainly on two assumptions:

*Assumption 1*: If further units of the product can be sold or billed at the same price, the institution's total revenues (sales) can be represented by the straight line *TR*, which begins at the origin. This would apply to an organization in a purely "competitive" industry, inasmuch as it is a fundamental assumption of pure competition that no one institution is large enough to influence the market price by offering or withholding its output. But the case may also be applicable to many organizations in other competitive situations (for example, oligopoly, where a few producers control the demand for many buyers) if the product can be sold without a break in the price over wide ranges of output. In fact, this is generally true in the health-care industry.

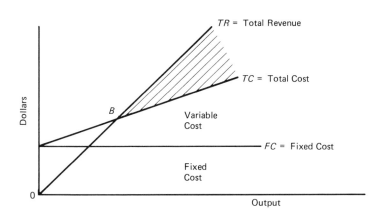

**Figure 4-29.** Break-Even Chart for Linear Systems

*Assumption 2*: If further units of productive services or inputs can be purchased at the same price per unit, that is, there are no price breaks, the costs would now be represented by a linear total-cost curve *TC*, which begins at the intersection of the fixed-cost line *FC* with the vertical axis. The production function must also be linear in these formulations. The assumption of a linear total-cost curve may also be quite reasonable within wide ranges of output. The resulting break-even chart in figure 4-29, developed from its theoretical counterpart assuming linear expense and sales relationships with output, thus reveals the profitability of operations at each output level within the institution's normal production range. Since the sales and cost curves are straight lines, there is only one break-even point, which occurs at *B*. The shaded area represents net profit, which is also shown by the *NR* line in figure 4-30.

The total-cost line of the chart shows what the total expenses would be for any given sales or billing volume according to the current expense schedule. From the chart, administration can read off net revenue or loss that would result from any output volume. The chart can be interpreted in the same manner irrespective of whether the output volume (the abscissa) is in physical units, in dollar values of usage or sales, or in percentage of capacity utilized. And of course the output volume in units, sales, or percentage of capacity at which the operation breaks even can also be determined from the graph, by dropping a perpendicular from the intersection of the *TR* and *TC* curves to the horizontal axis.

**Example**: A given hospital "manufacturing" facility, such as a dietary department having $40,000 in fixed costs, can produce certain items at $1.20 per unit irrespective of the volume produced, within a finite range. These items can be sold or billed for $2.00 per unit, the sales price being independent of the quantity sold. Furthermore, the hospital can sell all that it

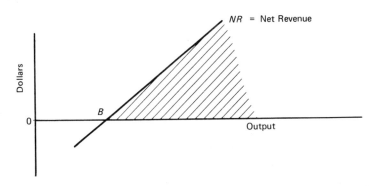

**Figure 4-30.** Net-Revenue Curves for Linear Systems

produces. At what level of production, then, will this hospital function break even?

The solution to this problem can be obtained graphically, numerically, or algebraically.

**Graphic Solution:** The income and the costs (in thousands of dollars) are shown on a scale along the ordinate or vertical axis of figure 4-31. The units produced (in thousands of units) are shown along the abscissa or the horizontal axis. The fixed-costs line is drawn next. In this case, this is a horizontal line at $40,000. This line is, of course, independent of the units produced. The variable costs are also linear in this case. Therefore, the income or total-revenue line, *TR*, emanates from the origin and rises at a slope of 2 to 1; that is, two units of revenue (vertical axis) are raised for each unit of sales or production (horizontal axis). Similarly, the total-costs line rises at a slope of 1.2 to 1, but it starts or has an intercept at $40,000, the fixed cost on the vertical axis.

The results are shown in figure 4-31, from which it can be noted that the *TR* and *TC* lines cross at 50,000 units.

**Numerical Solution:** The numerical solution is straightforward and is demonstrated in table 4-2. Assuming a given number of units produced and

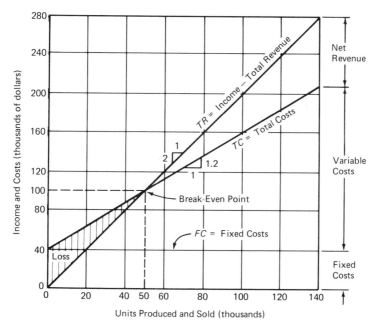

**Figure 4-31.** Graphical Solution of a Break-Even Problem

sold in column 1, multiply the value in this column by $1.20, the unit cost of production, to obtain the total variable costs listed in column 2. The total costs of column 4 are obtained by adding $40,000 to the total variable costs. The total income is, of course, obtained by multiplying by $2.00 the number of units of column 1. Net-revenue (-loss) figures are obtained by subtracting the figures in column 4 from those in column 5. Again, it can be seen that the break-even volume is 50,000 units.

### Limitations of Static Break-Even Analysis

In connection with this methodology as it is commonly used (break-even analysis is not readily applicable to multiproduct analyses), Weston and Brigham [14] say the following:

Break-even analysis is useful in studying the relations among volume, prices, and cost structure, and is thus useful for making pricing, cost control, and financial decisions. It has limitations, however, as a guide to managerial actions.

Break-even analysis is especially weak in what it implies about the sales possibilities for the "firm." Any given break-even chart is based on a contant selling price, so in order to study net-revenue possibilities under different prices, a whole series of charts is necessary, one chart for each price. Volume discounts can be handled by recognizing this fact in the variable-cost (VC) line, which becomes discontinuous under these conditions.

With regard to costs, break-even analysis is also deficient-the relations indicated by the chart do not obtain at all output levels. As sales increase, existing plant and equipment are worked to capacity; and both this situation and the use of additional workers and overtime pay causes variable costs to

**Table 4-2**
**Example of a Break-Even Numerical Solution**

| Units Sold (1) | Total Variable Costs (2) | Fixed Costs (3) | Total Costs (4) | Total Income (5) | Net Profit (Loss) (6) |
|---|---|---|---|---|---|
| 20,000 | $ 24,000 | $40,000 | $ 64,000 | $ 40,000 | $(24,000) |
| 40,000 | 48,000 | 40,000 | 88,000 | 80,000 | (8,000) |
| 50,000 | 60,000 | 40,000 | 100,000 | 100,000 | — |
| 60,000 | 72,000 | 40,000 | 112,000 | 120,000 | 8,000 |
| 80,000 | 96,000 | 40,000 | 136,000 | 160,000 | 24,000 |
| 100,000 | 120,000 | 40,000 | 160,000 | 200,000 | 40,000 |
| 120,000 | 144,000 | 40,000 | 184,000 | 240,000 | 56,000 |
| 140,000 | 168,000 | 40,000 | 208,000 | 280,000 | 72,000 |

rise sharply. Additional equipment and plant will be required, thus increasing fixed costs. Finally, over a period the products thus manufactured and sold will change in quality and quantity; such changes in product mix influence the level and slope of the cost function. In short, break-even analysis is useful as a first step in developing the basic data required for pricing and making financial decisions. More detailed analysis is required before final judgments can be made.

In general, of course, there is no reason that break-even analysis as a concept could not be applied to situations that are dynamic in nature, that is, where there exists an actual time dependency. This is in fact the case when the level of output being decided on will be maintained for extended periods of time or where a sizable amount of cash is tied up. When technological changes, either in product or in methods of production, are anticipated, or when shifts in the costs of production, capital, or unit revenues are expected, the static break-even analysis fails. There are many other dynamic situations in which it would be desirable to determine the point of break-even operations.

A fuller discussion of the dynamic applications of break-even analysis is given in [6].

## ABC Analysis

A close look at materials-transactions data often corroborates what materials managers call the *80/20 rule of thumb*—namely, 20 percent of the items account for 80 percent of the dollar usage value, or 20 percent of the items cause 80 percent of the headaches, such as stockouts. Good management practice must clearly address the big-dollar-volume categories or the "big-headache" categories in a disproportionate way. This gives rise to the so-called ABC analysis.

The main purpose of this technique is to distinguish those line items that have the most bearing on inventory costs, so that management can concentrate efforts on those items that promise the highest possible payoffs in terms of savings.

To achieve this objective, the dollar values of annual institutional purchases of line items are sorted and arranged in descending order. A computer program is often used to calculate the cumulative percentage of the annual institutional dollar purchases, for example, the percentage of total dollar purchase value resulting from $Y$ percent of the line items inventoried.

Figure 4-32 shows the ABC curve of standard-stock line items from one institution. The actual numbers from which the curve was drawn are given in table 4-3. Three classes of items can thus be identified:

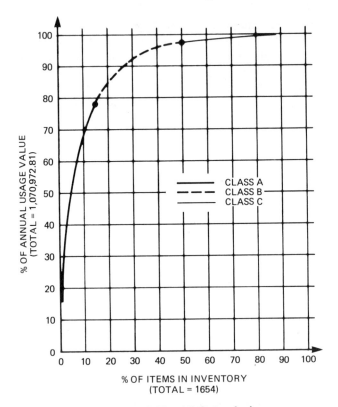

**Figure 4-32.** ABC Analysis

1. *Class A*—items that account for a high percentage (79 percent) of the total annual institutional-dollar-purchase value, and a low percentage (15 percent) of line items (items with their annual regional institutional purchases exceeding $992.19).
2. *Class B*—includes 25 percent of the line items and 20 percent of the total annual regional-dollar-purchase value (items whose annual regional purchases range from $121.12 to $992.18).
3. *Class C*—items that account for a very low percentage (1 percent) of the total annual institutional-dollar-purchase value and a very high percentage (50 percent) of line items (items whose annual institutional purchases are below $121.12.

In addition to giving management a better perspective of where the money goes, the ABC analysis is also useful is designing sampling plans for various ad hoc materials-management studies or for ongoing MMS audit and control procedures. Thus a 10- or 15-percent stratified random sample can be drawn up so as to reflect the relative importance of the *A* category

**Table 4-3**
**Sampling Strata and Numbers of Line Items**

| Aggregate Purchase Value (Strata) | Total Number of Line Items |
|---|---|
| $      0-200 | 975 |
| 200.01-400 | 194 |
| 400.01-600 | 123 |
| 600.01-800 | 74 |
| 800.01-1,000 | 41 |
| 1,000.01-1,200 | 41 |
| 1,200.01-1,400 | 22 |
| 1,400.01-1,600 | 23 |
| 1,600.01-1,800 | 15 |
| 1,800.01-2,000 | 9 |
| 2,000.01-2,200 | 13 |
| 2,200.01-2,400 | 10 |
| 2,400.01-2,600 | 14 |
| 2,600.01-2,800 | 10 |
| 2,800.01-3,000 | 8 |
| 3,000.01-3,200 | 4 |
| 3,200.01-3,400 | 11 |
| 3,400.01-3,600 | 3 |
| 3,600.01-3,800 | 8 |
| 3,800.01-4,000 | 3 |
| 4,000.01-8,000 | 32 |
| 8,000.01-12,000 | 10 |
| 12,000.01-16,000 | 5 |
| 16,000.01-24,000 | 2 |
| 24,000.01-64,000 | 0 |
| 64,000.01-68,000 | 1 |
| Total | 1654 |

items vis-à-vis those of *B* and hence *C* categories. Chapter 6 discusses the use of such approaches.

**Make or Buy**

Every hospital or clinic includes departments that use or consume materials that could be bought from outside vendors or manufactured in house. There are clearly many possibilities when all the materials and supplies consumed in an institution are considered. Fortunately, a very large share of such items are clearly not serious candidates for a make-or-buy decision. No hospital would consider manufacturing its own paper clips, pencils, or erasers. Moreover, some high-technology and proprietary items require a level of specialization in the manufacture that makes it uneconomical for a health-care-provider institution to consider such manufacture. Because of this fact, many items are bought, thus overlooking some real opportunities.

On the other hand, many consumables, such as food, have traditionally been manufactured within hospitals. Because of tradition and/or existing capacity to produce such items, opportunities for using outside vendors, in whole or in part, are often overlooked. A hospital dietary department or pharmacy uses many ingredients, some of which may be classed as raw materials, some as pre-prepared ingredients that can be bought either in bulk or in individualized portions, and some as finished-product supply items. To what extent should the institution devote its skills and effort to manufacturing, and which items should simply be bought are two key questions. Moreover, what constitute valid criteria for making these decisions is another issue of concern [15].

Make-or-buy decisions often involve both products and services. This is typically true in the dietary departments and at times in institutionally based pharmacies. A number of possibilities clearly exist. In the dietary department, for example, configurations range from the full in-house kitchen and distribution capability all the way to vendor-prepared and -dispensed foods.

Whenever service-related issues are involved in make-or-buy decisions, the least-cost decision rule must be viewed in expanded format. Additional criteria must be considered. Some of these are implied in the checklist for value analysis of contracted services, which appears in appendix 4C. The methodology best recommended for decisions involving choices between multiple alternatives using multiple criteria is, of course, the decision table, which is further discussed in chapter 5.

In addition to the checklist and audit procedures for contracted services, appendix 4C also provide a checklist for value analysis of contracted services and audit procedures for the use of value analysis in connection with contracted services.

### Calculation of Inventory-Related Unit Costs

Inventory-control models require some measure of system performance. Unless it is expressed totally in nonmonetary terms, this measure includes various unit-cost or cost parameters. The efficacy of any inventory-control decision rule in real-world settings largely depends on the accuracy and acceptability of the data used to estimate these cost parameters as well as on the assumptions made and the techniques used in developing such rules. A sophisticated decision rule can be developed by using elegant mathematical techniques with valid assumptions. However, this rule will remain merely a mathematical exercise as long as the cost parameters are not correctly measured or evaluated. The converse is also true; having accurate cost figures without a reliable inventory-replenishment rule will not remedy the situation. The combination of good cost-accounting and operations-research methodologies, in addition to good communication with the various administrators and health providers, is the essence of an effective and implementable inventory-control system.

A great deal of effort has been expended over many years on the development of inventory models, and a vast amount of literature exists. On the other hand, the problems associated with the evaluation of cost parameters used in the models or decision rules have received little attention in the operations-research literature. Few studies have been performed along these lines, although cost accounting has developed sophisticated ways of measuring direct costs. This can be attributed to the fact that the measurement of cost parameters is costly, difficult, and relatively unique for each institution.

This section will present some approaches that can be employed in evaluating the cost parameters required by the decision rules or models described earlier in the chapter. The parameters in question are:

1. Setup costs or order costs.
2. Inventory carrying costs.
3. Shortage costs.

The concepts that are discussed next are based on [16] and are followed by detailed worksheets.

## Setup or Ordering Costs

### Production-Setup Costs

The setup cost to be used in the various inventory models can be evaluated by the management-engineering department using standard industrial-engineering techniques, such as motion-and-time studies or predetermined micromotion standards and unit personnel costs [17].

### Ordering Costs

The ordering-cost figure can be obtained by time studies tracing the flow of an order from its inception in the user department or the purchasing function through, say, computer generation of a shipping invoice. The following cost components are typically found to be directly relevant to processing an order:

1. Clerical labor in the user and/or the purchasing departments.

It is customary to distinguish between ordering and setup costs. Ordering costs are relevant when outside suppliers are involved, whereas setup costs are relevant when the commodity is self-supplied or reprocessed. The basic format to establish either cost, however, is similar in nature as shown below:

(1) Salaries of all individuals involved in inventory management

    (a) Salaries (or full-time equivalents, if appropriate) per unit time of

        [a1]   Buyers/procurement officers.        $ _____

        [a2]   Clerical personnel in the procurement division.   $ _____

        [a3]   Receiving clerk and material-handling personnel.   $ _____

        [a4]   Stock-recording clerks.        $ _____

        [a5]   Accounting-department personnel responsible for accounts receivable and payment of vendors' bills.   $ _____

        [a6]   Providers/personnel (e.g., nurses, etc.) responsible for stock replenishment.   $ _____

    (b)   Total of [a1] through [a6]      $ _____

    (c)   Number of orders placed per unit time      _____

    (d)   Equivalent salaries per order (b) ÷ (c) $/order      _____

    (e)   Average number of different items in an order      _____

    (f)   Equivalent salaries per item per order (d) ÷ (e)      _____

(2) Other costs associated with placing orders ($/unit time)

    (a)   Communication

        [a1]   Telephone      _____

        [a2]   Telex      _____

        [a3]   Postage, etc.      _____

        [a4]   [a1] + [a2] + [a3]      _____

    (b)   Purchase or printing of order forms      _____

    (c)   Duplication (xeroxing, etc.) costs and other supplies      _____

    (d)   Add [a4] + (b) + (e)      _____

(e)  (d)÷(1c)  $/order  _____

(f)  (e)÷(1e)  _____

(g)  Order cost  $/item/order
      (1f) + (f)  _____

(3)  Setup cost

(a)  Time per setup and cleanup (man-hours)  _____

(b)  Labor Rate ($/man-hour)  _____

(c)  Costs incurred for equipment setup and cleanup
      $/setup
      (a) x (b)  _____

(d)  Costs incurred for startup scrap that results from the
      first few items produced ($)  _____

(e)  Other one-time costs associated with a batch of goods
      produced ($)  _____

(f)  Total of (c) through (e)  =============

*Numerical Example*

It is customary to distinguish between ordering and setup costs. Ordering costs are relevant when outside suppliers are involved, whereas setup costs are relevant when the commodity is self-supplied or reprocessed. The basic format to establish either cost, however, is similar in nature as shown below:

(1)  Salaries of all individuals involved in inventory management

(a)  Salaries (or full-time equivalents, if appropriate) per unit time of

[a1]  Buyers/procurement officers.  $  18,000

[a2]  Clerical personnel in the procurement division.  $  13,000

[a3]  Receiving clerk and material-handling personnel.  $  12,000

[a4]  Stock-recording clerks.  $  12,000

[a5]  Accounting-department personnel responsible
        for accounts receivable and payment of vendors'
        bills.  $  5,000

[a6]  Providers/personnel (e.g., nurses, etc.) responsi-
        ble for stock replenishment.  $  0

(b)  Total of [a1] through [a6]  $  60,000

| | | |
|---|---|---|
| (c) | Number of orders placed per unit time | 2,000 |
| (d) | Equivalent salaries per order (b) ÷ (c) $/order | 30 |
| (e) | Average number of different items in an order | 10 |
| (f) | Equivalent salaries per item per order (d) ÷ (e) | 3 |

(2) Other costs associated with placing orders ($/unit time)

| | | |
|---|---|---|
| (a) | Communication | |
| | [a1]　Telephone | 1,200 |
| | [a2]　Telex | 0 |
| | [a3]　Postage, etc. | 300 |
| | [a4]　[a1] + [a2] + [a3] | 1,500 |
| (b) | Purchase or printing of order forms | 500 |
| (c) | Duplication (xeroxing, etc.) costs and other supplies | 3,000 |
| (d) | Add [a4] + (b) + (e) | 5,000 |
| (e) | (d)÷(1c)　$/order | 2.5 |
| (f) | (e)÷(1e) | 0.25 |
| (g) | Order cost　$/item/order (1f) + (f) | 3.25 |

(3) Setup cost

| | | |
|---|---|---|
| (a) | Time per setup and cleanup (man-hours) | 3 |
| (b) | Labor Rate ($/man-hour) | 8 |
| (c) | Costs incurred for equipment setup and cleanup $/setup (a) x (b) | 24 |
| (d) | Costs incurred for startup scrap that results from the first few items produced ($) | 10 |
| (e) | Other one-time costs associated with a batch of goods produced ($) | 2 |
| (f) | Total of (c) through (e) | 36 |

**Figure 4-33.** Worksheet for Ordering- and/or Setup-Cost Calculations

2. Telephone and/or postage costs in the purchasing department.
3. Order entry cost in the purchasing department.
4. Keypunching costs in the purchasing department.

These components can be evaluated and then summed up to obtain an ordering cost per order. This ordering cost per order is then divided by the average number of different items per order to yield estimated average ordering cost per order per item. Figure 4-33 provides a worksheet for evaluating ordering and set up costs.

**Inventory Carrying Costs**

*Components of Inventory Carrying Costs*

Inventory carrying costs are those that are directly attributable to the amount, type, location, and so on of inventory carried and that increase in direct proportion to increase in inventory on hand and in the time for which inventoried items are held. Inventory carrying holding costs are at times expressed as a fraction or percentage of the dollar value of average inventory carried and at other times as actual dollars per unit of time. The former parameter multiplied by the dollar value of inventory gives the latter parameter. The following can be found to be more-or-less significant components of the inventory carrying cost. Acquisition of these data is discussed in chapter 6. The purpose of this section is to show how available data are used to arrive at accurate cost estimates for the parameters of the inventory-replenishment decision rules or models.

(1) = Cost of capital or (1)' = opportunity cost.

(2) = Clerical and administrative costs.

(3) = Handling or labor costs.

(4) = Storage or warehousing costs.

(5) = Insurance and taxes on inventory held.

(6) = Costs of depreciation, deterioration, and obsolence of inventory.

As an alternative to the cost of capital, some suggest that the opportunity cost (the cost of foregone opportunities) should be included in computing inventory carrying cost. Two alternative approaches to determine inventory carrying costs are shown next. In both cases, the unit carrying costs are expressed as a fraction of the average dollar inventory of materials held.

*Alternative 1*

In this method the number of turnovers of the inventory within a year is taken into consideration. If *TR* denotes the inventory turnover, then the inventory carrying cost per dollar invested in the inventory is given by the following formula:

$$\text{Inventory carrying cost} = \frac{(1) + [(2)/TR] + [(3)/TR] + [(4)/TR] + (5) + (6)}{\overline{I}}$$

where $\overline{I}$ is the dollar value of the average inventory carried throughout the year for that item or category of items. The numbers in parentheses correspond to the components listed earlier.

*Alternative 2*

Alternative 1 is a commonly used approach for determination of inventory carrying costs. It includes all those costs that are considered to be related to inventory and that tend to appear in institutional accounting records. The approach discussed in this section can be considered as an alternative. Suppose that at a point in time the problem is to choose from among several options an inventory system to replace what exists. In this case the institution is interested only in those costs that will directly respond to a change in the level of inventory carried, namely insurance, depreciation, and so on. In this case, then, the opportunity cost should be used instead of the cost of capital because the opportunity of investing the money in the best possible way, which may not be inventory, is foregone. Therefore, the following formula for computing the inventory carrying cost is suggested.

$$\text{Inventory carrying cost} = \frac{(1)' + (5) + (6)}{\overline{I}}$$

This formula does not include storage and handling costs. If these figures are significant, they can be added to the numerator. Figures 4-34 and 4-35 provide worksheets for evaluating the holding-cost parameters and the holding-cost respectively.

**Shortage Cost**

*The Nature of Shortage Cost*

Shortage cost is the cost incurred as a consequence of a stockout, that is, when the demand cannot be fully and immediately satisfied owing to a stock shortage. The problem of shortage-cost evaluation arises in:

1. Determining the total cost incurred by a selected inventory-control policy.
2. Determining the optimal parameters of an inventory policy where it is assumed that shortage cost is measurable and included in the decision model.
3. A situation where it is necessary to compare the cost of a stockout with the cost of eliminating that stockout by obtaining the items from elsewhere in the institution or from another institution.

Figure 4-36 provides a worksheet for calculating the shortage costs.

Among all inventory-control-cost parameters, the evaluation of shortage costs have received the least attention in the literature [18,19,20,21]. In the context of a health-care institution, shortage costs can be evaluated based on any one of three considerations:

1. Cost of expediting or emergency procedures.
2. Cost of substitution.
3. Cost of lost sales.

The shortage-cost-evaluation worksheets provided later in this chapter address each of these considerations.

*Substitutability of Materials*

In health-care services as anywhere, one can nearly always find different products, brands, or sizes to satisfy any particular need for materials. Functionally at least, substitutability of one item for another is often feasible. Housley [21] enumerates the following reasons for product substitution: (1) product unavailability, (2) product recall, (3) product change, (4) price hikes in the original item, (5) change in suppliers, and (6) product obsolescence. To this list one should add (7) product cost effectiveness; (8) product consolidation, for example, getting users to agree to some standardization; and (9) temporary stockout of products within the institution. All of the above reasons for product substitutions, with the exception of (9) and in some cases (1), give rise to long-term substitutability considerations. These should be addressed by standardization committees or their equivalents using some form of value or cost-effectiveness analysis of all feasible alternatives or options. Value analysis was discussed in chapter 2.

The needs for short-term substitutability arise whenever there is a temporary stockout for whatever reason. In this type of situation, consideration must be given to tradeoffs between costs on the one hand and the urgency of the need for the item on the other. A discussion of urgency issues follows this section. Clearly, whenever an item is substituted for another one, either a higher or lower cost has been incurred and a stockout situation

1. Cost of Capital

This cost parameter should reflect the cost of borrowing money and/or the cost of foregone opportunities, foregone earnings, and so on, if the capital that is tied up in inventory were invested elsewhere. For example, if the average annual inventory "book value"
is $1 million, what is the institution's cost of this tied up capital? The following steps for
calculating this cost of capital are based on a general model for the cost of capital discussed in [6].

(a)   Average book value of the inventory held in stock
     ($/unit time)                                            _____

(b)   Foregone return on investment

    [b1]   Return on available opportunities from commercial
             paper, government securities, etc, %               _____

    [b2]   Opportunity foregone [b1] x (a) $/$/ unit time       _____

(c)   The amount of capital raised through financing

    [c1]   The amount of *debt* capital of the

          (c1-1)   1st category of debt ($)              _____

          (c1-2)   2nd category of debt ($)             _____

              .
              .
              .

          (c1-m)   $m$th category of debt ($)           _____

          (c1-o)   Sum of (c1-1) through (c1-m) ($)      ==========

    [c2] [a]  The amount of (new) preferred stock less brokerage
           of the

          (c2-1)   1st category ($)                 _____

          (c2-2)   2nd category ($)               _____

              .
              .
              .

          (c2-n)   $n$th category ($)               _____

          (c2-o)   Sum of (c2-1) through (c2-n) ($)      ==========

    [c3] [a]  The amount of new common stock less the broker's
           commission ($)                       _____

    [c4] [a]  Add lines (c1-0) + (c2-0) + [c3]
           [This must equal line (a) above[ ($)     ==========

(d)   The interest rates

    [d1]   The interest rate paid on debt capital of the

          (d1-1)   1st category $/$/unit time          _____

[a]Applicable to some proprietory institutions only.

(d1-2)   2nd category $/$/unit time        _____

.                                          .
.                                          .
.                                          .

(d1-m)   $m^{th}$ category $/$/unit time

[d2] [a] The dividend rate committed to the preferred
stockholder of the

(d2-1)   1st category $/$/unit time        _____

(d2-2)   2nd category $/$/unit time        _____

.                                          .
.                                          .
.                                          .

(d2-n) $n^{th}$ category $/$/unit time     _____

[d3] [a] The dividend rate (investors' expectation rate) paid
on common stock $/$/unit time             _____

(e)   Cost of capital

[e1]   Debt financing component

(e1-1)   Multiply lines (d1-1)x(c1-1)
$/unit time                      _____

(e1-2)   Multiply lines (d1-2)x(c1-2)
$/unit time                      _____

.
.
.

(e1-m)   Multiply lines (d1-m)x(c1-m)
$/unit time                      _____

(e1-o)   Add lines (e1-1) through (e1-m)
$/unit time                      _____

(e1-p)   Divide lines (e1-o)÷(c1-o)[b]     _____

[e2] [a] Preferred stock component

(e2-1)   Multiply lines (d2-1)x(c2-1)
$/unit time                      _____

(e2-2)   Multiply lines (d2-2)x(c2-2)
$/unit time                      _____

.
.

(e2-n)   Multiply lines (d2-n)x(c2-n)
$/unit time                      _____

[a]Applicable to some proprietory institutions only.
[b]This is the cost of capital for institutions listing debt financing only.

(e2-o)   Add lines (e2-1) through (e2-n)
$/unit time                                    _____

(e2-p)   Divide lines (e2-o)÷(c2-o)            ===========

[e3]ᵃ Common stock component

(e3-p)   Copy amount in line [d3]              _____

[e4]    Add (e1-o) + (e2-o) + (e3-o) $/unit time    _____

[e5]    Add (c1-o) + (c2-o) + (c3-o) $/unit time    _____

[e6]    The cost of capital due to all forms of financing is
        [e4] [e5] $/$/unit time               ===========

(f)    Average dollar inventory held in stock    _____

(g)    Average cost of capital for money tied up in inventory
       [e6] x (f)   ($/unit of time)           _____

2. Insurance Cost

(a)    Average dollar value of inventory held from line 1(a)    _____

(b)    Insurance premium based on the average inventory held
       during the unit time period $/unit of time    _____

(c)    (b)÷(a)   $/$/unit time                  ===========

3. Storage, Handling, and Administrative Costs

(a)    Rental or equivalent of the warehouse and/or other storage
       space ($/unit time)                     _____

(b)    Depreciation on material handling equipment ($/unit time)    _____

(c)    Payroll to add materials management personnel for record
       keeping, warehousing, etc., of the inventory ($/unit time)    _____

(d)    (a) + (b) + (c)                          ===========

(e)    Average dollar value of inventory held in stock ($)
       from line 1(a)                           _____

(f)    (d)÷(e)                                  _____

4. Deterioration, Obsolescence, and Pilferage Cost

This cost is extremely difficult to determine even under the best practice of inventory
record keeping. Hence, often executive judgments may be used.

(a)    Deterioration and obsolescence cost ($/unit time)    _____

(b)    Pilferage cost ($/unit of time)          _____

(c)    (a) + (b)                                _____

(d)    Average dollar value of inventory held in stock ($)    _____

(e)    (c)÷(d)                                  ===========

ᵃApplicable to some proprietory institutions only.
ᵇThis is the cost of capital for institutions listing debt financing only.

*Numerical Example*

1. Cost of Capital

This cost parameter should reflect the cost of borrowing money and/or the cost of foregone opportunities, foregone earnings, and so on, if the capital that is tied up in inventory were invested elsewhere. For example, if the average annual inventory "book value" is $1 million, what is the institution's cost of this tied up capital? The following steps for calculating this cost of capital are based on a general model for the cost of capital discussed in [g] .

(a) Average book value of the inventory held in stock
    ($/unit time)                                                      *1,000,000*

(b) Foregone return on investment

    [b1]  Return on available opportunities from commercial
          paper, government securities, etc, %                         *0.16*

    [b2]  Opportunity foregone [b1] x (a)  $/$/ unit time              *160,000*

(c) The amount of capital raised through financing

    [c1]  The amount of *debt* capital of the

          (c1-1)  1st category of debt ($)                            *600,000*

          (c1-2)  2nd category of debt ($)                            *500,000*

                  .
                  .
                  .

          (c1-m)  $m^{th}$ category of debt ($)                        _____

          (c1-o)  Sum of (c1-1) through (c1-m) ($)                     *1,100,000*

    [c2] [a] The amount of (new) preferred stock less brokerage
             of the

          (c2-1)  1st category ($)                                    _____

          (c2-2)  2nd category ($)                                    _____

                  .                                                       .
                  .                                                       .
                  .                                                       .

          (c2-n)  $n^{th}$ category ($)                               _____

          (c2-o)  Sum of (c2-1) through (c2-n) ($)                    _____

    [c3] [a] The amount of new common stock less the broker's
             commission ($)                                           _____

    [c4] [a] Add lines (c1-0) + (c2-0) + [c3]
             [This must equal line (a) above[ ($)                     _____

(d) The interest rates

    [d1]  The interest rate paid on debt capital of the

[a]Applicable to some proprietory institutions only.

[b]This is the cost of capital for institutions listing debt financing only.

(d1-1)   1st category $/$/unit time                                    0.09

(d1-2)   2nd category $/$/unit time                                   0.10

.                                                                                  .

.                                                                                  .

.                                                                                  .

(d1-m)   mth category $/$/unit time                          _____

[d2][a] The dividend rate committed to the preferred
       stockholder of the

(d2-1)   1st category $/$/unit time                          _____

(d2-2)   2nd category $/$/unit time                         _____

.                                                                                  .

.                                                                                  .

.                                                                                  .

(d2-n)   nth category $/$/unit time                          _____

[d3][a] The dividend rate (investors' expectation rate) paid
       on common stock $/$/unit time                      _____

(e)   Cost of capital

    [e1]   Debt financing component

        (e1-1)   Multiply lines (d1-1)x(c1-1)
                 $/unit time                                        54,000

        (e1-2)   Multiply lines (d1-2)x(c1-2)
                 $/unit time                                        50,000

             .

             .

             .

        (e1-m)   Multiply lines (d1-m)x(c1-m)
                 $/unit time                                    _____

        (e1-o)   Add lines (e1-1) through (e1-m)
                 $/unit time                                      104,000

        (e1-p)   Divide lines (e1-o)÷(c1-o)[b]              0.0945

    [e2][a] Preferred stock component

        (e2-1)   Multiply lines (d2-1)x(c2-1)
                 $/unit time                                    _____

        (e2-2)   Multiply lines (d2-2)x(c2-2)
                 $/unit time                                    _____

             .

             .

             .

        (e2-n)   Multiply lines (d2-n)x(c2-n)
                 $/unit time                                    _____

[a]Applicable to some proprietory institutions only.
[b]This is the cost of capital for institutions listing debt financing only.

| | | |
|---|---|---|
| (e2-o) | Add lines (e2-1) through (e2-n) $/unit time | _____ |
| (e2-p) | Divide lines (e2-o)÷(c2-o) | _____ |
| [e3]<sup>a</sup> Common stock component | | |
| (e3-p) | Copy amount in line [d3] | _____ |
| [e4] | Add (e1-o) + (e2-o) + (e3-o) $/unit time | 104,000 |
| [e5] | Add (c1-o) + (c2-o) + (c3-o) $/unit time | 1,100,000 |
| [e6] | The cost of capital due to all forms of financing is [e4] [e5] $/$/unit time | 0.0945 |
| (f) | Average dollar inventory held in stock | _____ |
| (g) | Average cost of capital for money tied up in inventory [e6] x (f)   ($/unit of time) | 94,500 |

2. Insurance Cost

| | | |
|---|---|---|
| (a) | Average dollar value of inventory hold from line 1(a) | 1,000,000 |
| (b) | Insurance premium based on the average inventory held during the unit time period $/unit of time | 5,000 |
| (c) | (b)÷(a)  $/$/unit time | .005 |

3. Storage, Handling, and Administrative Costs

| | | |
|---|---|---|
| (a) | Rental or equivalent of the warehouse and/or other storage space ($/unit time) | 12,000 |
| (b) | Depreciation on material handling equipment ($/unit time) | 6,000 |
| (c) | Payroll to add materials management personnel for record keeping, warehousing, etc., of the inventory ($/unit time) | 60,000 |
| (d) | (a) + (b) + (c) | 78,000 |
| (e) | Average dollar value of inventory held in stock ($) from line 1(a) | 1,000,000 |
| (f) | (d)÷(e) | 0.78 |

4. Deterioration, Obsolescence, and Pilferage Cost

This cost is extremely difficult to determine even under the best practice of inventory record keeping. Hence, often executive judgments may be used.

| | | |
|---|---|---|
| (a) | Deterioration and obsolescence cost ($/unit time) | 80,000 |
| (b) | Pilferage cost ($/unit of time) | 20,000 |
| (c) | (a) + (b) | 100,000 |
| (d) | Average dollar value of inventory held in stock ($) | 1,000,000 |
| (e) | (c)÷(d) | 0.10 |

<sup>a</sup>Applicable to some proprietory institutions only.

<sup>b</sup>This is the cost of capital for institutions listing debt financing only.

**Figure 4-34.** Worksheets for Inventory-Holding-Cost Parameter Calculations

Calculation alternative 1 approach

(a)　Cost of capital

　　　From line 1(g) _____

(b)　Inventory turns ratio

　　　From records _____

(c)　Storage, handling, and administrative cost

　　　From line 3(d) _____

(d)　(c) ÷ (b) _____

(e)　Insurance cost

　　　From line 2(b) _____

(f)　Deterioration, obsolescence, and pilferage cost

　　　From line 4(c) _____

(g)　(a) + (d) + (e) + (f) _____

(h)　Average inventory

　　　From line 1(a) _____

(i)　Holding cost $/$/unit of time

　　　(g) ÷ (h) ══════════════

Calculation alternative 2 approach

(j)　Opportunity-foregone cost from line 1 [b2] _____

(k)　(j) + (e) + (f) _____

(l)　Holding cost (k) ÷ (h) ══════════════

*Numerical Example*

Calculation alternative 1 approach

(a)　Cost of capital

　　　From line 1(g) *94,500*

(b)　Inventory turns ratio

　　　From records *6*

| | | |
|---|---|---|
| (c) | Storage, handling, and administrative cost | |
| | From line 3(d) | *78,000* |
| (d) | (c) ÷ (b) | *13,000* |
| (e) | Insurance cost | |
| | From line 2(b) | *5,000* |
| (f) | Deterioration, obsolescence, and pilferage cost | |
| | From line 4(c) | *100,000* |
| (g) | (a) + (d) + (e) + (f) | *212,500* |
| (h) | Average inventory | |
| | From line 1(a) | *1,000,000* |
| (i) | Holding cost $/$/unit of time | |
| | (g) ÷ (h) | *0.21* |
| Calculation alternative 2 approach | | |
| (j) | Opportunity-foregone cost from line 1 [b2] | *160,000* |
| (k) | (j) + (e) + (f) | *265,000* |
| (l) | Holding cost (k) ÷ (h) | *0.265* |

**Figure 4-35.** Worksheets for Holding-Cost Calculations

has simultaneously been prevented, thereby assuring continuity of patient care. It must be recognized that in case of a price hike for functionally equivalent items, the long-term and short-term substitutability categorization can easily change. Therefore, identification of substitutable items with their characteristics and prices should always be available and kept current within a materials-management information system (MMIS).

There are several types of short-term substitutability.

**One-Way Substitutability**. Here the substitutability is unidirectional. This may take several forms:

1. One-item substitution for only one other item. This case may take several modes:
   a. Two or more smaller size items substituting for one larger size item;

(1)   Cost of shortage avoided by expediting or emergency procedure

    (a)   Number of units short of a given item during a given period (number of units/unit time).   _____

    (b)   Cost of special calls (personnel and communication) to the supplier(s).   $_____

    (c)   Cost of special packaging.   $_____

    (d)   Cost of special shipping.   $_____

    (e)   (b) + (c) + (d)   $_____

    (f)   (e) ÷ (a) in $/unit of an item/unit time.   _____

If the item is self-supplied (i.e., manufactured in house, it may be necessary to consider

    (g)   Cost of disrupting a planned production schedule.

        [g1]   Cost of clean-up and new equipment setup.   $_____

        [g2]   Cost of labor overtime.   $_____

        [g3]   [g1] + [g2]   $_____

    (h)   $[g^3]$ ÷ (a) $/unit of an item/unit time.   _____

(2)   Cost of shortage avoided by substitution

    (a)   Number of units short of a given item during a given period (number of units/unit time).   _____

    (b)   Per-unit price of the item.   $_____

    (c)   Per-unit cost of the substituting item, where the substitute is of a better quality or a larger quantity or size than the item originally required.   $_____

    (d)   Unit cost of substitution = (c) - (b) in $/unit of the item/unit time.   $_____

    (e)   Total cost of substitution (d) x (a).   _____

(3)   Cost of lost sales or cancellation

    (a)   Number of units of an item the order for which is cancelled because of shortage (in number of units/unit time).   _____

    (b)   The gross "profit" (not earnings per unit) that could have resulted had the shortage not occurred (the unit cost of lost opportunity) $/unit of the item/unit time.   $_____

(c) The experience factor (greater than one) to take account of the extent to which future sales are lost due to one-time shortage.

(d) (c) ÷ (d) in $/unit of the item/unit time.

### Numerical Example

(1) Cost of shortage avoided by expediting or emergency procedure

(a) Number of units short of a given item during a given period (number of units/unit time).                                    100

(b) Cost of special calls (personnel and communication) to the supplier(s).                                                            $    50

(c) Cost of special packaging.                                                                   $    30

(d) Cost of special shipping.                                                                    $    15

(e) (b) + (c) + (d)                                                                              $    95

(f) (e) ÷ (a) in $/unit of an item/unit time.                                                        0.95

If the item is self-supplied (i.e., manufactured in house, it may be necessary to consider

(g) Cost of disrupting a planned production schedule.

    [g1]  Cost of clean-up and new equipment setup.                         $    36

    [g2]  Cost of labor overtime.                                           $    28

    [g3]  (g1) + (g2)                                                       $    64

(h) (g) ÷ (a) $/unit of an item/unit time.                                                           0.64

(2) Cost of shortage avoided by substitution

(a) Number of units short of a given item during a given period (number of units/unit time).                                    100

(b) Per-unit price of the item.                                                                 $    1.00

(c) Per-unit cost of the substituting item, where the substitute is of a better quality or a larger quantity or size than the item originally required.                                         $    1.30

(d) Unit cost of substitution = (c) - (b) in $/unit of the item/unit time.                                                             $    0.30

(e) Total cost of substitution (d) x (a).                                                            30

| | |
|---|---|
| (3)   Cost of lost sales or cancellation | |
|    (a)   Number of units of an item the order for which is cancelled because of shortage (in number of units/ unit time). | 50 |
|    (b)   The gross "profit" (not earnings per unit) that could have resulted had the shortage not occurred (the unit cost of lost opportunity) $/unit of the item/unit time. | $   30 |
|    (c)   The experience factor (greater than one) to take account of the extent to which future sales are lost due to one-time shortage. | 1.1 |
|    (d)   (a) x (b) x (c)/(a) = (b) x (c) in $/unit of the item/unit time. | 33 |

**Figure 4-36.** Worksheet for Shortage-Cost Calculation

    for example, two 250-mg polycillin capsules can substitute for a 500-mg one.

    b.   A larger or more-specialized item substituting for a smaller or less-specialized one, for example, 8½″ × 14″ photocopier paper substituting for 8½″ × 11″ paper, or a large sterile surgical gown substituting for a disposable isolation gown.

2.   One item substituting for several items; for example, a 14″ x 17″ X-ray film can substitute for the 8″ × 12″, 10″ × 12″, or 11″ × 14″ sizes.

3.   Several items substituting for one item; for example, size 7 or 7½ sterile surgeon's gloves can substitute for a pair of medium sterile-procedure gloves.

**Two-Way Substitutability.** Here a substitute may be substituted for by yet another item, making the substitutability multidirectional. This takes various forms:

1.   Less than one unit of an item can substitute for another item; for example, less than one 1,500-ml unit of normal saline irrigating solution can substitute for a 1,000-ml one.

2.   One unit of an item can substitute for or be substituted for by one unit of another item, for example, single-fold paper hand towel and multifold paper hand towel.

3.   Two or more units of an item can substitute for a unit of another item, for example, two units of a 500-ml 5-percent dextrose in $H_2O$ intravenous solution can substitute for one unit of a 1,000-ml one.

    Substitutable items drawn from a stratified random sample of standard-stock items used by an HMO are listed in table 4-4 to illustrate the concept of one- and two-way substitutability.

*Urgency Requirements of Materials*

Materials-management systems in health-care-delivery institutions must reflect the critical elements and idiosyncracies of the delivery of health care. Medical staff and materials-management personnel consulted in several institutions provided the following insights. Medical staffs believed that this critical element could be summarized by the categorization of items according to urgency. In a multifacility health center, four categories of urgency were identified:

**Use-Location Urgency.** No stockout is allowed at a use location. These are the most urgent items and must be available to the materials users at all times. In case of a stockout at the use location, the demand for the item is lost and cannot be satisfied by interdepartmental transfers, mainly because the need is highly urgent or because the item can be found only in a single department. Examples are sterile laporatomy pack, chromic gut suture, and the largest-sized X-ray film (14″ × 17″).

**Facility-Location Urgency.** No stockout is allowed at a facility. These items have the second-highest urgency. Any given use location in a facility at a given time may experience stockout, since interdepartmental transfers can be used to satisfy these local stockouts. However, the item must be available in the facility as a whole—somewhere among all the use locations in the facility. In case of a stockout in the whole facility, the demand is lost and cannot be satisfied by interfacility transfers. Examples are nonsterile vinyl examination gloves, sterile maternity pad, 6-ounce specimen container, and sterile disposable hypothermic syringe.

**Regional-Location Urgency.** No stockout is allowed at the regional location—all the use locations of all the facilities. The items falling into this category have the third-highest urgency. Any given use location in a facility or any facility as a whole may experience stockouts at a given time. Interdepartmental and interfacility transfers can be used to satisfy these types of stockouts. However, the item must be available in the region as a whole.

If a stockout occurs in the region as a whole, the demand is lost and cannot be satisfied from other sources. Examples are PBZ 50-mg, telepaque tablets, and deluxe underpad liner.

**No Urgency.** Items for which stockouts are allowed at all levels—use locations, facility locations, and regional locations. These are the nonemergency items for which a temporary stockout is allowed. Examples are oral thermometer, interdepartmental envelopes, and examining-table paper.

**Table 4-4**
**Item Substitution**

| Catalog Number | Item Description | Is substitutable by: | Catalog Number | Item Description |
|---|---|---|---|---|
| 80-154507 | Film X-ray Gevaert Poly 10 × 12 125/pkg | ↑ [a] | 80-154704 | Film X-ray Gevaert Poly 14 × 17 |
| 80-154506 | Film X-ray Gevaert Poly 11 × 14 | ↑ | | |
| 80-154308 | Film X-ray Gevaert Poly 8 × 10 | ↑ | | |
| 25-034904 | Gown Isolation Disp W/Cuff 100 CS | ↑ | 25-035059 | Gown surgical sterile large |
| 85-171507 | Sponge Gauze 4 × 4 — 16 ply Nonsterile 2M/CS | ↑ | 85-171406 | Sponge Gauze 3 × 3 — 12 ply Nonsterile |
| 40-067507 | Towel Hand Paper Multifold 3750/CS | ↑ [b] | 40-067608 | Towel Hand Paper Single-Fold |
| | | | 05-004075 | Syringe Insul. Disposable 100-U W/26 G × 1/2 Ndl 5652 |
| 05-004059 | Syringe Insul. Disposable 100-U W/26 G × 1/2 Ndl | ↑ | 05-004307 | Syringe TB Disposable 100-U W/27 G × 1/2 Ndl |
| 45-074302 | Sol IV 5% Dex in Lact Ring 1000 ML | ↑ | 45-074401 | Sol. IV 5% Dex in Lact Ring 500 ML |
| 20-025907 | Cup Coffee Plastic W/Handle 7 oz. | ↑ | 20-026202 | Cup Styrofoam 6 oz. |
| | | | 20-026301 | Cup Styrofoam 8 oz. |
| 15-020608 | Cath. Tray Foley W/O Cath. Add-a-Poley | ↑ | 15-020509 | Cath. Tray W/14-16 FR Cath. Strl 20/CS |
| 30-048469 | Bicillin LA 1.2 Mu | ↑ | | Nonstandard Stock .6 Available |
| 45-077107 | Sol Irrigating Distilled Water 1500 ML | ↑ | 45-077206 | Sol Irrigating Distilled Water 1000 ML – 500 ML |
| 30-054517 | Capsules, Polycillin 500 Mg | ↑ | 30-054443 | Capsules, Polycillin 250 Mg |
| 65-129408 | Paper Xerox White 8 1/2 × 11 | ↑ | 65-129507 | Paper Xerox White 8 1/2 × 14 |
| 20-027358 | Packette Utensils Breakfast 555/CS | ↑ | 20-027408 | Packette Utensils Brunch & Dinner |
| 50-087603 | Tube Culture Disp. 13 × 100 MM | ↑ | 50-087504 | Tube Culture Disp. 12 × 75 MM |
| 30-040821 | Sodium Chloride Injection 30 ML 100/CS | ↑ | 45-076604 | Sol. IV Nor. Saline 250 ML |
| 05-000503 | Cannula IV Medicut Strl. 20G × 2 50/Ctn | ↑ | 05-000404 | Cannula IV Medicut Strl. 18G × 2 51/Ctn |

| Code | Item | | Code | Item |
|------|------|---|------|------|
| 85-161605 | Bandage Elas Rubber Reinforced 3 10/pkg | ↑ | 85-161506 | Bandage Elas Rubber Reinforced 2 |
| | | | 85-161704 | Bandage Elas Rubber Reinforced 4 |
| 75-147507 | Bag Bedside 2000/CS | ↑ | 40-065404 | Bag Paper 5 lb 500/pkg |
| | | | 31-051462 | Bottle Screwlock Amber Dr 16 |
| 31-051447 | Bottle Screwlock Amber 13 DR | ↑ | 31-051448 | Bottle Screwlock Amber DR 20 |
| 25-036503 | Sheet Pediatric 72 × 103 10/CS | ↑ | 25-036255 | Sheet Drape Sterile 60 × 84 |
| 60-097220 | Cannula Aspirator Disp 10 FR Airshield | ↑ | 60-097212 | Cannula Aspirator Disp 8 FR Airshield |
| | | | 60-097238 | Cannula Aspirator Disp 12 FR Airshield |
| 40-066303 | Cup Paper Waxed 4 oz. | ↑ | 20-026202 | Cup Styrofoam 6 oz. |
| | | | 20-126301 | Cup Styrofoam 8 oz. |
| 85-170903 | Sponge Ctn Fld Radiopaque Large 2M/CS | ↑ | 85-171000 | Sponge Ctn Fld Radiopaque Super 1M/CS |
| 05-001501 | Needle Hypodermic Disp Strl. 20G × 1 1/2 | ↑ | 05-001303 | Needle Hypodermic Disp Strl. 19 × 1 1/2 |
| | | | 05-001709 | Needle Hypodermic Disp Strl. 21 × 1 1/2 |
| 85-165002 | Binder Abdominal Surgical Small | ↑ | 85-165101 | Binder Abdominal Surgical Medium |
| 45-076653 | Sol. IV Nor Saline 250 ML .9% SOD | ↕ | 45-076604 | Sol. IV Nor Saline 250 ML |
| 45-077503 | Sol. Irrigating Normal Saline 1500 ML 6/CS | ↑ | 45-077602 | Sol. Irrigating Normal Saline 1000 ML |
| 45-077206 | Sol. Irrigating Distilled Water 1000 ML | ↑ | 45-077305 | Sol. Irrigating Distilled Water 500 ML |
| 50-085904 | Needle Vacutainer Mltpl Smpl 20G × 1 1/2 1M/CS | ↑ | 50-086001 | Needle Vacutainer Mltpl Smpl 21G × 1 1/2 100/pkg |
| 85-160508 | Bandage Adhesive Trnspt. 1 × 3 | ↑ | 85-160409 | Bandage Adhesive Transpt. 3/4 × 3 |
| 31-051421 | Bottle Screwlock Amber 7 DR | ↑ | 31-051447 | Bottle Screwlock Amber 13 DR — |
| | | | 31-051462 | Bottle Screwlock Amber 16 DR |
| 45-074005 | Sol. IV 5% Dex in H2O 1000 Ml | ↕ | 45-074104 | Sol. IV 5% Dex in H2O 500 Ml |
| 30-051737 | Suspension, Polycillin 250 Mg-200Mt | ↑ | 30-054566 | Suspension, Ampicillin 250 Mg-150 ML |
| 25-034003 | Diaper Poly Disposable 13 × 17 — 400 CS | ↑ | 25-036800 | Underpad Liner Deluxe 23 × 36 150/CS |
| 85-171208 | Sponge Cover 4 × 4 Sterile 25 | ↑ | 85-171107 | Sponge Cover 4 × 3 Sterile 25 |

**Table 4-4** *(continued)*

| Catalog Number | Item Description | | Catalog Number | Item Description |
|---|---|---|---|---|
| 85-171406 | Sponge Gauze 3 × 3 — 12 ply Nonstrl | ↑ | 85-171505 | Sponge Gauze 4 × 4 — 16 ply Nonstrl 2M/CS |
| 30-041688 | Apresoline 25 Mg | ↕ | 30-041704 | Apresoline 50 Mg |
| 60-100800 | Gloves Procedure Sterile Medium 50 Pr./Bx | ↑ | 60-101303 | Gloves Surgeons Sterile Size 7 |
| | | | 60-101402 | Gloves Surgeons Sterile Size 7 1/2 |
| 30-404821 | Sodium Chloride Injection 30 ML 100/CS | ↑ | 45-076604 | Sol. IV Nor. Saline 250 ML |
| 05-000909 | Infusion Set Scalp/Vein Strl. 21G 100/CS | ↑ | 05-001006 | Infusion Set Scalp/Vein Strl. 23G 100/CS |
| 50-087405 | Swab Culture Throat Sterile Swabs 200/CS | ↑ | 85-160201 | Applicator Cotton-Tip 6 Sterile 25 2M/CS |

aShows one-way substitutability in the direction shown.
bShows two-way substitutability in both directions.

**Level of Substitutability.** It must be noted that in categorizing items according to urgency, many items are assigned the facility-location or the regional-location urgency levels solely because one or more items can be used as substitutes in case of a stockout in a lower-urgency category, namely use-location or facility-location urgency levels. This is particularly true for the items with regional-location urgency. However, as mentioned earlier, in an ongoing system substitutability is a means by which stockouts are prevented on a temporary basis. In other words, short-term substitutability should be the exception rather than the rule in a well-designed MMS. It is therefore essential to consider each item in isolation from any substitutable items when considering its urgency requirements, even though substitutability is acceptable in a crisis. Again, in a smoothly operating environment, item characteristics and item costs should inhibit such actions on a regular basis. Thus, to strip the urgency categorization of its substitutability element, one needs to upgrade the assigned urgency of the items by one level and to remove their substitutability characteristic as a permanent trait. It must be emphasized that whenever there are any doubts about the urgency level of an item, the more-urgent category should be assigned.

### Substitutability, Urgency, and Costs

It can be proved mathematically that no matter how elaborate the inventory-control mechanisms, the possibility of a stockout will always exist unless, of course, an infinite supply of stock for all line items is available all the time at all the use locations (an impossibility from both logical and practical points of view). Short-term substitutability provides a backup for such developments, albeit not without a cost. The elements of such costs are:

1. *Extra material costs*: When a more-specialized or larger item, or more than one unit of an item, is substituted for a less-specialized or smaller item or only one unit of another item in the same use location, extra costs are incurred.
2. *Personnel inconveniences*: When the substitute for a stocked-out item is not found in its use location, and its urgency dictates its acquisition from other use locations in the same facility, the system is imposing undesired strain on the ultimate users.
3. *Personnel and transportation costs*: When an interfacility transfer is required for substituting an urgently needed item, the system incurs transportation- and materials-management-personnel costs.
4. *Other costs*: It is clear that when a temporary stockout persists for an urgent item, the urgency level may change. When this happens, a substitutable item must be found from other sources, other hospitals,

or other vendors. This gives rise to communication costs, materials-management-personnel costs, high air-freight or other transportation costs, and much inconvenience.

## Standardization

The discussions of substitutability and urgency in the preceding sections were clearly concerned with short-term or on-the-spot substitution for an out-of-stock item by another, generally more costly, item. In the longer range, all stocked items must be treated as potential candidates for substitution by more cost-effective products. Moreover, different products that serve identical, similar, or closely related functions, albeit in different departments, should be reviewed for possible standardization. Standardization tends to reduce inventories and to promote purchasing effectiveness through volume discounts and to promote efficiency through simpler and/or fewer orders and simpler bookkeeping. However, the process of standardization must be treated with care and attention to the needs and to some extent the wishes of the users.

Individual physicians and nurses may have good reason for insisting on one product over another. These should be heard and discussed, preferably by peers. Standardization committees having representatives from the various user constituencies are generally a good link between the materials-management function and the providers of health care.

In summary, the objective of standardization committees is to monitor and control all consumables, disposables, and reusables used within an institution, toward the end of containing costs while maintaining or upgrading the quality of care.

### Standardization Procedures and Processes

All new products being considered for use by the institution must be submitted to the director of materials management, or alternatively to the director of purchasing, by the advocates of that particular product, such as salespersons, physicians, nurses, administrators, or patients. The materials-management department, after performing the required initial screening of such items and (it is hoped) some form of value analysis, will submit these for consideration by the standardization committee. Either the materials-management department or the standardization committee should contact the concerned departments for any and all recommendations and comments. The concerned department should be provided with samples of the product, any literature pertaining to same, and/or briefings by the manufacturers' representatives. Based on this information from the materials-management department on the one hand, and that from the user departments on the other, the standardization committee can act either to accept or to reject the product, or to request a more extensive review and evaluation involving the use of the given product over a period of between thirty and ninety days. Finally, the standardization committee may need to act as a mediator between various user departments or individuals where differences exist that lead toward proliferation of product types.

Appendix 4B provides some additional thoughts on standardization in the form of a checklist for issues of standardization and in the form of audit procedures for standardization processes.

**Reusables**

No discussion of materials management in the health-care industry would be complete without addressing the issues associated with the management of resuables. Linen is clearly the most voluminous category of reusables, especially in hospitals. Owing to the high rate of inflation for basic materials such as petroleum and wood pulp (the ingredients in the manufacture of plastics and of paper, respectively), many of the trends toward the use of disposables may well be slowed if not reversed in the future. The ecologic impacts of disposal contribute to this countertrend through moral, economic, and regulatory considerations.

Reusables involve all the same purchasing, receiving, central-storing, use-location-stocking, and distribution activities as do consumables. In addition, however, resuables also involve *collection* and *production* (servicing), including quality-control activities.

Unfortunately, reusables, especially linen, do not have a 100-percent return rate. Specifically, linen-replacement costs are currently reported to range from 20 to 40 percent of the total cost of a hospital laundry and linen service. An estimated 80 percent of linen replacement is attributable to misuse, including theft [22]. The dollar value of linen noncontrol can be estimated by recognizing that laundry and linen services fall in a range close to the 2-percent level of hospital operating budgets. Thus, a hospital with a $10-million annual budget spends $200,000 annually on linen, with $40,000 to $80,000 being spent annually on replacements, of which $32,000 to $64,000 is the result of noncontrol. Thus it can be seen that there is some potential for saving in improving linen usage and control in most hospitals.

Consequently, the MMIS must be capable of addressing issues involved with the collection and production (servicing) activities of reusables as well as all the previously discussed consumables-related issues.

Therefore, timely and accurate data are needed on the return side as well as on the delivery and stock-status sides. The MMIS should capture and contain daily data involving all linen transactions for all use locations. These data can then be used for specifying restocking, production, replacement, and pickup and delivery requirements, as well as for charging each organizational unit for the linen placed for its use. The data can also be used to pinpoint problem areas in a timely way. Such information can, in fact, act as a deterrent to some misuse of linen. Specifically, an MMIS armed with proper decision rules and control ratios can print out daily delivery requirements based on the amount of soiled linen returned to the central laundry from each previously designated linen-use unit. If data show that a use unit needs additional linen, that unit can then be charged with the addition and an equal amount of new linen added to stock in the central laundry. Such data eliminate the need for periodic inventories, because the linen-in-use information is updated daily. Data also allow linen-replacement costs to be analyzed by use unit.

The MMIS can also print a laundry-production-requirements report based on such data. The number of washloads of each wash category or the exact number of pieces to be produced can thus be specified.

### Processing of Reusables[a]

The use-location-stocking decision rules for reusables are generically no different than those for consumables. However, the frequency and timing of pickups and deliveries of reusables must dovetail with several external constraints, such as nursing-station activities and laundry schedules. Moreover, the frequency of pickups must recognize the undesirability of inventorying soiled linen or dirty dishes at the use locations.

Whenever possible, servicing should be based on economic-lot-size formulations in consideration of setup as well as reorder and other costs. Management of reusables must therefore include the usual inventory considerations at the use locations. These, however, as will be further discussed in subsequent paragraphs, are compounded by the problem of inventorying the soiled materials. Reusables also pose significant manufacturing and logistical problems. The manufacturing issues involve in-process- as well as "finished"-goods inventory management in addition to the production-control and scheduling issues. The logistical problems of reusables, as indicated, must take into consideration the schedules of both the users and the producers while minimizing the combined costs of production and of inventory.

---

[a]Much of the information contained in this section was made available by Don Soth of the American Sterilizer Company.

An example of the flow of soiled materials through the various processing units is shown in figure 4-37.

As indicated earlier, the basic distinction between consumables and/or disposables, on the one hand, and reusables on the other, is that the latter must be returned for reprocessing. Thus, there is a *logistical* component as well as a *process* component of pickup and delivery. This section will address the issues involved in reprocessing.

To an ever-increasing extent, institutions are considering consolidation of reprocessing functions into central processing departments and/or into multi-institutional shared services. These are designed to facilitate the institutional requirements for complete processing of supplies and equipment for reuse, and at the same time to:

Conserve skills,

Improve response time and capability,

Minimize operating expenditures, and

Improve processing procedures

through the economics of scale. Skill conservation is thus achieved by delegating tasks from higher skill levels to lower skill levels and to machines. Response is improved by consolidating all processing of equipment and supplies. Operating expenditures are reduced by the utilization of mechanical transport (within the department) instead of manpower. Processing procedures are improved through the use of equipment that provides effective disinfection, sanitization, or decontamination of items. Additional skills and manpower economy may be achieved through inventory and distribution control, that is, planning for the availability of every supply item when the user needs it, and being able to document and evaluate that use.

The concept provides a materials-processing unit operated by people trained in sanitation, disinfection, and decontamination. These trained specialists relieve nurses and other skilled professionals from materials-processing tasks, thereby affording them more time for direct patient care.

The department layout and the equipment arrangements in central departments mitigate against unnecessary or duplicate actions. The principle of bringing the work to the workers is utilized, thereby increasing overall efficiency. Moreover, the aggregation of all processing functions offers additional advantages, which will be discussed later.

Central processing departments may include the following functions:

1. Washing and decontaminating of heat- and moisture-stable items.

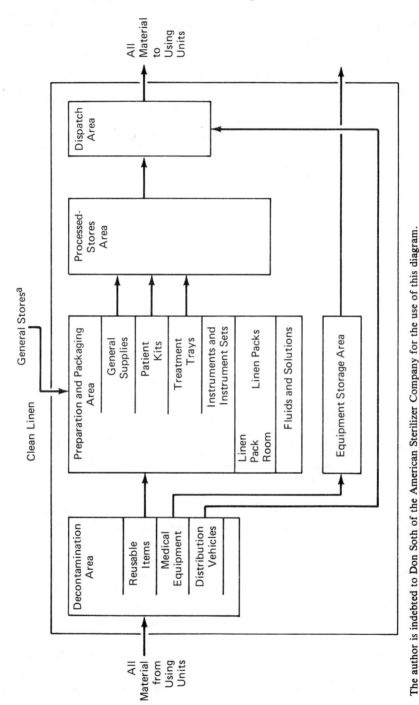

The author is indebted to Don Soth of the American Sterilizer Company for the use of this diagram.
[a]Not generally part of central processing department.

**Figure 4-37.** An Example of Central-Processing-Department Material Flow

2. Cleaning and disinfecting or decontaminating of heat- and/or moisture-sensitive items.
3. Manufacture of distilled water for rinsing purposes.
4. Sanitization and/or decontamination (and storage) of medical equipment.
5. Processing of distribution vehicles.
6. Preparation of linen packs for terminal sterilization.
7. Preparation and wrapping of instruments, instruments sets, utensil sets, treatment trays, and so on for terminal sterilization.
8. Wrapping, bagging or otherwise preparing items that do not require terminal sterilization.
9. Terminal sterilization (steam and gaseous sterilization).
10. Aeration of items sterilized by ethylene-oxide sterilant.
11. Storage of processed items.
12. Loading and dispatching of distribution vehicles.

They may comprise five separate but functionally integrated areas, such as:

1. Decontamination area
   a. General
   b. Equipment processing
2. Terminal processing and packaging area
   a. General
   b. Linen packaging
   c. Instrument packaging
   d. Solutions
3. Equipment-storage area
4. Processed-unit and stores area
5. Staging and dispatch area

A detailed discussion of recommended materials, processing procedures, and equipment is provided in appendix B at the end of this book.

## Retrieval and Recovery of Reusables and Recyclables

No discussion of reusables can be complete without addressing retrieval or recovery programs. Some costly items inadvertently end up in the trash during the day-to-day operations of complex systems such as hospitals or even clinics. Surgical implements, hot-water bottles, rubber pillows, and so on are very often deposited in laundry chutes or bins along with soiled linen. Laundry personnel, especially in shared-laundry organizations, are not in a position to distinguish good, expensive items from those intended as trash. Some costly materials are lost as part of the process of servicing or providing care. For example, according to M.R. Traska [23], radiology departments have traditionally been more-or-less negligent in letting much silver from photographic solutions go down the drain, even in those institutions that have silver-recovery systems in operation. "At $4.50 per troy ounce of silver, a typical 100-bed hospital should be able to recover $2000 per year." Clearly, a tertiary-care facility should be able to recover much more on a per-bed basis especially so since silver has inflated in price to $12 to 15 per troy ounce as of the writing of this book.

According to M.F. Anthony and G. Wilson [24], Johns Hopkins Hospital saved $22,352 in replacement costs during the first year after instituting an instrument-recovery program at the soiled-linen-sorting stations of a shared (cooperative) linen service. In spite of an awareness program within the hospital itself, $18,417 was recovered during the second year of the program. A fallout of this program was the reduction in linen-processing costs owing to the lower weigh-ins of what is supposed to be soiled linen.

Materials-usage teams or committees organized as part of, or working in conjunction with, standardization committees should be charged with identification of areas for potential savings resulting from retrieval and recovery programs. Materials-management personnel should provide technical input, in an advisory capacity, to the deliberations of these committees or teams.

Appendix 4C provides a checklist for evaluating the layout of central processing areas.

**Materials Distribution**

Flows of materials into and within a hospital or health center are depicted in figure 4-38 in a highly aggregated way. All materials are shown to arrive at the receiving dock and to be distributed via the stores department to the consumer or using departments either directly or through one or a number of processing departments. Consumer departments in turn send the reusables back for reprocessing and the waste for disposal. Figure 4-39 shows this information in a somewhat more deaggregated fashion. The added detail focuses attention on the complexities of the distribution, processing, and storage aspects of materials management in a health center and to some of the systems interactions therein.

If nothing else, these diagrams point to the extensive amount of materials handling that is involved and hence to the need for facilities layout so as to minimize the distances over which materials need be transported.

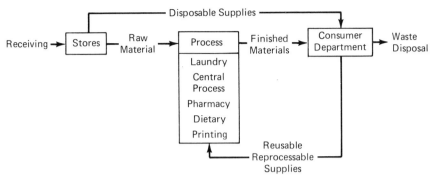

The author is indebted to Don Soth of the American Sterilizer Company for the use of this diagram.

**Figure 4-38.** Material Flow

The notion of a central processing center was discussed in an earlier section. Having most if not all of the receiving, storage, processing, and dispatching departments in physical proximity clearly minimizes the materials-transportation distances within the institutional-materials support function. Figure 4-40 depicts the relative allocation of space to materials-support-function units within a health center and the basic materials-flow interactions between such units.

*Materials Distribution and Pickup*

The materials-management function within a given institution must concern itself with the logistics of materials distribution and of pickup. Materials must be distributed to user units and picked up in turn for recycling or disposal. These pickups and deliveries must be performed in a timely fashion. In order to meet institutional objectives, they must be organized so as to maximize service, within the usual budgetary constraints. Alternatively, as shown in figure 4-41, this function must be organized so as to minimize costs in due consideration of maintaining the service levels agreed on by all as being acceptable. In either case, the logistics of pickup and delivery must consider the optimum frequency with which a user department or area will be serviced for any particular item or class of items. Clearly, the frequency with which supply shelves are restocked need not be the same as the frequency with which clean linen is delivered or picked up. Frequency is concerned with "how often." In a health institution, however, and especially in a hospital setting, it is not sufficient to be concerned merely with how often to pick up and deliver goods. Timing is an issue of equal concern. Schedules must therefore be developed to take into account the

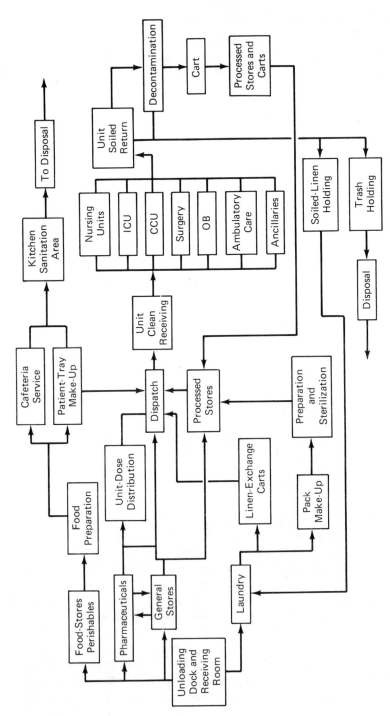

The author is indebted to Don Soth of the American Sterilizer Company for the use of this diagram.

**Figure 4-39.** Materials-Distribution Subsystem

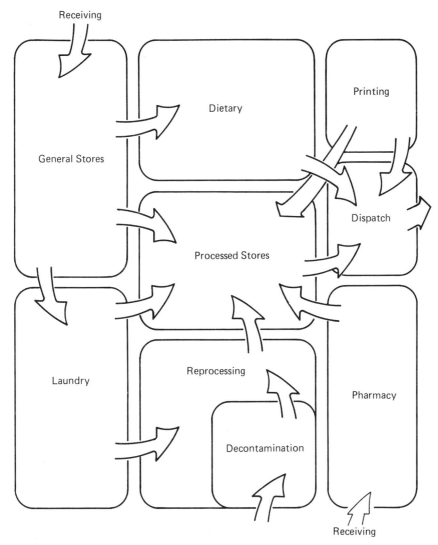

The author is indebted to Don Soth of the American Sterilizer Company for the use of this diagram.

**Figure 4-40.** Space Relationship—Material Support Services

desired frequencies of delivery. They must also consider the various constraints imposed by user departments on the one hand and by the availability of pickup and delivery personnel on the other. Nursing stations must adhere to certain schedules dictated by requirements of the time of day. This dictates, for example, feeding, medical-treatment, and linen-changing schedules.

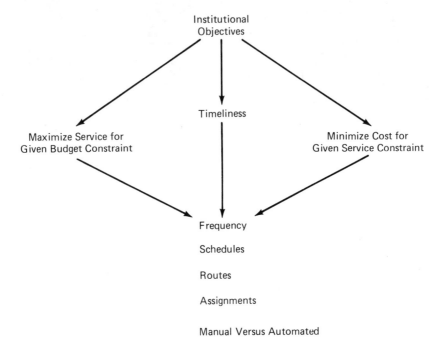

**Figure 4-41.** Transportation-Distribution Issues

Frequencies and schedules of pickups and deliveries dictate considerations of optimum routes of travel and of personnel assignments to such routes. To accomplish all this at minimum cost is not a trivial matter.

As indicated earlier, the frequency of deliveries and pickups is dictated by higher-order decisions, such as considerations of the economic ordering quantity, space availability, and so on. Similarly, schedules are often also user dictated. Given these considerations, management of distribution functions need good ways to develop each of the routes for each of the distribution persons. By routes we mean who, or what department, will be called on, and in what order, by each of the distribution persons on each of the "runs." Vehicle-routing or "traveling-salesman" decisions have been the subject of considerable investigation by theoreticians and practitioners of operations-research-management science for over a quarter of a century. This attention has resulted in a series of solution techniques that yield better or cheaper routes. Clarke and Wright [25] developed a methodology that yields good solutions to large-scale routing problems of the traveling-salesman type. Moreover, the Clarke and Wright technique can be executed relatively cheaply. C.L. Doll recently reported a "quick and dirty vehicle routing procedure" [26]. Doll's method seems to yield solutions that are not much worse than those that could be obtained by the more extensive technique cited earlier, yet the solutions can be obtained in a much more straightforward fashion.

Questions concerned with evaluation of pickup and delivery functions are delineated in a checklist provided in appendix 4C.

**References**

1. Chambers, J.C.; Mullick, S.K.; and Smith, D.D. "How to Choose the Right Forecasting Technique." *Harvard Business Review* (July-August 1971):45-74.
2. Reisman, A.; Gudapati, K.; Chandrasekaran, R.; Darukhanavala, P.; and Morrison, D. "Forecasting Short-Term Demand." *Industrial Engineering* 8 (1976):38-45.
3. Whybark, D.C. "A Comparison of Adoptive Forecasting Techniques." *The Logistics and Transportation Review* 8 (1972):13-26.
4. Chambers, J.C.; Mullick, S.K.; and Smith, D.D. *An Executive's Guide to Forecasting.* New York: John Wiley and Sons, 1974.
5. Wheelwright, S.C., and Makridakis, S. *Forecasting Methods for Management.* New York: John Wiley and Sons, 1977.
6. Reisman, Arnold. *Managerial and Engineering Economics.* Boston: Allyn and Bacon Publishing Company, 1971.
7. Harris, F. *Operations and Costs.* Factory Management Series. Chicago: A.W. Shore Company, 1915.
8. Hadley, G., and Whitin, T.M. *Analysis of Inventory Systems.* Englewood Cliffs, N.J.: Prentice-Hall, 1963.
9. Fairfield, E. Raymond. *Quantity and Economy in Manufacture.* Princeton, N.J.: D. Van Nostrand Company, 1931.
10. Arrow, K.J.; Harris, T.; and Marschak, J. *Optimal Inventory Policy.* Chicago: University of Chicago Press, 1951.
11. Whitin, Thompson M. *The Theory of Inventory Management.* Princeton, N.J.; Princeton University Press, 1953.
12. Javad, Shahriar. "Multi-echelon Inventory Systems in Health Care Delivery Organizations." Unpublished Ph.D. dissertation, Case Western Reserve University, 1980.
13. Westwick, C.A. *How to Use Management Ratios.* New York: John Wiley and Sons, Halsted Press, 1973.
14. Weston, J.F., and Brigham, E.F. *Managerial Finance.* New York: Holt, Rinehart and Winston, 1966.
15. Buffa, E.S. *Basic Production Management.* New York: John Wiley and Sons, 1971.
16. Reisman, Arnold; Dean, Burton V.; Oral, Muhittin; and Salvador,

Michael. *Industrial Inventory Control.* New York: Gordon and Breach, 1972.

17. Maynard, Harold B., ed. *Industrial Engineering Handbook.* New York: McGraw-Hill, 1971.

18. Yu, Chang S. "An Investigation of Stock Depletion Costs and its Effect on Inventory Control Models." Ph.D. dissertation, Washington University, 1964.

19. Schwartz, B.L. "A New Approach to Stock-out Penalties." *Management Science* 12 (1966):B538-B544.

20. Oral, Muhittin; Salvador, Michael; Reisman, Arnold; and Dean, Burton V. "On the Evaluation of Shortage Costs for Determining Inventory Control Policies." *Management Science* 18 (1972):B344-B351.

21. Housley, C.E. *Hospital Materiel Management.* Germantown, Md.: Aspen Systems Corporation, 1978.

22. Ellis, B. "Cost Containment in Laundry and Linen Service." *Hospitals*, March 16, 1978.

23. Traska, M.R. "Hospitals See Silver Recovery Benefit." *Modern Health Care* (February 1978).

24. Anthony, M.F., and Wilson, G. "Costly Materials Retrieved from Laundry Chutes" *Hospitals, JAHA*, May 16, 1978.

25. Clarke, G., and Wright, J.W. "Scheduling of Vehicles from a Central Depot to a Number of Delivery Points." *Operations Research* 12 (1964):568-581.

26. Doll, C.L. "Quick and Dirty Vehicle Routing Procedure." *Interfaces* (February 1980):84-85.

# Appendix 4A: Checklists and Audit Procedures for Decision Rules

### Checklist for MMS Decision Rules and Their Use

This section is based on "Checklist and Guidelines for Evaluating Purchasing and Materials Management Functions in Private Hospitals: Opportunities for Improving Hospital Purchasing, Inventory Management and Supply Distribution," part II, U.S. General Accounting Office, PSAD 79-58B, April 1979.

|  | *Comments (Provide data on "yes" answers. Explain "no" answers.)* | |
|---|---|---|
| *Questions* | *Yes* | *No* |
| A. Is ABC analysis used as a guide in setting safety-stock levels? ("A" items are high-dollar-value items, "B" the middle-dollar-value items, and "C" the low-dollar-value items)? | _____ | _____ |
| B. Are supplier lead time and the lead-time demand analyzed when reorder points are set? | _____ | _____ |
| C. Is economic-order-quantity theory applied? | | |
| D. If centralized distribution systems are used: | _____ | _____ |
|     1. Are nursing stations' and other departments' stock levels established by a central manager? | _____ | _____ |
|     2. Are nursing stations' and other departments' stock levels based on an analysis of usage or a forecast of future needs? | _____ | _____ |

|  | *Comments (Provide data on "yes" answers. Explain "no" answers.)* | |
|---|---|---|
| *Questions* | *Yes* | *No* |

3. Are nursing stations' and other departments' stock levels periodically reviewed and revised? _____ _____

4. Are nursing stations' and other departments' requests for additional medical-surgical supplies monitored? _____ _____

E. Is the pharmacy chief responsible for controlling pharmaceutical inventories, including departmental stocks? _____ _____

   1. Are there written procedures for the organization and management of the pharmacy inventory? _____ _____

   2. Is each item dated and priced when received? _____ _____

   3. Is there a catalog or formulary of pharmaceuticals stocked? _____ _____

   4. Is there a separate list of those items with expiration dates, and is this list reviewed regularly? _____ _____

   5. Is the inventory reviewed periodically to remove static, slow-moving, or obsolete items? _____ _____

F. If pharmacy staff replenish and/or purchase their own inventories, do they use ABC analysis to identify high dollar-volume items and to set priorities for purchasing and controlling pharmaceuticals? _____ _____

G. Does the pharmacy attempt to minimize its purchasing and inventory costs by:

   1. Systematically establishing reorder points, based on vendor lead time and safety-stock requirements, to minimize inventory on major items? _____ _____

| Questions | Comments (Provide data on "yes" answers. Explain "no" answers.) | |
|---|---|---|
| | Yes | No |
| 2. Using economic-order-quantity theory to control purchase volume and inventory for major items? | _____ | _____ |
| 3. Purchasing directly from the manufacturer when volume permits? | _____ | _____ |
| 4. Taking advantage of volume discounts? | _____ | _____ |
| H. Does the dietary department attempt to minimize its purchasing and inventory costs by: | | |
| 1. Systematically establishing reorder points and safety-stock requirements, to minimize inventory on major items? | _____ | _____ |
| 2. Using economic-order-quantity theory to control purchase volume and inventory for major items? | _____ | _____ |
| 3. Taking advantage of volume discounts? | _____ | _____ |

## Audit Procedures for Inventory-Control Policy

*Objective*: To determine whether inventory control methods are being complied with.

*Audit Steps*:

1. Obtain a current quantity list of all items in inventory and
   a. Determine whether this list is up to date with respect to actual inventory on hand.
   b. Verify that there is a means of cross-referencing items that may be available in floor stocks and central storerooms.

2. Check maintenance-service reports to verify
   a. That drug, food, and supply locations are properly maintained for refrigeration, safekeeping, lighting, and cleanliness.
3. Observe inventory procedures to
   a. Verify that all items are labeled by a responsible person.
   b. Check that inventory reports are made periodically and reviewed by the manager.
   c. Determine whether there is a quality-control system.
   d. Check whether professional supplies, maintenance supplies, and stationery supplies are properly separated.
4. Obtain at random some inventory requisitions and verify correctness of
   a. Summarization of quantities.
   b. Unit conversions.
   c. Prices used.
5. Review procedures to determine correctness of determining
   a. Consignments-in.
   b. Inventory in the hands of processors and suppliers.
   c. Inventory in warehouses, if any.
6. Check the records for
   a. Written approval for adjusting records for discrepancies in inventory.
   b. A signature of the person requisitioning or receiving materials.
   c. Written documents approving movement of materials from one department to another.
   d. Prenumbering of receiving reports.
7. Obtain written instructions for
   a. Taking physical inventory count.
   b. Identification to indicate supply items already counted.
   c. Handling merchandise on hand that is not hospital property.
   d. Sales to employees.
8. Verify that
   a. Persons independent of custodianship of physical inventories maintain inventory records.
   b. Persons independent of custodianship of physical inventories and inventory-record maintenance determine inventory-taking and -counting procedures.

**Audit Steps of MMS Decision Rules and Their Use**

This section is based on "Checklist and Guidelines for Evaluating Purchasing and Materials Management Functions in Private Hospitals: Opportunities for Improving Hospital Purchasing, Inventory Management and

Supply Distribution," part II, U.S. General Accounting Office, PSAD 79-58B, April 1979.

*Objective*: To determine whether all replenishments of materials within the institution are based on enlightened decision rules.

*Audit Steps*:

1. Discuss with responsible staff at all replenishment institutional levels and units how the reorder point and order quantity were established for each walkthrough item.
   a. For each item ascertain how the unit determines the safety factor and/or distribution lead time. Using the safety factor and lead time thus established, calculate and verify some of the unit's current reorder points. Determine the reason for any differences and assure that the methods used by the department or unit are consistent for all items.
   b. If the department or unit has not systematically established its reorder point, calculate what the reorder point should be and compare this to the reorder point used.
   c. If the department or unit uses a quantitative method such as economic-order-quantity (EOQ) theory to determine order quantities, verify its calculations. Determine that the required inventory ordering and carrying costs are calculated properly and include all relevant factors. Determine whether volume discounts are properly analyzed when purchase-order quantities are set.
   d. If the department or unit has not used economic-order-quantity theory for its high-dollar-volume items, calculate the EOQ for these items and compare it to the quantity currently ordered.
   e. Determine whether reorder points and order quantities are reevaluated at least once a year for each walkthrough item.
2. Discuss weaknesses in replenishment-decision procedures with the department or unit manager.

# Appendix 4B:
# Checklists and Audit
# Procedures for
# Standardization

## Checklist for Issues of Standardization

| Questions | Comments (Provide data on "yes" answers. Explain "no" answers.) Yes | No |
|---|---|---|
| A. Does the purchasing function have a written policy for utilizing the benefits of standardization? | ____ | ____ |
| B. If yes, is there a written policy that is applicable to central purchasing as well as decentralized purchasing units? | ____ | ____ |
|   1. Are both organizations brought together under one workable policy to achieve maximum benefits? | ____ | ____ |
| C. Is there an updated list of items presently standardized? | ____ | ____ |
|   1. Are brand and generic names of supplies cross-referenced? | ____ | ____ |
|   2. Are forms standardized? | ____ | ____ |
|   3. Is equipment standardized? | ____ | ____ |
|   4. Are spare-parts lists and inventories for standardized equipment maintained? | ____ | ____ |
|   5. Are food supplies standardized, using generic rather than brand names where possible? | ____ | ____ |
|   6. Are pharmaceuticals standardized, using generic rather than brand names where possible? | ____ | ____ |
|   7. Are uniforms standardized? | ____ | ____ |

|  | *Comments (Provide data on "yes" answers. Explain "no" answers.)* | |
|---|---|---|
| *Questions* | *Yes* | *No* |
| D.  Have users been contacted regarding issues of standardization? | _____ | _____ |
|     1. Do users agree with choice of standardized items? | _____ | _____ |
|     2. Are there provisions for exceptions to standardization policies among users? | _____ | _____ |
|     3. Do these exceptions require proper approval? | _____ | _____ |
|     4. Are there provisions for updating and changing items of standardization? | _____ | _____ |
|     5. Are users notified promptly of changes? | _____ | _____ |
| E.  Have the benefits of standardization been evaluated? | _____ | _____ |
|     1. Are cost benefits evaluated? | _____ | _____ |
|     2. Are quality benefits evaluated? | _____ | _____ |
|     3. Are space benefits evaluated? | _____ | _____ |
|     4. Are users aware of cost-benefit analysis? | _____ | _____ |
|     5. Are there provisions for future reevaluation of benefits to ensure that they do in fact still exist? | _____ | _____ |
| F.  Have committees been established to provide for ongoing use of standardization for fullest benefits? | _____ | _____ |
| G.  Are there routines to ensure compliance with standardization procedures? | _____ | _____ |
|     1. Do these routines provide for periodic audits of inventories as well as orders placed? | _____ | _____ |
|     2. Are results of audits communicated to those possessing authority? | _____ | _____ |
|     3. Are standardization routines reestablished if not in compliance? | _____ | _____ |

*Questions*                                          *Yes*          *No*

H.  Are there provisions to contact other
    organizations to determine if additional
    areas can be standardized?                   _____        _____


**Audit Procedures for Issues of Standardization**

*Objective*:  To determine whether standardization is used to achieve significant benefits such as cost savings and inventory reduction.

*Audit Steps*:

1.  Determine that there is an updated list of items presently standardized.
    a.  Verify that brand and generic names are corss-referenced.
    b.  Verify that the following types of items are included for standard-
        ization: forms, supplies, equipment, spare parts, and uniforms.
2.  Physically inspect the storage areas and major floor stocks to determine
    that standard procedures listed herein are indeed being followed.
    a.  For items not standardized, calculate the monetary savings and in-
        ventory reduction that could have been achieved if a single brand
        and type was obtained from the lowest-priced source.
    b.  If the institution has a standardization committee, review its
        minutes to determine the extent of effort to standardize these items.
    c.  Determine that standardization policies are applied consistently.
    d.  Discuss observations with the manager.
3.  Verify that users are aware of standardization procedures.
    a.  If a standardization committee is not established, recommend that
        one be established. Include users.
    b.  Verify that users are notified promptly of changes.
    c.  Verify that users agree with standardization of items. Reconcile
        discrepancies.
    d.  Verify that changes require proper approval.
    e.  Review procedures to determine whether there are provisions to con-
        tact other organizations to determine if additional areas can be stan-
        dardized.

     f.  Determine whether benefits of standardization have been adequately communicated to users as well as management.
4. Determine that results of standardization have been evaluated with regard to improvements such as cost benefits, quality benefits, and space benefits.
5. Verify that there is a procedure for future reevaluation of benefits to ensure that they do in fact still exist.
6. Review with management observations, and
     a.  Identify any obstacles to standardization and determine what is being done to eliminate them.
     b.  Ascertain and evaluate the reasons for not standardizing.

# Appendix 4C: Checklists and Audit Procedures for Processing, Handling, and Value Analysis

**Checklist for Evaluating the Layout of Central Processing Areas**

| Questions | Comments *(Provide data on "yes" answers. Explain "no" answers.)* | |
| --- | --- | --- |
| | *Yes* | *No* |
| **A. Space:** | | |
| 1. Is space assigned to the MMS used to maximum cost effectiveness? | _____ | _____ |
| 2. Has planning for new space been considered? | _____ | _____ |
| 3. Does contemplated space have physical restrictions? | _____ | _____ |
| 4. Are aisles carrying their loads to best advantage? | _____ | _____ |
| 5. Are locations properly founded? | _____ | _____ |
| 6. Are files located to best advantage? | _____ | _____ |
| **B. Work:** | | |
| 1. Does it travel in a straight line? | _____ | _____ |
| 2. Do some employees have to wait for work to arrive? | _____ | _____ |
| 3. Is there piling up or congestion? | _____ | _____ |
| 4. Is there unnecessary searching for records? | _____ | _____ |
| **C. People and equipment:** | | |
| 1. Is each person allowed sufficient space? | _____ | _____ |
| 2. Has room been allowed for more personnel? | _____ | _____ |
| 3. Is each person in the best location? | _____ | _____ |

|  | Comments (Provide data on "yes" answers. Explain "no" answers.) | |
| --- | --- | --- |
| *Questions* | *Yes* | *No* |

4. Are the employees comfortable and satisfied? _____ _____

5. Is equipment doing the job adequately? _____ _____

6. Are the proper tools in the proper places? _____ _____

D. Environment:
 1. Is the light adequate? _____ _____
 2. Are the proper colors being used? _____ _____
 3. Are the atmospheric conditions at maximum efficiency levels? _____ _____
 4. Is noise being isolated, absorbed, and dampened? _____ _____
 5. Do the chairs hold the stationary employees correctly and fit surroundings? _____ _____
 6. Are the best desks being used? _____ _____
 7. Is the office at maximum utility? _____ _____

**Checklist for Evaluating Pickup and Delivery Functions**

A. Are orders and delivery times scheduled? _____
 1. How frequent is delivery? _____
 2. What is the order-to-delivery lag time? _____

B. Are printed forms complete and specific? _____
 1. Are there provisions to indicate the following:
  a. Quantity needed in units? _____ _____
  b. Order unit? _____ _____
  c. Size? _____ _____
  d. Description of item? _____ _____
  e. Delivery location? _____ _____
  f. Stock number? _____ _____

|  | *Comments (Provide data on "yes" answers. Explain "no" answers.)* | |
| --- | --- | --- |
| *Questions* | *Yes* | *No* |

C. Is a catalog provided that lists all available items by category with stock numbers and stocking units for each? _____ _____
   1. Does each ordering location have a catalog? _____ _____

D. Is there provision to go directly to central supply to have (emergency) orders filled in person? _____ _____

E. Is there automatic backordering for supplies not available? _____ _____
   1. What is the average backorder length? _____

F. Are there specified delivery locations and means of informing requisitioner that items are "in"? _____ _____

G. Is there a provision for returning goods that are delivered in error or are faulty? _____ _____

**Checklist for Evaluating Material Handling**

A. Are the following work practices being followed:
   1. Manual handling of materials is eliminated wherever possible. _____ _____
   2. Distances over which material is handled are reduced to a minimum. _____ _____
   3. Transfers of material from one place to another are avoided wherever possible. _____ _____
   4. Workplaces are arranged so as to reduce the amount of lifting, bending, and reaching required on the part of employees. _____ _____

| | Comments |
| | *(Provide data on* |
| | *"yes" answers.* |
| | *Explain "no"* |
| | *answers.)* |

| *Questions* | *Yes* | *No* |
|---|---|---|
| 5. Gravity is utilized wherever possible to move materials. | _____ | _____ |
| 6. Mixing of materials of different types and sizes is avoided wherever possible, thus keeping the sorting of materials to a minimum. | _____ | _____ |
| 7. A number of items are moved as a unit rather than individually. This can be accomplished through the use of material-handling equipment such as containers, trays, carts, skids, trucks, and so on. | _____ | _____ |
| 8. Equipment such as hand trucks, platform trucks, pneumatic tubes, chutes, and so on are considered for use in those work situations where employees are required to handle materials having considerable weight, or where materials must be moved over long distances. | _____ | _____ |
| 9. When material-handling equipment is employed, an adequate maintenance program is established to ensure the continued availability of the equipment. | _____ | _____ |
| 10. The handling method that is employed (whether manual or mechanical) is a simple and safe method for personnel to use. Factors such as floor surfaces, ceiling height, door openings and clearances, aisle space, and elevator capacity should be investigated when considering the use of mobile handling equipment. | _____ | _____ |

**Checklist for Value Analysis of Contracted Services**

|  | *Comments (Provide data on "yes" answers. Explain "no" answers.)* | |
|---|---|---|
| *Questions* | *Yes* | *No* |
| A. Can the hospital control and monitor the service? | _____ | _____ |
| B. Can the hospital itself provide this service? | _____ | _____ |
| C. Can the contractor provide the service more effectively? | _____ | _____ |
| D. Can the contractor provide the service more economically? | _____ | _____ |
| E. Does the contractor have enough data on the hospital to update and improve his or her services when possible? | _____ | _____ |
| F. Are this specific contractor's service costs lower than other contractors' service costs? | _____ | _____ |
| G. Has this contract service displaced personnel? | _____ | _____ |
| H. If so, is there a procedure to call back this personnel if needed? | _____ | _____ |
| I. Does this contract service increase direct and indirect costs in other departments and for other contracted services? | _____ | _____ |
| J. Does the contract provide for growth of service? | _____ | _____ |
| K. Does this specific contractor provide adequate supervision? | _____ | _____ |
| L. Will contract service personnel have a detrimental effect on the attitude of hospital personnel? | _____ | _____ |

| *Questions* | *Yes* | *No* |
|---|---|---|
| M. Is this contract service unionized? | _____ | _____ |
| N. Can inessential parts of the contracted service be eliminated? | _____ | _____ |
| O. Is this service essential to hospital activities? | _____ | _____ |

**Audit Procedure for Evaluating the Use of Value
Analysis for Contracted Services**

*Objective*: To determine whether value analysis has been applied to contracted services.

*Audit Steps*:

1. Select a contracted service and ask the hospital personnel involved whether
   a. This service is essential to hospital activities.
   b. The hospital itself can provide this service.
   c. Inessential parts of the service can be eliminated.
2. Obtain the invoices from this contracted service and determine
   a. What the cost would be if the hospital would provide this service itself.
   b. The savings involved in replacing the contracted service with another contracted service or in using the hospitals' own services.
3. Determine whether
   a. The hospital is adequately monitoring the contracted service.
   b. The contractor is gathering data with which to improve his services.
4. Review the hospital's files for documentation on
   a. Other competitive contractors' prices and services.
   b. Exactly what the present service contract involves legally.
   c. Special services that only this contractor can provide.

5. Analyze the impact of this contract service with respect to
   a. Effect on hospital-personnel attitudes.
   b. Indirect costs that involve other departments.

6. Review written procedures with the managers on actions taken
   a. If this service were to cease without notice.

# 5

## Techniques for MMS Improvement and Control Studies

Materials-management systems (MMS) involve people, information, and materials. Figure 5-1 shows the various basic activity categories involving people, information, and/or materials in a materials-management system. Thus decisions are made by people, although in some cases repetitive decisions, such as replenishment, may be relegated to a good materials-management information system (MMIS), providing of course for the possibility of management overrides. Movement in an MMS, on the other hand, involves people and information as well as materials, whereas storage generation and disposal are activities that essentially involve materials and information.

In [1], a *system* was defined as a set of resources—personnel, materials, facilities, and/or information—*organized to perform designated functions in order to achieve desired results.* Clearly, the MMS falls within the scope of that definition. And because that definition places emphasis on having the resources organized to perform designated functions in order to achieve desired results, it is necessary first to determine what the desired results are and then to assure that the resources are properly organized so that the designated functions can be accomplished and the system achieve the results desired of it. Chapter 2 addressed the question of goal setting within an organization in the section dealing with a discussion of management by objectives. The sections of that chapter dealing with purchasing, receiving, inspection, warehousing, and so on addressed questions of the designated functions of those particular components or functions of a materials-management system. This chapter will go a little further in the direction of satisfying the definition of a system, by addressing the various systems and procedures necessary to perform MMS activities involving people, information, and materials.

### Graphic Techniques for MMS Improvement and Control Studies

The various professions practicing systems analysis have, over the years, developed and standardized a number of graphic tools for describing materials-management systems. Some of the techniques that have withstood

---

This chapter is based on chapter 3 of a companion volume: Arnold Reisman, *Systems Analysis in Health-Care Delivery* (Lexington, Mass.: Lexington Books, D.C. Heath and Company, 1979).

| Resources | Activities | | | | |
|---|---|---|---|---|---|
| | Decisions | Movement | Storage | Generation | Disposal |
| People | X | X | O | O | O |
| Information | X | X | X | X | X |
| Materials | O | X | X | X | X |

X — Yes
O — No

**Figure 5-1.** MMS Activities Involving People, Information, and/or Materials

the test of time and are used extensively as aids in materials management will be presented and discussed in this section. The others are extensively discussed in a companion volume [1]. Table 5-1 provides a summary of the techniques included, the information they display, and their use. All these charts are succinct statements describing in operationally meaningful terms the essence of the systems they depict. They are based on detailed observations and systematic recording and analysis of processes within the system defined by the analyst.

In generating the operator-oriented charts, such as the operator, "simo," man-flow process, multiple-activity, assembly, and operation-process charts, the analyst must be able to break the job down into a set of meaningful components. What is meaningful depends on the scope and/or import of the job itself and on the costs of doing the analysis and the benefits to be gained therefrom. It is folly to invest $X$ dollars in the analysis of a job if the potential savings is $\wedge X$, where $\triangle X$ over the life cycle of the job is of the same order of magnitude as $X$ itself. There are, of course, extenuating circumstances, such as resource constraints and meeting deadlines. The numerical value of the study-cost $X$, of course, depends on the level of detail that the analyst becomes concerned with and on the sophistication of the methods used both in the description and the design or redesign of the job. When the same job is performed by a large number of operators or over an extended period of time, detailed time-and-motion or work-sampling studies might be justified in securing these data. Methods for doing this are discussed in chapter 6 and more extensively in [2]. On the other hand, when the number of operators doing a job are few and/or the job does not have a long life cycle, simply breaking the job into tasks that are distinguishable from one another will suffice. Moreover, task analysis can be used as a first approximation to the more detailed data- and information-collection methods. The literature of job analysis and evaluations is extensive [2-13].

**Table 5-1**

**Classification, Information Displayed, and Use of Tools for Systems Description and Analysis**

| Model | Information Displayed | Use |
|---|---|---|
| Operator charts | Relationship of the activity of the hands | Man analysis |
| Micromotion or "simo" charts | Time relationship of the activity of the hands | Man analysis |
| Man-flow process charts | Worker movement and activity sequence | Sequence and distance-traveled analysis |
| Product-flow process charts | Relationship of operations, transports, storage, and inspections | Flow analysis |
| Two- and three-dimensional product-flow process charts | Relationship of machinery and equipment | Layout analysis |
| Procedure flow charts | Relationship of paperwork operations | Analysis of paperwork flow |
| Sequence-analysis charts | Relationship of departmental areas in process layout | Layout analysis, process layout |
| Operation-process chart | Relationship of productive operations and parts | Flow analysis |
| Routing sheet | | Planning and control |
| Logic diagram | Sequence of logical questions relevant to a decision process | Decision making |
| Assembly charts | Relationship of assembled parts | Flow analysis |
| Flow chart | Sequence relationship of operations, storage, and so on | Flow analysis |
| Geneology tree | Hierarchical relationship of system components | System-structure analysis |
| Decision tree | Sequential relationship of series of decisions | Decision anaylsis |
| Incidence table | Interactions of functional arrays | Correlation analysis |
| Precedence diagram | Precedence relationship of activities | Planning |
| Precedence matrix | Precedence relationship of activities | Planning |
| Bill of materials | Parts requirements for finished product | Inventory control, planning, assembly |
| Explosion chart | Part-requirements aggregation for several products | Inventory control, planning, assembly |
| Input-output table | Interactions of functional arrays | System analysis and redesign |
| Gantt charts | Time relationships of orders, inventories, machine-time allocations | Schedule and load analysis |
| Information-process charts | Relationship of operations, storage retrieval, and so on | Information-flow analysis |
| Network charts | Precedence relationship of activities | Planning |
| PERT charts | Precedence relationship of activities with probabilistic times | Planning and control |
| PERT cost diagrams | Precedence relationships of activities with costs and probabilistic times | Planning and control |

Source: Arnold Reisman, *Systems Analysis in Health-Care Delivery.* (Lexington, Mass.: Lexington-Books, D.C. Heath and Company, 1979).

Reference [1] provides illustrative examples of task definitions for a repetitive short-cycle-time job, such as that of a hospital cafeteria worker, and for other jobs at a much more sophisticated and complex level.

In the cases of the operation-process, the assembly, and the product-flow charts, the focus in the order stated shifts more and more from the operator to the product. Nevertheless, the task analysis, definition, and documentation is still a generally useful if not mandatory step in generating the respective charts.

Starting with the procedure flow and moving through the logic diagram, the focus shifts from physical acts to the more abstract notions of decision making. In the logic diagram questions are raised and, depending on the answers given, decisions are made as to how to proceed. These charts are like traffic cops, guiding either the worker, the product, or the machine through the maze of decisions and actions in the more complex jobs which, although repetitive, are not identically so. That is, every job may be different depending on the permutations and combinations of answers to the questions raised. It is difficult to say much about the job cycle time for which these charts are applicable. The standard operating procedure for ordering equipment in an organization may involve a number of workers and their supervisors. It may take several calendar days or weeks to process. However, a complex procedure requiring the search for, retrieval of, and manipulation of data, and the printing of a report, may require seconds of computer time if fully mechanized.

*Operator Charts*

Operator charts are appropriate when the task has a short cycle time and the volume to be produced is low to moderate. The operator charts analyze the motions of each hand into components of reach, grasp, transport, position, assemble, and so forth, and place each hand's activities in parallel columns in order to describe how the two hands work together, as seen in figure 5-2.

Small circles indicate manipulative activity, large circles indicate reaches and transports of material, and a simple connective line indicates that the hand is idle. Figure 5-2 shows a completed operator chart for tasks performed by a hospital-cafeteria worker.

Operator charts can also display a time scale. Thus the relative value of each activity can be appraised. These time data may come from standard time values for motions such as reach, grasp, move, and position, or from detailed time studies of the operation being analyzed.

*Micromotion Analysis or Simo Charts*

Using micromotion analysis the operation can be broken down into elements called *therbligs*, which represent a finer breakdown than do the

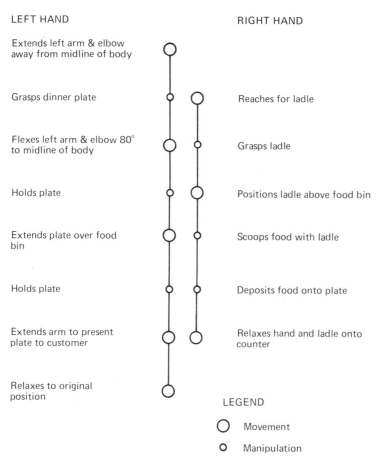

LEFT HAND                                    RIGHT HAND

Extends left arm & elbow
away from midline of body

Grasps dinner plate                          Reaches for ladle

Flexes left arm & elbow 80°
to midline of body                           Grasps ladle

Holds plate                                  Positions ladle above food bin

Extends plate over food
bin                                          Scoops food with ladle

Holds plate                                  Deposits food onto plate

Extends arm to present
plate to customer                            Relaxes hand and ladle onto
                                             counter

Relaxes to original
position                                     LEGEND

                                    ◯    Movement

                                    ₒ    Manipulation

Arnold Reisman, *Systems Analysis in Health-Care Delivery* (Lexington, Mass.: Lexington Books, D.C. Heath and Company, 1979).

**Figure 5-2.** Operator Chart: Tasks Performed by a Hospital-Cafeteria Worker

elements in the operator charts; and the results are plotted against a time scale so that the exact simultaneity of the two hands working together can be examined. The resulting chart is often called a *simo chart* because it shows this relationship. The data for the chart are gathered by means of motion pictures. Time in thousandths of a minute is measured by placing a clock in the camera field or by using a synchronous motor drive on the camera so that each frame of the film represents one thousandth (or some fraction thereof) of a minute. In either case, a special movie projector is used to analyze the film. The analyst can thus advance the film one frame at a time to obtain the elapsed times for the therblig elements by the clock readings or from the frame counter on the projector. A simo chart for opening a corrugated case is shown in figure 5-3.

## SIMO CHART

Sheet No.     Of                                                    Film No.

| Operation | Open Case for casing 2½ # corn meal | | | | | Date |
|---|---|---|---|---|---|---|
| | | | | | | Operation No. |
| Part Name | | | | | | Part No. |
| Operator's Name and No. | | | | | | Chart by     CBS |

| Left Hand Description | Symbol | Time | Thousandths of min. | Time | Symbol | Right Hand Description |
|---|---|---|---|---|---|---|
| Grasp case | G | 5 | | 5 | G | Grasp case |
| Upright case | TL | 5 | | 6 | TL | Upright case |
| R. to end flap | RL&TE | 4 | | 5 | RL&TE | R. to end flap |
| Grasp flap | G | 2 | —20— | 5 | G | Grasp flap |
| Open case | TL | 15 | | 10 | TL | Open flap & case |
| Fold over flap | TL | 3 | | 6 | TL&RL | fold over flap |
| R. to side flap | TE | 3 | | 5 | TE | To side flap |
| Close flap | G&TL | 3 | —40— | | | |
| Regrasp to close flap | G | 6 | | 2 | TL | Close flap |
| | | | | 14 | TE&G | To case bottom |
| Case to conveyor | TL | 23 | —60— | | | |
| | | | | 14 | TL | Case to conveyor |
| R. to end flap | RL&TE | 5 | | 2 | RL&TE | To end flap |
| Bend over flap | TL | 8 | —80— | 8 | TL | Bend over flap |
| R. to side flap | TE | 5 | | 5 | TE | To side flap |
| Bend over flap | G &TL | 12 | | 12 | G&TL | Bend over flap |
| | | | —100— | | | |

From: E.S. Buffa, *Models for Production and Operations Management* (New York: John Wiley and Sons, 1963). Reproduced by permission.

**Figure 5-3.** Micromotion Analysis or Simo Chart for Opening a Corrugated Case

*Man-Flow Process Chart*

The man-flow process chart is useful when the procedure is done repetitively with short-or intermediate-range cycle time. This chart describes in sequence all the tasks (activities) that need to be performed by the operator, all the destinations to which he or she will need to travel in performing the procedures, and all the locations of and reasons for any waiting on the part of the operator. Moreover, the chart normally also provides an indication of the distances. Figure 5-4 is a fairly typical example of a man-flow process chart. It indicates all the activities, travel (with distances included) destinations, and reasons for waiting for a pharmacy clerk receiving, filling, and delivering prescriptions in an outpatient clinic. Figure 5-5, on the other hand is an example of a more advanced man-flow process chart. In addition to the three usual actions—activities, movements, and waiting—this format delineates five activities, for example, operations, transportation, inspection, delay, and storage. Inspections and storage are the two activities that are explicitly considered in the format of figure 5-5. They are, of course, lumped in the activity heading of figure 5-4. Significantly, however, this preprinted format provides information about the quantity of items involved in each task, the task time, and the "why" analysis, including the what, where, when, who, and how of each task. Finally, the format provides space for stating the results of the man-flow process redesign, for example, the before-and-after number of operations, distances traveled, and time taken.

*The Product-Flow Process Chart*

The product-flow process chart, as the name implies, traces the flow of the product through the various activities that transform some aspect of it. Figure 5-6(a) and (b) schematically show, in sequence, all the components of the process. The figure describes the locations of storage and/or activities and the destinations, as well as distances traveled, for all movements of the product. The processes of hemostat sterilization and utilization are described in figures 5-6(a) and (b) on two-dimensional floor plans of the areas where the processes take place. These processes are also shown in a product-flow process chart superimposed on an isometric sketch of a multifloor (three-dimensional) layout of the department in figure 5-7.

*The Procedure Flow Chart*

The procedure flow chart (figure 5-8) is somewhat more abstract than the operator, man-flow process, and product-flow process charts that preceded it. The preceding charts focus on the tangible operator or product. This

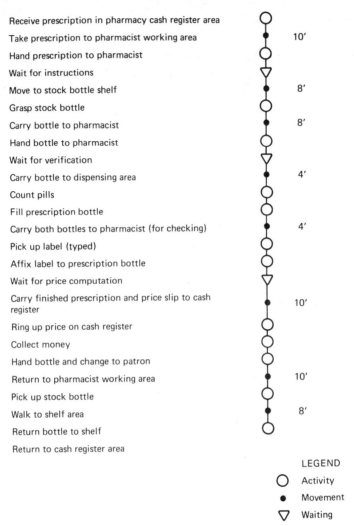

Receive prescription in pharmacy cash register area
Take prescription to pharmacist working area     10'
Hand prescription to pharmacist
Wait for instructions
Move to stock bottle shelf     8'
Grasp stock bottle
Carry bottle to pharmacist     8'
Hand bottle to pharmacist
Wait for verification
Carry bottle to dispensing area     4'
Count pills
Fill prescription bottle
Carry both bottles to pharmacist (for checking)     4'
Pick up label (typed)
Affix label to prescription bottle
Wait for price computation
Carry finished prescription and price slip to cash register     10'
Ring up price on cash register
Collect money
Hand bottle and change to patron
Return to pharmacist working area     10'
Pick up stock bottle
Walk to shelf area     8'
Return bottle to shelf
Return to cash register area

LEGEND

◯   Activity

●   Movement

▽   Waiting

Arnold Reisman, *Systems Analysis in Health-Care Delivery* (Lexington, Mass.: Lexington Books, D.C. Heath and Company, 1979).

**Figure 5-4.** Man-Flow Process Chart for Pharmacy Clerk's Role in an Outpatient Clinic—Function: To Receive, Fill, and Deliver Prescriptions

chart, on the other hand, focuses on the procedures that must be performed, in sequence, by man and/or machine in order to perform a service that is the sum total of the procedural components. This instrument is sometimes referred to as the paperwork flow chart, and, as the name implies, is often used to describe, specify, or prescribe the flow of documents,

| FLOW PROCESS CHART | | | | | | | | NO. 1 | | PAGE NO. 1 | | | NUMBER OF PAGES 1 | | | |
|---|---|---|---|---|---|---|---|---|---|---|---|---|---|---|---|---|

PROCESS  Obtain patient blood sample. Typical tray method using elevator

[X] MAN OR [ ] MATERIAL

CHART BEGINS  Leaving laboratory Venipuncture area
CHART ENDS  Returning to lab. Venipuncture

CHARTED BY  Tom Lamphier
DATE  8/10/70

ORGANIZATION

SUMMARY

| ACTIONS | PRESENT | | PROPOSED | | DIFFERENCE | |
|---|---|---|---|---|---|---|
| | NO. | TIME | NO. | TIME | NO. | TIME |
| ○ OPERATIONS | 25 | – | 25 | – | – | – |
| ⇨ TRANSPORTATIONS | 24 | – | 16 | – | 8 | – |
| □ INSPECTIONS | – | – | – | – | – | – |
| D DELAYS | 2 | – | 2 | – | – | – |
| ▽ STORAGES | | | | | | |
| DISTANCE TRAVELED (feet) | 1,028 | – | 879 | – | 149 | – |

| STEP NO. | DETAILS OF METHOD [ ] PRESENT [ ] PROPOSED | OPERATION | TRANSPORTATION | INSPECTION | DELAY | STORAGE | DISTANCE (feet) | QUANTITY | TIME | ANALYSIS (why?) WHAT WHERE WHEN WHO HOW | NOTES | ANALYSIS ELIMINATE COMBINE SEQUENCE CH'NGE PLACE PERSON IMPROVE |
|---|---|---|---|---|---|---|---|---|---|---|---|---|
| 1 | Walk to elevator | ○ | ● | □ | D | ▽ | 272 | 1 | – | | Carry tray | |
| 2 | Wait for elevator | ○ | ⇨ | □ | ● | ▽ | – | 1 | – | X | Possibility of taking stairs | X |
| 3 | Travel in elevator | ○ | ● | □ | D | ▽ | – | 1 | – | X | —"— | X |
| 4 | Walk to nursing station | ○ | ● | □ | D | ▽ | 22 | 1 | – | | Carry tray | |
| 5 | Imprint patient labels | ● | ⇨ | □ | D | ▽ | – | 8 | – | | | |
| 6 | Walk to room area | ○ | ● | □ | D | ▽ | 48 | 1 | – | | Carry tray | |
| 7 | Walk into patient room | ○ | ● | □ | D | ▽ | 2 | 1 | – | | —"— | |
| 8 | Prepare equipment | ● | ⇨ | □ | D | ▽ | – | 1 | – | | | |
| 9 | Obtain patient specimen | ● | ⇨ | □ | D | ▽ | – | 1 | – | | | |
| 10 | Aside specimen and equipment to tray | ● | ⇨ | □ | D | ▽ | – | 1 | – | | | |
| 11 | Repeat x7 lines | ○ | ● | □ | D | ▽ | 91 | 1 | – | | | |
| | 7 to 10 for | ● | ⇨ | □ | D | ▽ | – | 1 | – | | | |
| | additional | ● | ⇨ | □ | D | ▽ | – | 1 | – | | | |
| | specimen in area | ● | ⇨ | □ | D | ▽ | – | 1 | – | | | |
| 12 | Walk to next room area | ○ | ● | □ | D | ▽ | 116 | 1 | – | | | |
| 13 | Walk to elevator | ○ | ● | □ | D | ▽ | 56 | 1 | – | | Carry tray | |
| 14 | Wait for elevator | ○ | ⇨ | □ | ● | ▽ | – | 1 | – | X | Possibility of taking stairs | X |
| 15 | Travel in elevator | ○ | ● | □ | D | ▽ | – | 1 | – | X | —"— | X |
| 16 | Walk to laboratory Venipuncture area | ○ | ● | □ | D | ▽ | 272 | 1 | – | | Carry tray | |
| | | ○ | ⇨ | □ | D | ▽ | | | | | | |
| | | ○ | ⇨ | □ | D | ▽ | | | | | | |
| | | ○ | ⇨ | □ | D | ▽ | | | | | | |

From T. Lamphier, "Flow Charting Speeds Hospital Work," *Industrial Engineering* 2 (November 1970):50-53.

**Figure 5-5.** Blood-Sample-Collection Flow-Process Chart

forms, and so on necessary to facilitate some physical activity or to produce an end document.

Symbols specifically designed for use in a procedure flow chart are shown in [1], as is a nongraphic verbal specification for doing the same thing. The graphics format, however, can be handled through the more

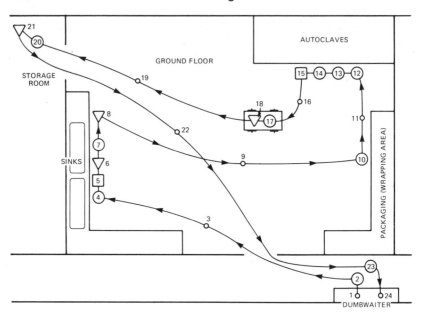

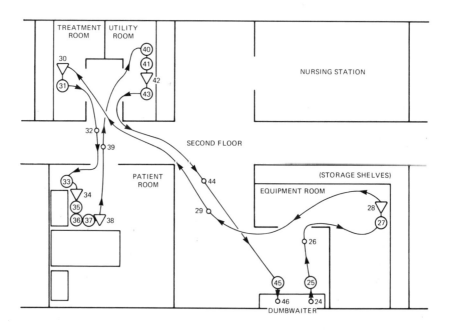

Arnold Reisman, *Systems Analysis in Health-Care Delivery* (Lexington, Mass.: Lexington Books, D.C. Heath and Company, 1979).

**Figure 5-6.** Product-Flow Process Diagram for Hemostat Sterilization in Two Dimensions

generally applicable and standard flow-charting symbols discussed later in this chapter.

## Operation-Process Charts

Like the procedure flow chart, the operation-process chart (figure 5-9) focuses on the procedures necessary to provide a service that, although routine in process, is not routine in product. Moreover, both are applied to jobs that require human judgment or professional expertise at some points in the process. Specifically, among the many routine clerical and mechanical activities or tasks there are also some decisions, such as "select proper intravenous (IV) solution" or "verify proper strength of formula before delivering," that require some professional judgment or expertise.

## The Assembly Chart

The assembly chart (figure 5-10) is useful for short-, medium-, or relatively long-cycle-time procedures that are performed repetitively, intermittently, or continuously. It clearly describes what needs to be put together and how to create a "subassembly." It then does the same for all subassemblies and, in sequence, delineates how to assemble the final product. Normally, assembly charts do not convey information on the task time, work-center location, part and/or subassembly number, specification, or identification. However, there is no reason that any or all of the preceding items of information cannot be superimposed on the diagram where warranted.

## Routing Sheet

A routing sheet (also called operations-route or specification sheet) describes the processing steps or operation sequences required to make each part. Routing is broadly applicable to a variety of institutional environments. For example, routing information must be determined for patient processing, materials distribution, and so on. The routing sheet often shows the order in which the operations are to be completed. Although routing frequently identifies specific facilities at which given operations will be performed, output scheduling is not involved because (clock) arrival times of the "jobs" at the facilities are not indicated [1].

## The Logic Diagram

The logic diagram guides the human "operator" or the machine (with intelligence) through a series of questions to one of a number of end states

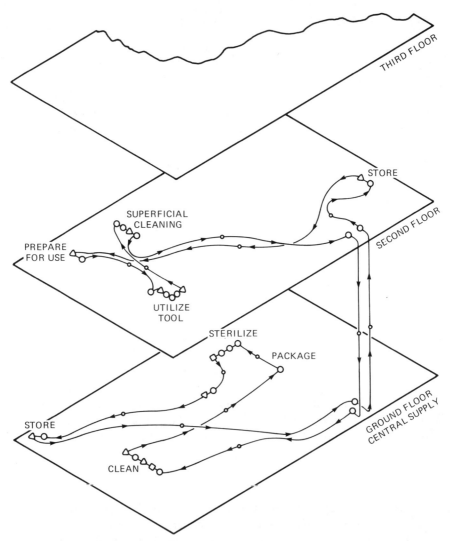

Arnold Reisman, *Systems Analysis in Health-Care Delivery* (Lexington, Mass.: Lexington Books, D.C. Heath and Company, 1979).

**Figure 5-7**. Product-Flow Process Diagram for Hemostat Sterilization and Utilization in Three Dimensions

depending on the responses to each question. Figure 4-12 depicts its use in describing a procedure for calculating the economic order quantity (EOQ) when quantity discounts are offered. Clearly, its intended user is a relatively professional human operator performing a repetitive job, albeit one that is not identical in all cases of cycles.

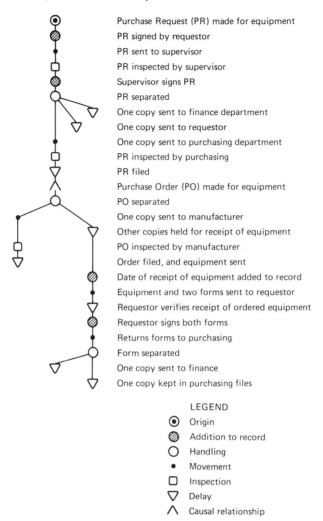

Purchase Request (PR) made for equipment
PR signed by requestor
PR sent to supervisor
PR inspected by supervisor
Supervisor signs PR
PR separated
One copy sent to finance department
One copy sent to requestor
One copy sent to purchasing department
PR inspected by purchasing
PR filed
Purchase Order (PO) made for equipment
PO separated
One copy sent to manufacturer
Other copies held for receipt of equipment
PO inspected by manufacturer
Order filed, and equipment sent
Date of receipt of equipment added to record
Equipment and two forms sent to requestor
Requestor verifies receipt of ordered equipment
Requestor signs both forms
Returns forms to purchasing
Form separated
One copy sent to finance
One copy kept in purchasing files

LEGEND
◉  Origin
◎  Addition to record
○  Handling
•  Movement
□  Inspection
▽  Delay
∧  Causal relationship

Arnold Reisman, *Systems Analysis in Health-Care Delivery* (Lexington, Mass.: Lexington Books, D.C. Heath and Company, 1979).

**Figure 5-8.** Procedure Flow Chart for Ordering Office Equipment

The logic diagrams can also be used in systems where man interacts with machine by following a predefined logic to reach any one of a number of end points or conclusions, having started with a given set of facts or data, or having made a number of judgmental decisions. Similarly, many repetitive decisions can be mechanized and a computer used to respond, based on information it finds in its files, to each of a number of questions that are raised by the programmed logic.

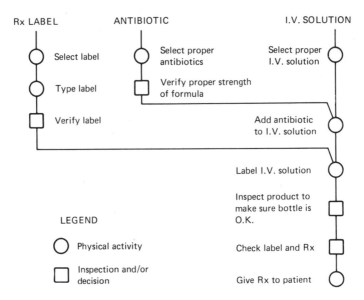

Arnold Reisman, *Systems Analysis in Health-Care Delivery* (Lexington, Mass.: Lexington Books, D.C. Heath and Company, 1979).

**Figure 5-9.** Operation Process Chart of Intravenous-Solution Prescription

*Flow Charts*

Information-handling problems in modern digital computers can be charted much as can the body movements and activities of an operator, the flow of material or of people, and the systems and procedures of paper work However, the charting techniques that have evolved in the computer world have some unique characteristics. Each of the major computer manufacturers has over the years developed, adopted, published, modified, and advocated flow-charting conventions. These conventions have differed from one computer manufacturer to the next, creating a proliferation of nomenclature and techniques.

In 1966, under the sponsorship of the Business Equipment Manufacturers Association, the American National Standards Institute (ANSI) published *A Standard of Flowchart Symbols for Information Processing*. The stated scope of this standard is to prescribe and define the symbols used on flow charts to represent the sequence of operations and the flow of data and paperwork of information-processing systems. The standard does not cover (1) identifying, descriptive, or explanatory information written inside or adjacent to a symbol; or (2) pictorial flow charts that use pictures or drawings to depict a system.

Definitions of terms and standard flow-chart symbols are indicated in

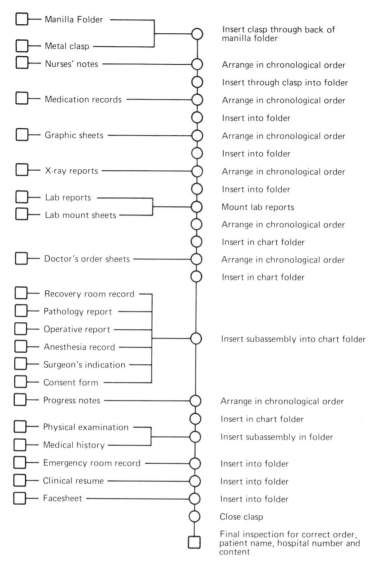

Arnold Reisman, *Systems Analysis in Health-Care Delivery* (Lexington, Mass.: Lexington Books, D.C. Heath and Company, 1979).

**Figure 5-10.** Assembly Chart of a Medical Record after Patient Discharge

table 5-2 and figure 5-11, respectively, with permission of the association. In addition, N. Chapin [14] provides an excellent tutorial on flow charting using the ANSI standard. Among many helpful *insights* and hints, he shows ways of laying out a chart. Some of this information is reproduced in figure 5-12. He also shows a flow diagram with identifications, using the basic and

| Input/Output | Process | Flowline | Annotation |
|:---:|:---:|:---:|:---:|

Punched Card            On Line Storage

Magnetic Tape            Off Line Storage

Punched Tape            Decision

Document            Predefined Process

Manual Input            Auxiliary Operation

Display            Manual Operation

Communication Link

Connector

Terminal

Reproduced with permission from "American Standard Flowchart Symbols for Information Processing," X3.5-1966, American Standards Association.

**Figure 5-11.** Summary of Flow-Chart Symbols

specialized outlines, with and without connectors and cross-referencing schemes.

## Genealogy Trees

It is often desirable to identify all the components of a system, giving full visibility to the system hierarchy. The traditional organization charts, figures 2-1 and 2-2, are good and well-known examples. Here one is able to identify very succinctly not just the formal organizational structure (for example, the divisions and departments, and the lineage of reporting), but also the names of individuals who fill the positions indicated.

## Table 5-2
## Standard Definitions for Terms Used in Charting Information Processes

**Analysis.** The investigation of a problem by a consistent method and its separation into related units for further study.

**Annotation.** An added descriptive comment or explanatory note.

**Automatic Data Processing.** The manipulation of data within a machine to solve a problem by using stored program techniques.

**Auxiliary Operation.** An operation performed on equipment not under direct control of the central processing unit.

**Auxiliary Storage.** Storage that supplements the primary storage.

**Bidirectional Flow.** Flow that can extend over the same lines in either or both directions.

**Central Processing Unit.** The component of a computing system that contains the arithmetic, logical, and control circuits of the basic system.

**Communication Link.** The means for automatically transmitting information from one location to another.

**Connector.** A means of representing on a flow chart the junction of two lines of flow or a break in a single line of flow.

**Data.** A representation of information in the form of words, symbols, numbers, letters, characters, digits, and so on.

**Decision.** A processing operation to determine further action based on the relationship of similar items of data.

**Display.** A visual representation of data.

**Document.** A medium of which information is recorded in a form for human usage, such as a report sheet or pages of a book.

**Flow-Direction Function.** The indicating of the sequence of available information and executable operations.

**Flow Chart.** A graphical representation of the definition, analysis, or solution of a problem where symbols are used to represent operations, data, flow, equipment, and so on.

**Flow Line.** A means of connecting flowchart symbols on a flow chart.

**Function.** A specific purpose or a characteristic action.

**Information.** The meaning assigned to data by the known conventions used in its representation.

**Information Processing.** The processing of data representing information and the determining of the meaning of the processed data.

**Input/Output.** A general term for the equipment, data, or media used in the entering or recording function, commonly abbreviated I/O.

**Input/Output Function.** The making available of information for processing and the recording of the processed information.

**I/O.** An abbreviation for input/output.

**Magnetic Tape.** A continuous medium coated with a magnetic substance on which data is recorded.

**Manual Input.** The entry of data into a computer or system by direct manual manipulation of a device.

**Manual Operation.** The processing of data in a system by direct manual techniques.

**Medium.** The material on which data is recorded, such as tape, cards, or paper.

**Normal Direction Flow.** The direction of flow from left to right or top to bottom.

**Off-Line Storage.** Storage not under control of the central processing unit.

**On-Line Storage.** Storage under direct control of the central processing unit.

**Operation.** The process of executing a defined action.

**Predefined Process.** A named process consisting of one or more operations or program steps that are specified elsewhere, such as a subroutine or logical unit.

**Problem Definition.** A term associated with both the statement and solution phase of a problem and used to denote the transformation of data and the relationship of procedures, data, constraints, environments, and so on.

**Processing.** A term including any operation or combination of operations on data, where an operation is the execution of a defined action.

**Processing Function.** The process of executing a defined operation or group of operations.

**Punched Card.** A card that is punched with a combination of holes to represent letters, digits, or special characters.

**Punched Tape.** A continuous-recording medium in which data is punched.

**Table 5-2** *(continued)*

**Random Sequence.** A sequence not arranged according to any prescribed order.

**Represent.** To use one or more characters or symbols to depict a well-defined concept.

**Reverse-Direction Flow.** The direction of flow other than left to right or top to bottom.

**Symbol.** A unit representation for characteristics, relationships, transformations, graphics, and so on.

**System.** A collection of men, machines, and methods required to accomplish a specific objective.

**Terminal.** A point in a system or communication network at which information can either enter or leave.

**Transmit.** To transfer information from one location to another.

Reproduced with permission from "American Standard Flowchart Symbols for Information Processing," X3.5-1966, American Standards Association.

The same graphic approach can be used in such disparate applications as grouping families of different materials (sutures, syringes, and so on) or grouping categories of workers in a materials-management hierarchy.

*Decision Trees*

The concept of decision trees has been used extensively in formalizing administrative and diagnostic decisions. Essentially, they are used for graphically delineating a series of decisions and/or outcomes that occur in a branching sequence, as shown in figure 5-13. This example serves to illustrate the set of questions that might be raised when one contemplates delegating a task. Corresponding to every question, all feasible answers or outcomes are delineated. The decision maker then follows that path within the tree that would provide him with the most enlightened decision. One possibility at all decision stages is, of course, to terminate the process.

A decision tree illustrating the process undergone by a health center in delineating the alternatives to satisfy the needs for additional plant capacity is shown in [1]. Clearly, a number of options are open to the decision maker. These include adding new facilities, adding to or improving existing plant and equipment, converting use of space, and so on. For each of these basic options there exists a number of secondary options. Thus new facilities can be added at a number of alternative sites or locations and under a number of financial arrangements (lease, buy, and so forth).

*Decision Tables*

The decision table is extremely useful whenever a choice must be made between several feasible alternatives (projects, candidates, products, programs, and the like), and especially when the choice must be based on a number of criteria.

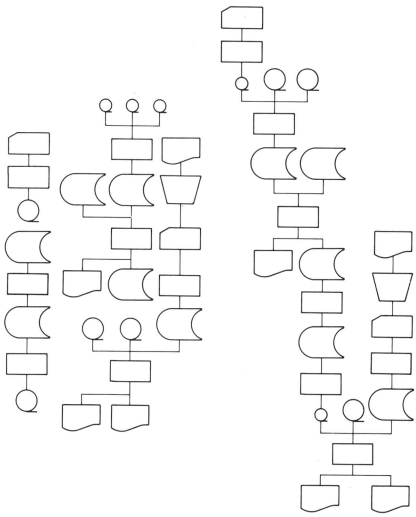

**Figure 5-12.** Example of a Tight and an Open Layout of a System Chart for the Same System

The decision table is essentially based on weighted scoring. Specifically, each criterion is preassigned a weight using any one of a number of possible scales [1]. Each alternative is then rated using some numerical scale on each of the criteria. These individual ratings are then multiplied by the weights corresponding to the respective criteria, and the products are summed for each alternative. The alternative with the highest score is then judged the prime candidate. Examples of the use of decision tables are given in [11], [12], and [15].

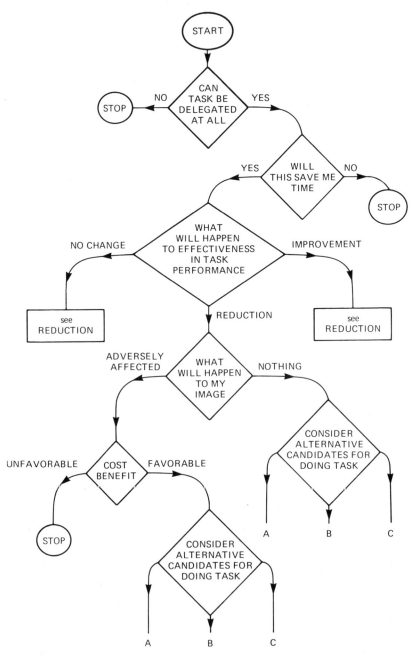

Arnold Reisman, *Systems Analysis in Health-Care Delivery* (Lexington, Mass.: Lexington Books, D.C. Heath and Company, 1979).

**Figure 5-13.** Task Delegation

| Factors | Weight | Vendor 1 | | Vendor 2 | | Vendor 3 | | Vendor 4 | | Vendor 5 | |
|---|---|---|---|---|---|---|---|---|---|---|---|
| | | Rtg. | Wtd. Rtg. | Rtg. | Wtd. Rtg. | Rtg. | Wtd. Rtg. | Rtg. | Wtd. Rtg. | Rtg. | Wtd. Rtg. |
| Cost | .161 | 5.0 | .805 | 4.0 | .644 | 3.0 | .483 | 2.0 | .332 | 1.0 | .161 |
| Software capability | .153 | 3.2 | .490 | 3.0 | .459 | 3.2 | .490 | 3.4 | .520 | 3.4 | .520 |
| Reliability (technical) | .136 | 3.0 | .408 | 3.6 | .490 | 3.2 | .435 | 2.6 | .354 | 2.8 | .381 |
| Turnaround time | .122 | 3.0 | .366 | 3.0 | .366 | 3.0 | .366 | 3.0 | .366 | 3.0 | .366 |
| Compatibility (hardware) | .109 | 3.0 | .327 | 3.0 | .327 | 3.2 | .327 | 3.0 | .327 | 3.0 | .327 |
| Compatibility (software) | .112 | 1.8 | .202 | 1.8 | .202 | 2.2 | .246 | 2.6 | .291 | 2.2 | .247 |
| Expansion potential | .109 | 2.0 | .218 | 2.0 | .218 | 2.0 | .215 | 2.0 | .218 | 2.0 | .218 |
| Stability (business) | .095 | 3.0 | .285 | 3.0 | .285 | 3.0 | .285 | 3.0 | .285 | 3.0 | .285 |
| Total weighted Score | | | 2.5 | | 3.0 | | 2.8 | | 2.7 | | 2.5 |

**Figure 5-14.** Computer-Service Selection-Decision Table

Decision tables could be used in selecting vendors for prime contracts or for contracted services. Figure 5-14 shows an example of a decision table used in selecting a computer-service bureau to process materials-management information. Among the factors used by this particular organization were (1) costs of the services provided and (2) the vendor's software capability, namely the vendor's ability to accept the data in the form collected and to process it into the kind of reports requested. The technical reliability of the vendor's hardware and software was of concern. Next, the institution was definitely interested in the turnaround time (the lapsed time between data submission and report availability) and in the compatibility of the vendor's hardware and software with other computer systems used by the institution. The institution was also interested in the potential for MMIS expansion, namely, generation of new kinds of reports and collection of additional types of data. Finally, because of the relatively high rate of computer-service business failures, the institution was concerned with the business stability of the vendor.

| CONSULT DESK / PRIMARY DESK | ALLERGY | CARDIOLOGY | CARD. FUNC. LAB | | | | | | | EMI SCAN |
|---|---|---|---|---|---|---|---|---|---|---|
| 1. ALLERGY | | | | | | | | | | |
| 2. CARDIOLOGY | | | | | | | | | | |
| 3. DENTAL | | | | | | | | | | |
| | | | | | | | | | | |
| | | | | | | | | | | |
| | | | | | | | | | | |
| | | | | | | | | | | |
| 28. UROLOGY | | | | | | | | | | |

Arnold Reisman, *Systems Analysis in Health-Care Delivery* (Lexington, Mass.: Lexington Books, D.C. Heath and Company, 1979).

**Figure 5-15.** Incidence Matrix

*Incidence Table*

The incidence table or matrix is used to show which elements in an array of functions, procedures, or products interact with which element of some other or the same array of functions, procedures, or products. For example, in establishing a route and schedule for runners who pick up and deliver materials in a large referral group practice, the question of the level of interaction between the departments was raised. First, an incidence matrix such as the one shown in figure 5-15 was used to answer the question on a yes-no basis. Later, data were collected to establish the level of such interactions by monitoring actual origins and destinations of materials being picked up and delivered.

*Precedence Diagram*

When there are several sequencing options based on and/or allowed by the process technology, a precedence diagram can be drawn to clarify such flexibility. Figure 5-16 depicts a precedence relationship. It is clear from this figure that activity *B* can be performed at the same time that activity *C* is in progress, but that both must await the completion of activity *A*.

*Precedence Matrix*

The information contained in the precedence diagram figure 5-16 can also be depicted in matrix form, as shown in figure 5-17. The digital format of such matrixes allows them to be easily incorporated into computer routines used in manpower scheduling or in control-materials-requirements planning and scheduling.

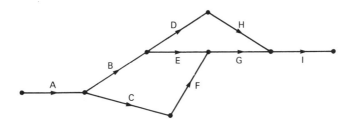

Arnold Reisman, *Systems Analysis in Health-Care Delivery* (Lexington, Mass.: Lexington Books, D.C. Heath and Company, 1979).

**Figure 5-16.** Precedence Diagram

| → | A | B | C | D | E | F | G | H | I |
|---|---|---|---|---|---|---|---|---|---|
| A |   | 1 | 1 | 0 | 0 | 0 | 0 | 0 | 0 |
| B | 0 |   | 0 | 1 | 1 | 0 | 0 | 0 | 0 |
| C | 0 | 0 |   | 0 | 0 | 1 | 0 | 0 | 0 |
| D | 0 | 0 | 0 |   | 0 | 0 | 0 | 1 | 0 |
| E | 0 | 0 | 0 | 0 |   | 0 | 1 | 0 | 0 |
| F | 0 | 0 | 0 | 0 | 0 |   | 1 | 0 | 0 |
| G | 0 | 0 | 0 | 0 | 0 | 0 |   | 0 | 1 |
| H | 0 | 0 | 0 | 0 | 0 | 0 | 0 |   | 1 |
| I | 0 | 0 | 0 | 0 | 0 | 0 | 0 | 0 |   |

Arnold Reisman, *Systems Analysis in Health-Care Delivery* (Lexington, Mass.: Lexington Books, D.C. Heath and Company, 1979).

**Figure 5-17**. Precedence Matrix

*Bills of Material*

The bill of materials is frequently shown on design or manufacturing drawings in industry. It specifies all the parts required to make a finished component or item and details the number of parts per item and the quantities of materials required by each part. Those parts that are to be purchased are indicated.

This concept can also be used in health services in whatever form is likely to be most useful. An example of a bill of materials in preparing IV solutions is shown in figure 5-18.

*Explosion Chart*

When several different end products share parts, an explosion chart is used to identify the aggregation of part requirements. This chart is a compilation of bills of materials for end products having common parts. It is a matrix of demand for parts based on parts "explosion" of end-use product demands.

Thus in figure 5-19 $D$ represents the demand for end-product $I$. This in turn requires three units of item $A$ and nothing else, whereas to satisfy the demand $D_2$ it is necessary to have three of each part $A$, $B$, and $C$. The raw sums $R_A$, $R_B$, and so on represent the total number of each part required to satisfy all the demands $D_1$, $D_2$, and so on for the end products 1, 2, and so on, respectively.

| | AMPHOTERICIN B (mg) | HYDROCORTISONE (mg) | LIDOCAINE (mg) | HEPARIN (unit) | ERYTHROMYCIN (mg) | DOPAMINE (mg) | POTASSIUM CHLORIDE (mEq) | AMINOPHYLLINE (mg) | CALCIUM GLUCONATE 10% (ml) | FOLIC ACID (mg) | SOLU B FORTE (ml) | SODIUM BICARBONATE (mEq) |
|---|---|---|---|---|---|---|---|---|---|---|---|---|
| 1. D5W 1000ml | 20 | 50 | 25 | | | | | | | | | |
| 2. D5W 300ml | 50 | 15 | | 1000 | | | | | | | | |
| 3. NaCl 0.5 100ml | | 5 | | | 1000 | | | | | | | |
| 4. D5W 2500ml | | | | 2500 | | 1000 | | | | | | |
| 5. D5W 360ml | | | | | | | 10 | 360 | | | | |
| 6. D5NaCl 0.9 1000ml | | | | | | | 10 | | 10 | | | |
| 7. D5W 1000ml | | | | | | | 20 | | | 1 | 10 | 88 |
| 8. D5W 1000ml | | | | | | | 20 | | | 1 | 10 | 44 |
| 9. D5NaCl 0.2 1000ml | | | | | | | 10 | | | | | |
| 10. D5W 200ml | 50 | 50 | 25 | | | | | | | | | |
| 11. D5W 400ml | 50 | 75 | | 1000 | | | | | | | | |
| 12. D5W 500ml | 50 | 50 | | 1000 | | | | | | | | |
| 13. D5W 250ml | | | | 250 | | 500 | | | | | | |
| 14. D5W 200ml | | 50 | 25 | | | | | | | | | |
| 15. D5NaCl 0.2 1000ml | | | | | | | | | | 1 | 10 | |
| 16. D5W 360ml | | | | | | | 20 | 360 | | | | |
| 17. D5NaCl 0.2 1000ml | | | | | | | 30 | | 10 | | | |
| 18. D5NaCl 0.45 1000ml | | | | | | | 20 | | | 1 | 10 | |
| 19. D5W 1000ml | | | | | | | 20 | | | 1 | | 88 |
| 20. D5W 50ml | | | | | 250 | | | | | | | |
| TOTAL REQUIRED | 220 mg | 295 mg | 75 mg | 5750 units | 1250 mg | 1500 mg | 160 mEq | 720 mg | 20 ml | 5 mg | 40 ml | 220 mEq |

Arnold Reisman, *Systems Analysis in Health-Care Delivery* (Lexington, Mass.: Lexington Books, D.C. Heath and Company, 1979).

Numbers 1 through 20 are large volume intravenous solutions.

D 5 W = Dextrose 5% in water
NaCl 0.5 = Sodium choloride 0.5% in water
D5NaCl 0.9 = Dextrose 5% in sodium chloride 0.9%
D5NaCl 0.2 = Dextrose 5% in sodium chloride 0.2%
D5NaCl 0.45 = Dextrose 5% in sodium chloride 0.45%

All the preceding solutions are available commercially in IV bottles or bags and are ready to administer to a patient.

The drugs listed along the top are additions to the IV solutions.

Large-volume intravenous solutions are used for fluid replacement or as a vehicle for administration of a drug.

**Figure 5-18.** Bill of Materials for IV Solutions

| ITEM | FINISHED PRODUCTS | | | | | |
|------|---|---|---|---|---|---|
|      | 1 | 2 | 3 | 4 | | PART PRODUCTION REQUIREMENTS |
| A | 3 | 3 | 0 | 0 | | $R_A$ |
| B | 0 | 3 | 0 | 0 | | $R_B$ |
| C | 0 | 3 | 1 | 5 | | $R_C$ |
| | | | | | | |
| | | | | | | |
| | | | | | | |
| DEMAND | $D_1$ | $D_2$ | $D_3$ | $D_4$ | | |

Arnold Reisman, *Systems Analysis in Health-Care Delivery* (Lexington, Mass.: Lexington Books, D.C. Heath and Company, 1979).

**Figure 5-19.** Explosion Chart

*Origin-Destination Tables*

Institutions and groups of institutions often are faced with the transportation or movement of patients, materials, and information to and from various locations or nodes in a network of such nodes. The extent of such movement in terms of some units (people, pounds, cubic feet) so moved may be of interest in the location of facilities (the nodes) vis-à-vis one another; in the design of the means for such movement, for example, the number of movers (trucks, workers, pneumatic tubes, conveyor belts, and so on); in the frequencies and the schedules of pickup and delivery; and so forth. A simple way of presenting such two-directional movement is through the use of an origin-destination table, where the rows represent the various nodes or points where movement originates and the columns represent the various destination points. Thus the numbers entered into the cells of such a table represent the quantity of units moved from the node represented by the row of the cell in question to the node represented by the column of the same cell. Clearly, the diagonal cells, for example, the cells whose row and column designations are identical, need not be filled out. Moreover, the table need not be square, since there may be more or fewer origin nodes than destination nodes.

Origin-destination tables are very closely related to input-output tables, discussed next. Indeed, the example in figure 5-20 can be viewed as an origin-destination table where the pickup departments (the rows) are the source nodes and the deliver-to departments (the columns) are the destinations for materials in a large group practice or clinic.

| CONSULT DEPT. ⟋ PRIMARY DEPARTMENT | 1. ALERGY | 2. CARDIOLOGY | 3. CARD. FUNC. LAB | | | | | | | EMI SCAN |
|---|---|---|---|---|---|---|---|---|---|---|
| 1. ALERGY | $C_{1,1}$ | $C_{1,2}$ | $C_{1,3}$ | | | | | | | |
| 2. CARDIOLOGY | $C_{2,1}$ | $C_{2,2}$ | $C_{2,3}$ | | | | | | | |
| 3. DENTAL | $C_{3,1}$ | $C_{3,2}$ | $C_{3,3}$ | | | | | | | |
| | | | | | | | | | | |
| | | | | | | | | | | |
| | | | | | | | | | | |
| ⋮ | | ⋮ | | | | | | ⋮ | | ⋮ |
| | | | | | | | | | | |
| 28. UROLOGY | $C_{28,1}$ | $C_{28,2}$ | $C_{28,3}$ | | | | | | | |

**Figure 5-20.** Input-Output Matrix

*Input-Output Table*

The input-output table is useful whenever a number of organizational units, departments, or work centers interact with each other through flows of patients, information, workers, or materials. The input-output table was originally developed for national and regional economic planning.

An example of an input-output table is given in figure 5-20. As mentioned earlier, this table can be used to indicate the extent of interactions in terms of materials needing to be picked up and delivered between the various departments.

Thus if the row represents the "from" or origin department, then entry in any one cell represents the number of items to be picked up in the row department for delivery to the respective column departments. Specifically, the number $C_{2,3}$ denotes the number of items sent by the cardiology department to the cardiofunction laboratory. Some of the $C_{i,j}$s will be zero or very small, and others will be extensive. The results of such data collection and analysis can be used to establish schedules and routes for the, "runners," such as materials-handling personnel. Tables such as these contain a great deal of information for analyzing existing systems as well as for designing decision rules for allocating resources.

The incidence table, precedence matrix, explosion chart, and input-output tables are designed to show, in a compact manner, the interrelationships that exist between the various units in a multiproduct, multidepartment, or multiactivity system network. In addition to the obvious advantages of compactness of display, these formats also lend themselves readily to mathematical and computer manipulations. Such manipulations are often the prerequisite for analysis of the existing system and for its redesign or modification.

The various versions of the Gantt (named for its developer, Henry L. Gantt), PERT (program evaluation and review technique), and CPM (critical path method) charts that follow are intended for project planning and control. The projects may range all the way from the design and fabrication of a piece of hardware or the development and installation of new systems and procedures, through the design and construction of a new facility, to major research and development undertakings.

### Gantt Charts

In planning operations, production, research and development projects, and the like, the administrator must allocate the various available capacities (resources) to the desired output. He must plan for the best use of facilities and resources and then control the operations in accordance with these plans. The most widely used device for such work is the Gantt chart.

The concept of the Gantt chart is simple. Listed vertically are the various resources or capacities that must be allocated, or orders to which resources are to be apportioned. The horizontal axis represents the time made available for this work. Allocation is accomplished by assigining the times necessary for performance of the given tasks to the available and required resources by trial and error until some feasible fit is discovered. This then becomes the plan for the time span covered by the chart. The chart may also be used as a control device on performance. As time passes and scheduled underperformance or overperformance is recognized, the various allocations can be shifted to conform with the new information at hand.

A large number of variations of the basic concept of Gantt charts are in use today. Pegboards with different-colored pegs used to represent the symbols and a vertical string showing the current data are quite common. Racks in which order cards can be placed opposite each capacity are a simple variation. Also in common use is a board with capacities in the left-hand column and clips strung out horizontally opposite each capacity. Paper tapes, the length of which corresponds to the time requirements for an order, are prepared and clipped opposite the capacities. A fit is obtained by moving the paper tapes around. Rescheduling is simplified by this device.

In summary, the Gantt chart depicts the work to be done. It has a time scale across the bottom of the chart that depicts the specific tasks relative to the entire project. The Gantt chart shows the relationships among the milestones within the same task, but not the relationships among the milestones contained in different tasks. This can best be illustrated by figure 5-21. Each of the circles (milestones) represents the accomplishment of a specific phase of the total undertaking, and each rectangle represents a task.

*PERT Charts*

The program evaluation and review technique (PERT) is a method of minimizing trouble spots—procedural bottlenecks, delays, and interruptions in large projects by determining critical activities before they occur, so that various parts of an overall job can be coordinated. It is basically a planning and control technique that utilizes a network to complete a predetermined project or schedule. A technique of this type helps to facilitate the communications functions in the organization by reporting favorable as well as unfavorable developments before they happen. In effect, PERT tries to keep managers apprised of all critical factors and considerations that bear on their decisions. From this standpoint, it often is a valuable managerial tool in decision making.

**Transformation of a Gantt Chart to a PERT Network**. The Gantt milestone chart discussed earlier is in itself a milestone in the development of PERT. Modification of Gantt's milestone chart to show the interrelationships among all milestones in a project is achieved in three steps. The first step calls for a removal of the rectangles. As indicated in figure 5-22, these are replaced by arrows connecting the milestones.

The second step calls for adding the relationships among the milestones for the various tasks, as shown in figure 5-23. Here several milestones must

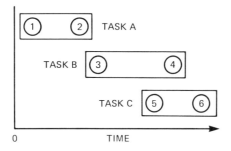

Arnold Reisman, *Systems Analysis in Health-Care Delivery* (Lexington, Mass.: Lexington Books, D.C. Heath and Company, 1979).

**Figure 5-21.** Gantt Milestone Chart

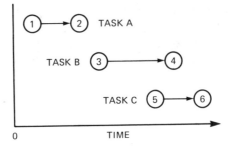

Arnold Reisman, *Systems Analysis in Health-Care Delivery* (Lexington, Mass.: Lexington Books, D.C. Heath and Company, 1979).
**Figure 5-22.** Gantt Chart with Rectangles Removed and Replaced with Arrows

precede other milestones. For example, milestone 5 cannot be started before milestones 1 and 3 are completed. This type of relationship is true for all other cases in the illustration. It should be noted that milestone 1 is the starting point and milestone 6 the ending point of the project.

In the final step, shown in figure 5-24 the term *task* is dropped since all the relationships, regardless of the task involved, are shown by arrows. Further, the horizontal time scale of the Gantt chart is dropped and replaced with individual time on each of the arrows. The transformation from the Gantt chart to a PERT network is now complete. All interrelationships among the milestones are made visible. The project is viewed as an integrated whole, rather than as a number of tasks. Each leg of the network is assigned its own expected time value and a PERT-time chart is the result, as shown in figure 5-25. This transformation permits the use of a network for large and complicated projects and may utilize statistics and/or notions of probability for determining estimated completion dates. The steps utilized in preparing a PERT-time-project network for planning and control are given in [1].

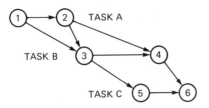

Arnold Reisman, *Systems Analysis in Health-Care Delivery* (Lexington, Mass.: Lexington Books, D.C. Heath and Company, 1979).
**Figure 5-23.** Gantt Chart Partially Transferred to a PERT Network

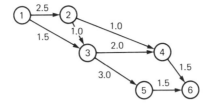

Arnold Reisman, *Systems Analysis in Health-Care Delivery* (Lexington, Mass.: Lexington Books, D.C. Heath and Company, 1979).

**Figure 5-24.** Complete Transformation of Gantt Chart to a PERT Network

In the development of complex networks involving many people, machines, and materials, it is often desirable to use a computer for the calculations. There are many standard computer packages available for doing this. A computer employing a PERT packaged routine provides a method of checking actual progress against the schedule. It can determine the slack times in the network as of certain points in time. This allows management to shift resources, if possible, and to rearrange subnetworks and like items in an attempt to complete the project in the shortest feasible time. Also, such packages can print an event report (going from the first event to the last), a latest-allowable-time report, and departmental reports for events.

In networks made up of approximately 100 activities or more, a computer application with a weekly updating of changes to produce a new critical path and related reports is desirable from both the accuracy and economy points of view. Moreover, most projects do not follow original plans, and revisions must take place each time an activity exceeds its planned time or is completed in less than its planned time. This can play havoc with manual methods.

**PERT-Cost Charts.** The PERT-cost technique is an expansion of PERT that integrates cost data with time data. It allows for tradeoffs between time and costs.

In applying PERT-cost, it is essential to make two time and cost estimates for each activity in the network—a normal estimate and a crash estimate. The normal estimate of time is analogous to the expected-time estimate. Normal cost is the cost associated with finishing the project in the normal time. The crash-time estimate is the time that would be required if no costs were spared in trying to reduce the project time. Crash cost is the cost associated with doing the job on a crash basis in order to minimize completion time. A companion volume [1] provides a detailed example of the use of PERT-cost charts for making time-cost tradeoffs in project management.

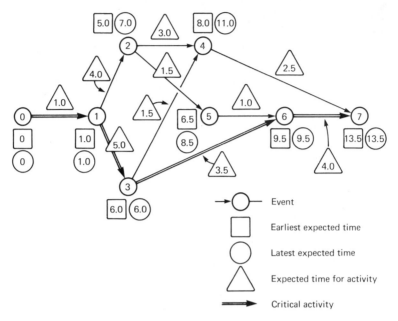

Event

Earliest expected time

Latest expected time

Expected time for activity

Critical activity

Arnold Reisman, *Systems Analysis in Health-Care Delivery* (Lexington, Mass.: Lexington Books, D.C. Heath and Company, 1979).

**Figure 5-25.** PERT Network: Earliest Expected and Latest Allowable Times, $T_E$ and $T_L$, Respectively

## *Development of a Generalized Systems Flow Chart*

Many, if not all, of the flow charts discussed in this chapter can be incorporated into the framework of a general network, as indicated in figure 5-26. The operations-function boundaries contain *n* nodes called *operations*, which are interconnected by a number of flows. Crossing the boundaries of the operations function are a set of *l* inputs and *m* outputs. It should be evident that this network reduces to the operator chart shown in figure 5-2 by recognizing first that each hand constitutes an operations system. The inputs are the various parts in the bin. The operations are the activities, such as "grasp bolt from bin 2," symbolized by the larger circles, as well as the "carry's" symbolized by the smaller circles. The outputs, of course, are the finished assemblies.

The man-flow-process and product-flow-process charts are clearly special cases of figure 5-24, where the operations are the various entries indicated by circles, triangles, or squares. It should be noted that figures 5-4, 5-6, and 5-7 represent single-path networks where all operations are in a simple sequence. Unlike its predecessors in the chapter, the procedure-flow diagram, figure 5-8, is also a special case allowing for some branching of activities. The operations process and the assembly charts, on the other hand,

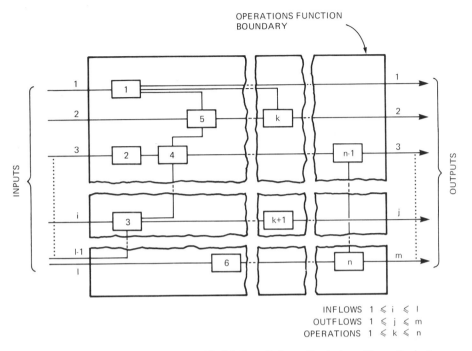

Arnold Reisman, *Systems Analysis in Health-Care Delivery* (Lexington, Mass.: Lexington Books, D.C. Heath and Company, 1979).

**Figure 5-26.** Operations-Function-Flow Schematic

generally have a number of inputs and sometimes a number of outputs as well. The logic diagrams often, although not exclusively, start with one initial state; exhibit much branching, including at times internal looping or feedback; and conclude with one or more end points. Clearly, the decision points exhibited by the diamond-shaped boxes of the logic diagram figure 5-12 are a specific type of node in the network of figure 5-26.

One could proceed to show that in the precedence diagrams and in the PERT networks the various branches have embedded in them specific operations. Moreover the nodes, that is, circles, of the PERT diagram represent milestones or completions of the activities described by the branches.

*Simulation**

Alternative *configurations* for materials-management systems were discussed in chapter 2 of this book. Chapter 3 discussed a number of issues

---

*This section is based on A. Reisman, "Simulation: An Emulator of Systems," in *Systems Analysis in Health-Care Delivery* by A. Reisman (Lexington, Mass.: Lexington Books, D.C. Heath and Company, 1979).

associated with choices of proper materials-management information systems, and chapter 4 discussed alternative decision rules that can be used in managing replenishments of inventories at the various stocking locations. Finally, most of this chapter was dedicated to presenting a number of techniques for analyzing or documenting various aspects of the MMS. This section will discuss computer-aided simulation, a technique that has been found extremely useful for emulating existing or projected MMS configurations, systems, and procedures.

Among its many attributes, simulation provides a vehicle for describing the dynamics of the many complex interrelationships among the MMS components and between the MMS and the various institutional units it serves or interacts with. It allows management to see with great clarity, at relatively low cost, and within a highly compressed time frame the impact on the system outputs of any changes in materials information or timing inputs to the MMS, in or modifications in MMS internal policies. Simulation is often referred to as the "laboratory for decision makers." As a laboratory it can be used with equal ease to emulate existing systems behavior or to simulate systems behavior subsequent to any design or redesign. It is therefore often also used as a training device much like the "Link" trainer, a flight simulator that was used to train pilots for night or "blind" flying during and after World War II.

Webster's dictionary defines *simulation* as an act of "assuming the appearance of, without the reality." If one were to paraphrase Webster's definition by saying, "to simulate is to attain the essence of, without the reality," then one would obtain the essential difference between the scientific and lay meanings of the word simulation.

According to Deacon [16], simulation is "a general field of activity having to do with the design, building, manipulation and study of models; 'a simulation' or 'a simulation exercise' being an experiment performed upon a model."

In the field of management science, simulation is seen as "the science of employing computational models as description for the purposes of (1) learning, (2) experimenting, (3) predicting in management problems" [17]. Magar [17] offers yet another, simpler definition of simulation as "the act representing some aspects of the real world by numbers, or other symbols, that can be easily manipulated in order to facilitate its study." He also indicates quite correctly that "in this sense, simulation is one of the oldest analytical tools."

Any or all of these definitions are quite acceptable for the purposes of this book.

### Types of Simulation

There is no complete and fully adequate scheme for classifying types of simulation. However, an attempt toward taxonomy was made when Magar offered two classification schemes. The first scheme classifies different types of simulation on the basis of the degree of abstraction from the real-life system, operation, or procedure enjoyed by the model being manipulated. Under this scheme, the focus is on the model being simulated and its relationship to its real-life counterpart. The other classification scheme is based on the objectives or purposes to be served by the simulation. This latter approach is more relevant to discussions of materials management.

Some of the categories of simulation usage objectives are as follows:

1. *Analysis or evaluation.* Simulation provides the vehicle for emulating real-life system behavior. It makes it possible to evaluate:
   a. The effectiveness of the system as it currently operates. Specifically, it is possible to evaluate the idle time of equipment and of the economics of the operation, the number of patients processed, or the amount of inventory turned over.
   b. The dynamics of the response of the existing system to changes in the external influences, such as patient-visit volume and/or pattern.
   c. The dynamics of the response of the existing system to changes in the internal variables or parameters, such as equipment failure and personnel no-shows.
   d. The intermediate and long-term operating levels, such as revenues and costs.
   e. The sensitivity of the system behavior and/or output to incomplete or imperfect knowledge regarding systems parameters, such as holding or shortage costs in inventory control, or cost of borrowed capital (mortgages) in investment decisions.
2. *Synthesis or design.* Simulation provides a laboratory or a "testbed" for pretesting the effects of:
   a. New decision rules or policies in existing organizations, such as alternative supplies-replenishment policies for central stores; alternative policies for scheduling clinic patients; and alternative frequencies, schedules, and routes for pickup and delivery trucks.
   b. Changes in organizational structures, such as redesigning manpower configurations, truck-fleet organization, and so on.
   c. Designing new organizations, for example, their configurations, which include the size and mix of the workforce.
3. *Training.* Simulation has traditionally been used for training purposes. War games and the "Link" trainers for nighttime or blind flying are only a few examples of simulation not necessarily aided by computers. Management games, however, are recent examples of the use of simulation for training.
4. *Demonstration.* Simulation is a very powerful device for demonstrating to management how their systems currently operate, how management thinks they operate, and how they will operate if the recommended

changes are instituted. Simulation also can be and has been used to track the behavior of proposed systems and procedures on actual and current data while the old systems are still operative.

### Attributes of Computer-Aided Simulation

Among the various attributes of simulation are:

1. *Time compression*. Through the use of simulation, one can compress or expand real time. The effect of a given policy decision on the actual system might not be felt fully for months or even years. However, the same effect could be studied through simulation in a matter of seconds or minutes. Moreover, the effect of alternate decisions could be similarly pretested and compared. On the other hand, short-order effects, such as an unusually large order for a manufacturing operation, a minor epidemic, or a major industrial accident, can often be scrutinized best if their effect through time can be expanded. This is also possible through simulation.

2. *Pretesting*. Simulation provides the vehicle that can be used to experiment with, test, and evaluate new systems with speed and accuracy and to propose changes in existing systems before having to make firm commitments.

3. *Economy*. Simulation allows for experimentation which often is far more economical than tests on the actual systems or even prototypes. This economy is reflected in both time and money.

4. *Reproducibility*. Simulation allows one to reproduce an experiment performed on a model at different times and in different locations.

5. *Replication*. Simulation allows for the replication of experiments under different conditions. A noteworthy example of this is the replication of economic time-series data, which just could not be accomplished without simulation.

However, it is worthwhile to note here that simulation may also have the following disadvantageous attributes:

1. High costs of modeling and programming. Whenever possible, it is often cheaper to obtain a mathematically derived or analytical solution than to have a simulation model developed and programmed for computer solution.

2. It is often costly to run simulation programs on a computer. This is especially true for models that are large or that must be solved for many numerical values of key variables or parameters.

3. Simulation will rarely yield the optimal solution. Even when the solution so obtained is the best possible solution, it is difficult to establish that this is so, whereas there is rarely any doubt about analytically derived optima.

4. It is at times difficult to validate a simulation model in terms of its faithfulness in reproducing the real system.

The most important and useful tools of simulation are the advanced computers. Had computers not been developed to today's levels, simulation would not be a useful and applicable approach to the study of systems. The various techniques for computer-aided simulation and their applications in health-care and other institutions are discussed in a variety of books and journals (see the Further Readings in Simulation listed at the back of [1]).

## References

1. Reisman, Arnold. *Systems Analysis in Health-Care Delivery*, Lexington, Mass.: Lexington Books, D.C. Heath and Company, 1979.
2. Ireson, W. Grant, and Grant, Eugene L. *Handbook of Industrial Engineering and Management*, 2d ed. Englewood Cliffs, N.J.: Prentice-Hall, 1971.
3. Taylor, F.W. *Scientific Management*. New York and London: Harper and Brothers (3d rev. by the publishers), 1947.
4. Lytle, C.W. *Job Evaluation Methods*, 2d ed. New York: Ronald Press, 1954.
5. Maynard, H.B., ed. *Industrial Engineering Handbook*, 2d ed. New York: McGraw-Hill, 1963.
6. Karger, D.W., and Bayha, F.H. *Engineered Work Measurement*, 2d ed. New York: Industrial Press, 1965.
7. Lott, M.R. "Wage Scales and Job Evaluation." *Management and Administration*, May 1925.
8. Benge, E.J. "Gauging the Job's Worth." *Industrial Relations* 3, nos. 2, 3, 4.
9. Livy, B. *Job Evaluation: A Critical Review*. New York: Halsted-Wiley, 1975.
10. Kress, A.L. National Trades Association Bulletin no. 3, parts I-VII of the Industrial Relations Policies and Procedures. Also, *Job Rating Manual and Hourly Job Rating Plan*. NEMA Industrial Department, 1953.
11. American Association for Industrial Management. *Job Rating Manual*. Melrose Park, Pa., 1969.
12. Dean, B.V.; Reisman, A.; and Svestka, J.A. "Job Evaluation Upholds Discrimination Suit." *Industrial Engineering* 3 (March 1971):28-31.
13. Dean, B.V.; Reisman, A.; and Svestka, J.A. "Guilty of Job Discrimination?" *Automation* 18 (July 1971):51-54.
14. Chapin, N. "Flow Charting with the ANSI Standard: A Tutorial." *Computing Surveys*, June 1970, pp. 119-143.

15. Reisman, Arnold. *Managerial and Engineering Economics*. Boston: Allyn and Bacon Publishing Company, 1971.
16. Deacon, A.R.L. *Simulation and Gaming: A Symposium*. American Management Association, AMA-55, 1961.
17. Magar, V.D. "Simulation, Its Forms and Applications." Unpublished papers, January 1965.

# Appendix 5A: Checklist for Evaluating MMS Systems and Procedures

|  | Comments (Provide data on "yes" answers. Explain "no" answers.) | |
|---|---|---|
| *Questions* | *Yes* | *No* |
| A. Do inventories include: | | |
|    1. Materials and supplies for use of health providers? | _____ | _____ |
|    2. Maintenance parts and supplies for service units, such as dietary? | _____ | _____ |
|    3. Stationary stock and administrative supplies? | _____ | _____ |
| B. Are there written inventory or stocking procedures for each type of material mentioned in question A? | _____ | _____ |
| C. Are the inventory procedures supervised by a responsible person(s)? | _____ | _____ |
| D. Are there written instructions for: | | |
|    1. Good physical arrangement of stock? | _____ | _____ |
|    2. Identification of stock by persons responsible for the stock? | _____ | _____ |
|    3. Determining quantities on hand, and on order. | _____ | _____ |
|    4. Determining quantities and timing of reorders. | _____ | _____ |
|    5. Verification of individual counts? | _____ | _____ |
|    6. Control of inventory tags or sheets? | _____ | _____ |
|    7. Segregation and description of slow moving, obsolete, or damaged items? | _____ | _____ |
|    8. Determining merchandise on hand that is not hospital property? | _____ | _____ |

| | *Comments (Provide data on "yes" answers. Explain "no" answers.)* | |
|---|---|---|
| *Questions* | *Yes* | *No* |
| E.   Are materials requisitions signed by the persons receiving the material? | _____ | _____ |
| F.   Are receiving reports under numerical control? | _____ | _____ |
| G.   Is there a procedure for investigating and adjusting differences between dollar amounts in perpetual-inventory records and the controlling account records? | _____ | _____ |

# 6

# Data Collection

## Types of Data

Whenever a materials-management system (MMS) or some subset thereof is being documented, analyzed, redesigned, controlled, or queried, some form of data collection is needed. Some of these data can be secured in hard form, for example, transactions that are counted or measured; quantities of items ordered, shipped, or used; number of patients serviced, supplies received, or units produced; and so on. Similarly, some system parameters may be obtained in hard form, for example, unit costs of personnel, space, supplies, and the like; number of people staffing a particular department; number of central supply rooms; investment in plant or equipment; and so on.

At the other extreme, it is not uncommon to find that system-information input requirements are unavailable in hard form or are uncollectable. Some typical examples are the cost of stockouts of supplies (for example, the cost of not having an item "on the shelf" when a health worker needs it) and the cost of patients' waiting time.

Between these two extremes there is a broad spectrum of data classes that can be collected in hard form, but at a cost. The costs range from trivial to prohibitive. Also, there are classes of data that, although collectable at some cost, require time for collection. The collection time span may be prohibitive from the point of view of the project or of the organization for which the data are needed. Then there are information inputs that by their very nature simply cannot be counted or measured, regardless of time and cost. Yet these inputs may very well be key to the success of, say, an MMS study. The analyst needs to be flexible and broad based in designing a data-collection process.

When it is possible and economical to obtain hard data by counting or measuring, this is preferable. The choice in such cases is between taking a census and conducting a survey (sampling). The size of the total "population" or amount of data collected is a tradeoff between the manageability (that is, the work required to collect, process, and interpret the data once secured) and the level of statistical significance or confidence desired for

This chapter is based on A. Reisman, "Data Collection," in *Systems Analysis in Health-Care Delivery*, by A. Reisman, Chapter 5 (Lexington, Mass.: Lexington Books, D.C. Heath and Company, 1979).

the results. When the costs of data collection and/or processing are related to sample size and are significant, then the tradeoffs are between costs and statistical significance.

At the other extreme, when data are by nature not collectable, then recourse is made to obtaining subjective judgments from the most knowledgeable people available. One extreme for obtaining subjective judgments is to get a single expert to express his or her opinion. The other extreme is to obtain a formal consensus from a well-designed panel of knowledgeable people using some formal, interactive, consensus-seeking process, such as the Delphi method [1,2,3,4]. Clearly, interviews, questionnaires, and so on, taken on either a census or a survey basis, are midrange possibilities. If necessary for the systems study, even the highly subjective data bits mentioned earlier can be quantified—not measured, not counted, but, yes, quantified. The remainder of this chapter will present the various techniques of data collection within the objective-subjective spectrum for the purposes of system description, evaluation, and valuation. As indicated in [3], much of this discussion is also applicable to forecasting demand for services, cash flows, and so on.

**Means for Data Acquisition**

*Census*

In the acquisition of data regarding any population, two approaches can be pursued. Information may be obtained by taking a complete enumeration of the characteristic of the population about which data are sought. This is called *taking a census*. Alternatively, a section of the population can be selected from which the population characteristic of interest can be inferred from the sample characteristic. This is referred to as *taking a sample* or *survey sampling*. Examples of both these approaches abound in practice. Where the population is finite, a census may be taken. A *physical inventory* or a complete count of all sutures or surgical gloves at a given location or facility is an example of a census. For a large population, say, the membership in a large health-maintenance organization (HMO), only a sample may be required for establishing characteristics of the user population.

Although a complete census might be prohibitively expensive in terms of both time and money, it does possess special advantages in some situations, such as in the testing of hospital-based equipment for electrical safety. In such cases, taking a complete census could be beneficial for the following reasons: (1) data for small population units can be obtained; (2) acceptance by regulatory agents and by health workers is better secured; (3) bias of coverage may be easier to check and reduce; and (4) sophisticated sampling techniques need not be used.

*Sampling Procedures*

Essentially there are two kinds of sampling procedures: *nonprobability sampling* and *probability sampling.* In nonprobability sampling, probabilities cannot be assigned to the units objectively, and hence the reliability of the sample results in terms of probability cannot be determined. Some examples of this procedure are *judgment sampling* and *quota sampling.* In judgment sampling, an expert selects a representative sample according to his or her expert subjective judgment. For example, a purchasing agent may be asked to select 10 vendors from a group of 200 for purposes of estimating the average delivery lead time of all the vendors in a given category. He or she may select 10 vendors who are thought to be representative of all the vendors, according to his or her own expert subjective judgment. Thus the reliability of the results depends on judgment and not on objective criteria such as probability theory. This, of course, does not imply that the method is of no use; in some cases it may be necessary to use this method, the results may be good, and the procedure may be economical. In *quota sampling,* more explicit instructions are provided about what to select. Thus in order to estimate the utilization of health services and hence the average materials usage by groups (about equal in size) of enrollees in an HMO, the surveyor may specify that the field worker select six families from each group. He may further specify that of the six selected, two should be from the upper-income bracket, two from the middle-, and two from the lower-income bracket, if that is the approximate ratio of the income brackets in the group. Subject to these conditions, he would leave any further selection process up to the field worker.

*Survey Sampling*

As mentioned before, survey sampling deals with the selecting and observing of a part (sample) of the population in order to make inferences about the population. A sample can have several advantages over a complete census: (1) economy in expenditure is generally assured since only a fraction of the aggregate is being handled; (2) speed and timeliness are greater then in a complete census for the same reason; (3) feasibility is generally greater because, for instance, if the observation is "destructive," as in destructive testing of equipment components, a census is not practical; and (4) quality and accuracy are in most cases better because there are many situations in which money simply cannot buy the trained personnel required for a good census. Because sampling plays such a large part in our lives—indeed, our knowledge, actions, and even attitudes are based to a large extent on samples—the principal steps involved in survey sampling are elaborated here:

1. Decide on the objectives of the survey.
2. Clearly define the population to be sampled.
3. Ascertain the data to be collected.
4. Specify the degree of precision desired (see [5] for the various objective tests available for establishing the precision or confidence levels of a sample).
5. Choose the method of measurement.
6. Construct the list of sampling units by dividing the population into appropriate parts.
7. Select the sample. (Stratification of the population to be sampled may often be necessary. This is discussed later in this chapter.)
8. Pretest the methodology.
9. Organize the field work, including data collection.
10. Summarize and analyze the data collected.
11. Make provisions to record the information gained for future surveys.

In summary, it may be said that the field worker is given definite quotas to fill and that these quotas are determined (by the surveyor) to a certain extent from the population characteristics so that the quota sample will be representative of the population.

In contrast to the preceding methods, *probability sampling*, as its name suggests, is objective and based on the laws of probability. Operationally, the sample is obtained in successive draws of a unit, each with a known probability of selection assigned at the first draw. Several refinements of this technique have been designed. One is *simple random sampling* (SRS), in which an equal probability of selection is assigned to each unit of the population at the first draw. The method implies an equal probability of selecting any unit from among the available units at subsequent draws. Thus, if the number of units in the population is $N$, the probability of selecting any unit at the first draw will be $1/N$, the probability of selecting any unit from among the available units at the second draw is $1/(N-1)$, and so on. A practical procedure to follow in selecting a simple random sample would be to (1) identify the $N$ units by preparing a list of $N$ units in the population and serially numbering them, (2) select different numbers from a table of random numbers (tables of random numbers are generally available [6]), and (3) take for the sample the units whose numbers correspond to those drawn from the table of random numbers. This procedure has been widely used in work-sampling surveys, equipment-utilization studies, and so on.

Another approach is called *stratified random sampling*. In this technique the population is divided first into nonoverlapping subpopulations called *strata*. Simple random samples are next selected from each stratum, and these are finally combined into a single sample to estimate the population parameters. Many real-life situations call for the use of this technique rather than for simple random sampling. The first and basic reason for this is that it may increase precision. (The conditions under which greater precision is assured form part of the statistical theory of sampling, which is beyond the scope of this text.) A second reason is that information concerning individual strata may be desired. Finally, it may make data collection easier for either physical or administrative reasons. A very practical case in which stratified random sampling could profitably be applied is given below.

Suppose it is desired to estimate the frequency of orders, delivery lead times, stockouts, and so on of consumables in a hospital. It is known that the majority of items have a small or middle-sized unit dollar value and/or small activity—there are few very expensive and/or highly used items. It is also known that these very-high-dollar-value items account for a substantial amount of the total annual expenditures. In other words, the dollar-value distribution of items is highly skewed. If the SRS procedure is applied to such a distribution, there is a chance that either none or too many of the very-large-dollar-value items may be included in the sample. As a result, the sample may not adequately represent the population. Alternatively, if stratified random sampling is done, the items would be divided into small-, medium-, and large-dollar-value groups. A certain number of items would then be selected from each of the three groups by simple random sampling, and the average inventory-management data would be estimated from this combined sample. Statistical theory does indeed confirm that in such a situation, stratified random sampling is more truly representative of the population than is simple random sampling.

A quick, economical modification of SRS is called *systematic sampling*. In contrast to the former method, in which units are drawn randomly, in the latter only the first unit is randomly drawn. Every subsequent draw is made according to a predetermined pattern. The result is a time- and effort-economical method of sampling, which under certain situations is more efficient than simple random sampling. For example, suppose a purchasing-department manager wants to know whether users of a health plan prefer one standard product used in delivery of care to another. Suppose further that there are 50,000 subscriber users, and that the manager wishes to select a random sample of 1,000 subscribers to investigate this problem. Using systematic sampling he picks up his list of 50,000 names and selects the first name at random from the first 50 names. Suppose this procedure results in the selection of the twentieth name. Then, starting with this name he would select every fiftieth name from his list; that is, he would select numbers 20, 70, 120, 170, . . . , 49, 970.

A fourth important approach to probability sampling is called *cluster sampling*. In this method the sampling units that are to be selected are initially arranged in clusters, and a random sampling of these clusters is done.

An example will make this clear. Suppose an estimate of the weekly expenditure on prescription drugs of families in New York City is desired. To use simple random sampling, it is necessary to have a list of these families. For all practical purposes, this is impossible to get. A similar problem is faced in systematic sampling. To apply stratified random sampling, New York City must be stratified so that similar income groups are in the same situation, if possible. This is at best a time-consuming and difficult task. Thus intuitively it can be seen that it would make the sampling survey easier in terms of preparation, cost, and administration if the sampling units to be selected were in clusters. For example, suppose New York City is divided into $M$ voting districts. Each voting district may be seen as a cluster of families. Then a random sampling of $m$ voting districts is selected. (The number in the sample $m$ is, of course, smaller than the number $M$ of voting districts.) In other words, instead of selecting families one at a time, $n$ groups of families are selected, with each group living in the same voting district. Random samples of $n_1, n_2, \ldots, n_m$ families are selected from each of the $m$ districts, and the sample sought is $n = n_1 + n_2 + \ldots + n_m$. When sampling units are selected in this fashion, a list is needed only of the $m$ voting districts and of the families in the $m$ voting districts that were selected. Furthermore, since the families that have been selected are clustered in voting districts, they will be easier to visit than if scattered throughout the population. Thus the overall administration of the sampling plan is also easier. In many cases, this reduction in cost and ease of administration allows a selection of a larger sample than would be the case if SRS were used, and this larger sample may more than compensate in terms of precision for the use of cluster sampling.

The preceding discussion by no means exhausts the list of sampling techniques available to the researcher or manager of materials. Methods such as multistage sampling, stratified cluster sampling, and replicated sampling are used in practice. All these techniques are modifications or extensions of the four basic probability-sampling techniques discussed earlier.

*Example of Stratified Random Sampling*

In the study concerned with the management of consumables and/or disposables for a large multifacility health center, it was necessary to collect hard transactions data for a sample of the 1,700 or so items the center handled as standard stock. Some items were much more expensive than others. Some moved in large quantities per any unit of time, while others experienced small movement in any given year. The hard data required are as follows:

1. Replenishment orders from the warehouse to the vendors.
2. Warehouse receipts.
3. Orders from the facility's central supply to the warehouse.
4. Central supply receipts.
5. Orders from departments to either the warehouse or the facility's central supply.
6. Departmental receipts.

The stratification and sampling technique used for selecting the items for which the transactions data were kept is described next. In order to see which items are controlling the investment in the inventory, an *ABC* analysis was performed. This classification was also used for the sampling plan and ultimately for the optimal control of inventory:

*Class A*: Items that account for a high percentage of the annual dollar usage value, usually a low percentage of items.

*Class B*: Items that account for a very low percentage of annual dollar usage value, usually a high percentage of items.

*Class C*: The remaining items.

The results of the ABC analysis are shown in figure 6-1.

Since a working unit of 1,700 items was unmanageable and expensive for purposes of the study, a stratified random sample consisting of 170 items was selected from the standard-stock items. This constituted about 10 percent of the number of items and accounted for 60 percent of annual purchase value. Following the sampling plan, most of the items were selected from group *A*, with the fewest items chosen from group *C*. The sample was enriched by other items so that it accurately represented all items carried in the inventory.

This sample of items was traced through the inventory-flow process and used for the analyses that were performed. The size of the sample was 10 to 15 percent of the total number of items, and it is shown in table 6-1.

*Work Measurement*

The term *work measurement* applies to all techniques that are used to arrive at a time value for the accomplishment of work. By far the most common applications of work-measurement techniques are to be found in production-type jobs such as those in the laundry, dietary, and housekeeping departments. This is true because such jobs must of necessity use standard-

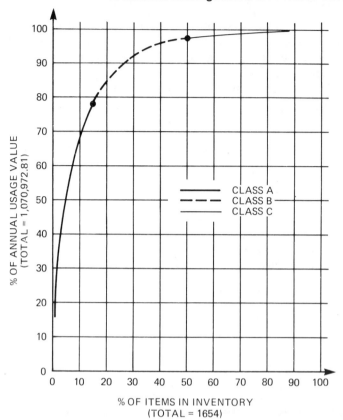

Arnold Reisman, *Systems Analysis in Health-Care Delivery* (Lexington, Mass.: Lexington Books, D.C. Heath and Company, 1979).

**Figure 6-1.** *ABC* Usage-Analysis Curve

ized materials, tools, and methods in order to produce identical operations. It therefore becomes a condition of work measurement that the exact criteria for which the standard was originally set must be maintained throughout the usefulness of the standard. Brief descriptions of the more common techniques of work measurement follow.

1. *Predetermined human work times.* In this technique, "basic" movements of hand and body members are assigned time values on the order of fractions of a second, and the time necessary to perform a given unit of work is built up by addition of these times. This technique is valuable in detailed job planning and estimating. It requires skilled personnel, and it has found its greatest application in production shops with appropriate volume to justify the expense.

2. *Stopwatch time study.* This is the technique most widely used at present in work measurement. In this type of measurement, a careful methods

**Table 6-1**
**Distribution of the Detailed Sampling-Plan Purchase Values of Items**

| Usage Value ($) | Frequency of Items | Number of Items to be Sampled | Ratio Used for for Sampling |
|---|---|---|---|
| 0-200 | 975 | 20 | 1/50 |
| 200.01-400 | 194 | 10 | 1/20 |
| 400.01-600 | 123 | 6 | 1/20 |
| 600.01-800 | 74 | 7 | 1/10 |
| 800.01-1,000 | 41 | 7 | 1/6 |
| 1,000.01-1,200 | 41 | 7 | 1/6 |
| 1,200.01-1,400 | 22 | 4 | 1/5 |
| 1,400.01-1,600 | 23 | 5 | 1/5 |
| 1,600.01-1,800 | 16 | 4 | 1/4 |
| 1,800.01-2,000 | 9 | 2 | 1/4 |
| 2,000.01-2,200 | 13 | 3 | 1/4 |
| 2,200.01-2,400 | 10 | 3 | 1/3 |
| 2,400.01-2,600 | 14 | 4 | 1/3 |
| 2,600.01-2,800 | 10 ⎫ | 5 | 1/2 |
| 2,800.01-3,000 | 8 ⎪ | | |
| 3,000.01-3,200 | 4 ⎪ | | |
| 3,200.01-3,400 | 11 ⎬ | All | 1 |
| 3,400.01-3,600 | 3 ⎪ | | |
| 3,600.01-3,800 | 8 ⎪ | | |
| 3,800.01-4,000 | 3 ⎪ | | |
| 4,000.01-6,800 | 50 ⎭ | | |

description is made of a task, and the task is then subdivided into elements for timing. An observer watches the task as it is performed and notes the time taken to accomplish it. The observer may then "rate" the observed times; this simply means that he adjusts the observed time to some standard of performance. Sometimes rating is not done, but rather a fixed proportion of the observed time is taken as standard.

3. *Elemental times or standard data.* This technique consists of the tabulation of elements from stopwatch time study according to physical characteristics of the workpiece and the building up of time standards by combining these elements. In using elemental times or standard data in this manner, less-precise results are obtained, but the expense of work measurement is also less.

4. *Historical or statistical data.* This technique is widely used in those work situations where it is felt that detailed studies are not justified because of variations in jobs received or because the expense involved seems too great for the possible savings in labor or better management. Very simply, some physical characteristics of the product or job are related to the time it has taken in the past to do jobs with similar characteristics. No detailed methods description is made, but such standards are a great deal better than no standards at all.

5. *Subjective overall evaluation.* This term may be applied to the common situation in which management and supervision make use of past experience and tradition to determine employee workloads. There is no measurement in the commonly accepted sense of the word.

It is immediately apparent that wide differences exist in work-measurement techniques. These differences lie in the degree of detail of methods description, the precision of the result, the degree of subjective judgment involved, the timing device used, the skill and experience of the technician performing the measurement, and the cost.

In any given situation, there are no hard and fast rules governing the use of a particular technique. Each management must use its own judgment in the matter, realizing that many of the techniques are somewhat versatile and that the conditions surrounding the use of the various techniques should be considered before an attempt is made to select a particular one. Further discussion of work-measurement and job-evaluation methods can be found in [7], [8], and [9].

*Work Sampling*

Work sampling is a measurement technique for the quantitative analysis, in terms of time, of the activities of people, of equipment, or of any observable state or condition of an operation or process. It is a technique that is particularly useful in the analysis of nonrepetitive or irregularly occurring activities, where no complete methods and frequency descriptions are available. It is also an extremely useful device with which to make an inexpensive overall survey of office, workroom, or service activities. Such a preliminary study can help in evaluating the need for further studies, and it may serve to establish work and/or compensation standards. Because it is extremely convenient, possesses known reliability, and operates without recourse to the stopwatch or subjective judgments of "effort" or "performance," work sampling has found wide acceptance in current managerial practice.

Essentially, a work-sampling study consists of a large number of observations taken at random intervals. In this process the state or condition of the object of study is noted and classified into predefined categories of activity pertinent to the particular work situation. From the proportions of observations in each category, inferences are drawn concerning the total work activity under study. As an oversimplified example, if a group of maintenance men are observed to be "waiting" in one-third of the observations made of their activity, a manager might draw the inference that better scheduling or supervision rather than increased crew size represents the most fruitful area for improvement.

The underlying theory in work sampling is that the percentage of observations recording a man or machine as idle, working, or in any other condition reflects, to a known degree of accuracy, the average percentage of time actually spent in that state or condition. If observations are randomly distributed over a sufficiently long period of time, this theory is held to be true regardless of the nature of the observed activity. An essential condition for using the technique, therefore, is that observations be taken at random. *Randomness*, in the sampling sense, requires that the time interval selected for observation has a likelihood equal to that of any other time interval. There is no apparent order to the times of observation, and thus observation time is independent of all other observation times. Finally, the entire period of time over which samples are taken must be subject to selection as the random times of observation are drawn. The exact degree of reliability of the study can be regulated very simply by varying the number of observations made.

The procedure for the taking of a work-sampling study divides itself naturally into three phases. The phases and tasks are as follows:

1. Preparing for work sampling:
   a. Deciding on the objectives of the study.
   b. Establishing and recording quantitative measures of production and so on with which results of the study may be correlated.
   c. Selection and training of personnel.
2. Performing work sampling:
   a. Classifying into categories the activities to be studied.
   b. Designing the necessary forms.
   c. Developing properly randomized times of observations.
   d. Observing activity and recording data.
3. Evaluating and presenting the results of work sampling:
   a. Evaluating the validity of data.
   b. Evaluating the reliability of data.
   c. Presenting and analyzing data.
   d. Planning for future studies.

As an example, work sampling was used to review the unavoidable-delay allowance of 8.5 percent for laundry personnel. For sampling purposes, the work was divided into three states: (1) the idle state owing to unavoidable delays, (2) the idle state for any reason other than unavoidable delays, and (3) the working state. An unavoidable delay was identified whenever

1. The worker was talking to a supervisor.
2. Lack of material occurred.

3. Maintenance or repair of equipment was taking place.
4. There was a general disruption of service.

Any activity not falling into the working or unavoidable-delay states was classified as unaccounted-for time. Personal time, fatigue allowances, and other special allowances were included in this category.

A tally sheet was developed for recording observations. Then the observers were trained to identify the three states easily from the observed postures of the workers. The specific people to be observed were chosen randomly.

In order to have sufficient accuracy it was found that the number of observations had to exceed 4,300. Based on this estimate, 45 observations of five workers per observation were taken each day for twenty days. A different schedule for observations was made every day by referring to a table of random numbers.

After 4,500 observations the total for the three states showed the following proportions:

| States | Observations | Percentages |
|---|---|---|
| Unavoidable delay | 374 | 8.3 |
| Unaccounted-for time | 293 | 6.5 |
| Working time | 3,833 | 85.2 |
| Totals | 4,500 | 100.0 |

Thus the existing unavoidable-delay allowance appeared to be correct.

In conclusion, it must be pointed out that to be effective, work sampling must be done properly. Objectives must be set that are attainable through the use of the technique. Management must lend its support to the study and must make proper use of the results. If these conditions are met, a work sampling becomes a convenient, reliable, and economical tool for managers to appraise their operations. Work sampling is discussed in greater detail in [10].

As indicated earlier, whenever hard or objective data are uncollectable, recourse must be made to subjective inputs or judgments. Various techniques for doing this have been developed and used. Most if not all of them are discussed in chapter 5 of [11].

**References**

1. Helmer, O. *Convergence of Expert Consensus Through Feedback.* Santa Monica, Calif.: Rand Corporation, 1964.

2. Pill, J. "The Delphi Method: Substance, Context, A Critique and an Annotated Bibliography." *Socio Economic Planning Sciences* 5 (1971): 57-71.

3. Reisman, A. *Managerial and Engineering Economics.* Boston: Allyn and Bacon, 1970.

4. Mantel, S.J., Jr.; Service, A.; Reisman, A.; Koleski, R.A.; Blum, A.; Dean, B.V.; Reich, R.; Jaffee, M.; Reiger, H.; Ronis, R.; and Rubinstein, J. "A Social Service Measurement Model." *Operations Research* 23 (1975):218-240.

5. Hoel, P.G., and Jessen, R.J. *Elementary Statistics for Business and Economics.* New York: John Wiley and Sons, 1971.

6. Hayes, E.H., and Romig, H.G. *Modern Quality Control.* Encino, Calif.: Bruce Publishing, 1977.

7. Maynard, H.B.G.; Stegmerten, G.J.; and Schwab, J.L. *Methods Time Measurement.* New York: McGraw-Hill, 1948.

8. Buffa, E.S. *Basic Production Management.* New York: John Wiley and Sons, 1971.

9. Barnes, R.M. *Motion and Time Study: Design and Measurement of Work*, 6th ed. New York: John Wiley and Sons, 1968.

10. Barnes, R.M. *Work Sampling.* Dubuque, Iowa: W.C. Brown Company, 1956.

11. Reisman, Arnold. *Systems Analysis in Health-Care Delivery.* Lexington, Mass.: Lexington Books, D.C. Heath and Company, 1979.

# Selected References: Purchasing and Materials Management

The American Hospital Association publishes the *Hospital Literature Index* on a quarterly basis.

## Purchasing

Aljian, George. *Purchasing Handbook*, 3rd ed. New York: McGraw-Hill, 1973.

Ammer, Dean S. *Purchasing and Materials Management for Health Care Institutions.* Lexington, Mass.: Lexington Books, D.C. Heath and Company, 1975.

Ammer, D.S. *Hospital Materials Management: Neglect and Inefficiency Promote High Costs of Care.* Boston, Mass.: Northeastern University, 1975.

Bellettini, J. Suppliers should share the blame for soaring hospital costs. *Hospital Purchasing Management* 3 (January 1978):15-16.

Blaes, S.M. Emerging legal responsibilities in hospital purchasing and materials management. *Hospital Purchasing* 21 (July-August 1977).

Boergadine, L.C. Prudent buyer. *Hospital Financial Management* 32 (February 1978):4.

Bremhorst, P.J. What you should expect from a salesperson. *Purchasing Administration* 1 (May-June 1977).

Burton, G.D. Purchasing performance: Best way to get it is to measure it. *Hospital Purchasing Management* 2 (January 1977):11-14.

Buying groups change the rules for winning vendor performance. *Hospital Purchasing Management* 2 (June 1977):13-15.

Campbell, G.R. How to organize a successful centralized purchasing program. *Hospitals, JAHA* 51 (December 1977):16, 91, 94-95.

Can every supplier be a prime vendor? *Hospital Purchasing Management* 2 (August 1977):8-10.

Certification: Sellers stampede; buyers, central service supers inch toward it. *Purchasing Administration* 1 (March-April 1977):12-13.

Dowst, S. Performance measurement: Job evaluation takes more than numbers. *Purchasing*, July 26, 1977, p. 26.

Engelman, R.M. Hospital "cap" planners call for careful buyers. *Medical Products Salesman* 8 (June 1977):5.

Esta, D. Leasing: Look at the bottom line. *Hospital Purchasing Management* 3 (January 1978):10-12.

Forward buying: When do rewards outweigh risks? *Hospital Purchasing Management* 3 (January 1978):3-4.

Friedman, W.R., Jr. Role of the purchasing manager in the changing hospital environment. *Osteopathic Hospitals* 21 (October 1977):15-18.

Group purchasing: Old idea gains wide acceptance, new methods boost effectiveness. *Hospital Purchasing Management* 2 (May 1977):5-16.

Heinritz, Stuart F., and Farrell, Paul V. *Purchasing: Principles and Applications*, 5th ed. Englewood Cliffs, N.J.: Prentice-Hall, 1971.

Henry, J.B., and Roenfeldt, R.L. Evaluation of advantages and cost measurement methodology for leasing in the health care industry. *Medical Instrumentation* 11 (January-February 1977):44-47.

Hodgins, B. Must low price mean low quality? *Dimensions in Health Service* (Canada) 54 (October 1977):28.

Housley, C. Stockless purchasing makes dollars and sense. *Dimensions in Health Service* (Canada) 54 (May 1977):24-26.

_____ . Make the most of your suppliers. *Dimensions in Health Service* (Canada) 54 (April 1977):18.

_____ . Case for centralized purchasing. *Dimensions in Health Service* (Canada) 54 (March 1977):20-21.

Joslen, R.A., and Schinderle, D.R. Measuring effectiveness of the purchasing functon. *Michigan Hospitals* 13 (October 1977):13-18.

King, J.G. Group purchasing: A cost containment tool. *Topics in Health Care Financing* 3 (September 1977):19-38.

Kohn, J. Rising prices trim 1977 savings for group buyers: Connecticut. *Modern Healthcare* 7 (April 1977):52-53.

Lauzon, C. Expectations and realities—purchasing style. *Hospital Administration* (Canada) 19 (January 1977):48-49.

Lee, Lamar, Jr., and Dobler, Donald W. *Purchasing and Materials Management*, 3rd ed. New York: McGraw-Hill, 1977.

Levinson, P. Group purchasing has made progress but we cannot afford complacency. *Hospital Purchasing Management* 2 (May 1977):17.

Maddison, L.W. Is there a case for leasing? *Hospital Administration* (Canada) 19 (September 1977):27.

McLaren, A. Harshness of the Tanstaafl: (There ain't no such thing as a free lunch). *Food Management* 12 (March 1977):15-16.

Negotiation: The art and science of making optimum use of your bargaining power. *Hospital Purchasing Management* 2 (October 1977):17.

Nevers, M.R. Purchasing and central supply: It's a marriage of convenience. *Purchasing Administration* 1 (July-August 1977):6.

O'Connell, J.A. Purchasing in the health care field. *Office* 87 (January 1978):86.

Plowden, M.D. We need prudent government even more than "prudent buyers." *Purchasing Administration* 1 (March-April 1977):32-33.

Pollard, T. Growth and development of a group purchasing program: Bellevue, Wash. *Hospitals, JAHA* 51 (May 1977):89.

Powell, P.B. Reduce costs through effective purchasing. *Health Services Manager* 10 (February 1977):9-10.

Product evaluation: Leadership from purchasing is essential to success. *Hospital Purchasing Management* 2 (December 1977):4-10.

Purchasing manager and his job. *Hospital Purchasing Management* 2 (November 1977):3-11.

Rubin, R. Prime vendors can bring $$$ savings. *Purchasing Administration* 1 (July-August 1977):24.

Shaughnessy, S. Back-door ordering: The problem of controlling salesman access. *Purchasing Administration* 1 (May-June 1977):1.

Tabaka, A.V. Seal the loopholes in your purchase order "boilerplate." *Hospital Purchasing Management* 2 (January 1977):15-16; (February 1977):15-16.

Trafas, C.J. Wilmington Medical Center: Write clear specs and let purchasing negotiate equipment contracts. *Hospital Purchasing Management* 2 (March 1977):10.

Twenty-one purchasing price indexes: How to use them, how they are compiled. *Hospital Purchasing Management* 2 (September 1977):10-20.

Unique view: From buying's other side. *Purchasing Administration* 1 (July-August 1977):15.

Vendor performance: Getting better but still not good enough. *Hospital Purchasing Management* 2 (June 1977):7-12.

Wheeler, D.L. Negotiating and bidding for good results. *Hospitals, JAHA* 51 (June 1977):125.

When do purchasing groups violate antitrust laws? *Hospital Purchasing Management* 2 (September 1977):4-5.

Wooldridge, M.G. Prime vendor benefits. *Hospital Administration* (Canada) 19 (January 1977):42.

Yuen, J.Y.S. Group pharmaceutical purchasing means savings and quality. *Dimensions in Health Service* (Canada) 54 (October 1977):37-38.

_____ . Group purchasing means savings and quality. *Dimensions in Health Service* (Canada) 54 (October 1977):37-38.

## Materials Management

Ammer, Dean S. *Hospital Materials Management: Neglect and Inefficiency Promote High Costs of Care.* Boston: Bureau of Business and Economic Research, Northeastern University, 1974.

_____ . *Materials Management,* 3rd ed. Homewood, Ill.: Richard D. Irwin, 1974.

American Hospital Association (AHA). *Readings in Materials Management*. Chicago: AHA, 1973.

Banister, R. Hospital laundry and linen services. *Hospital Development* 5 (November-December 1977):21-22.

Batty, G.R. Plan ahead for good material management. *Hospital Administration* (Canada) 19 (August 1977):18.

Board of directors compiles cost containment checklist. *Hospital Purchasing* 21 (July-August 1977):4-5.

Boehmer, N. Reducing lost charges: Daily cart exchange system. *Purchasing Administration* 1 (May-June 1977):11.

Bolz, E., et al. Is your materials management organization obsolete? *Hospital Purchasing Management* 2 (December 1977):17-20.

Bunetta, Joan M., and Slowiak, Paul. *Material Management Procedural Manual*. Rantoul, Ill.: Hospital Logistics Management, 1974.

Emerzian, A.D. Joseph. *Organizational Forms for Effecting Patient and Material Movement*. Atlanta: Institute of Health Administration, Georgia State University, 1976.

Engelman, R. Hospital materiels managers: The new buying professionals. *Medical Products Salesman* 8 (July 1977):1.

Fox, M.S., et al. New charge system reduces losses for patient-billed items. *Hospitals, JAHA* 51 (November 1977):105-106, 108.

Greene, E.A. Product recalls: More of them, but more ways to handle them. *Purchasing Administration* 1 (July-August 1977):18-19.

Guide to the Medical Device Act. *Purchasing Administration* 1 (March-April 1977):29.

Gunn, Thomas William. *Material Movement Systems Analysis: An Operational Researched Model Which Synthesizes Total Material Movement for the Health Sciences Centre at McMaster University in Hamilton, Ontario, Canada*. Ann Arbor, Mich.: CHI Systems, 1971.

Henning, W.K. Managing materials in today's hospital. *Hospitals, JAHA* 51 (June 1977):82-86.

Housley, C.E. *Hospital Materiel Management*. Germantown, Md.: Aspen Systems Corporation, 1978.

————. Telling the materiel management story. *Dimensions in Health Service* (Canada) 54 (November 1977):22-24.

————. Budgeting for materiel management. *Dimensions in Health Service* (Canada) 54 (October 1977):30-33.

————. Materiel management: let the consumer be the judge. *Dimensions in Health Service* (Canada) 54 (September 1977):40-41.

————. Job description for the materiel manager. *Dimensions in Health Service* (Canada) 54 (August 1977):24-26.

————. Establishing total materiel management. *Dimensions in Health Service* (Canada) 54 (July 1977):18.

————. Distributing the goods the right way. *Dimensions in Health Service* (Canada) 51 (June 1977):103-105.

————. Pharmacist as materiel manager. *Dimensions in Health Service* (Canada) 54 (February 1977):12-13.

————. Materiel management means savings and space. *Dimensions in Health Service* (Canada) 54 (January 1977):11-12.

Iglehart, J.K. Cost and regulation of medical technology: Future policy directions. *Milbank Memorial Fund Quarterly/Health and Society* 55 (Winter 1977):25-59.

Jones, Robert M. *Material Transportation—System Overview Analysis.* Ann Arbor, Mich.: Community Systems Foundation, 1971.

Kowalski, J. Comprehensive materials management: St. Mary's Medical Center, Racine, Wisc. *Hospital Progress* 58 (March 1977):76-83.

Kutilek, R.J., et al. An inexpensive model for a materials management system. *Hospital Topics* 55 (September-October 1977):42-45.

LeGwin, L.C., Jr. Waste containment committees can work. *Southern Hospitals* 45 (September-October 1977):10-11.

Leventhal, E. Computers in future of material management. *Hospital Administration* (Canada) 19 (August 1977):26.

Lo, J.S., et al. A simple cost control format in clinical laboratories. *Clinical Biochemistry* 10 (August 1977):164-167.

Meyer, E.M. Hospitals, manufacturers fuzzy about who's liable in testing new technology. *Modern Healthcare* 7 (August 1977):48.

Moore, G.G. Save on transportation costs. *Hospital Central Service* 11 (January-February 1977):5.

Norris, F.S., et al. Guidelines for defining and disposing of medical waste. *Aviation, Space and Environmental Medicine* 49 (January 1978):81-85.

Order central concept: Unusual approach to paperwork saves nurses time and the hospital money. *Hospital Topics* 55 (July-August 1977):26-29.

Perkins, John H. *Principles and Methods of Sterilization in Health Sciences*, 2nd ed. Springfield, Ill.: Charles C. Thomas, 1973.

Priest, J.L. Gummed labels save time, increase revenue. *Hospital Financial Management* 32 (January 1978):38-39.

Riggs, J.L. *Production Systems: Planning, Analysis, and Control.* New York: John Wiley and Sons, 1976.

Soth, D.G. Material management systems for linen inventory control proposed. *Laundry News* 3 (January 1977):3.

Self-sticking labels help Mt. Auburn (Mass.) Hospital hold on to charges. *Hospital Purchasing Management* 2 (April 1977):14-16.

Schabracq, A. Materiel management: What it is. *Hospital Administration* (Canada) 19 (August 1977):19.

Stadnik, J.K. How to measure materials management effectiveness. *Hospital Purchasing Management* 2 (February 1977):4-6.

Starr, M.K., and Miller, D.W. *Inventory Control: Theory and Practice.* Englewood Cliffs, N.J.: Prentice-Hall, 1962.

Thueson, J. Hospitals' programs and progress in cost containment reported. *Hospitals, JAHA* 51 (September 1977):131-132, 134, 136.

White, A.F. Materiel management: How it works. *Hospital Administration* (Canada) 19 (August 1977):19.

**Inventory**

Accurate inventory system requires work, but results are rewarding. *Laundry News* 3 (September 1977):9.

Ammer, D.S. Have a continuing audit process in your storeroom. *Hospital Purchasing Management* 2 (August 1977):2.

Branch, G.R. Cost control and inventory management in central service. *Texas Hospitals* 33 (July 1977):22-25.

Brown, R.G. *Decision Rules for Inventory Management.* New York: Holt, Rinehart and Winston, 1967.

Buchan, J. and Koenigsberg, E. *Scientific Inventory Management.* Englewood Cliffs, N.J.: Prentice-Hall, 1963.

Buffa, E.S. *Production-Inventory Control Systems: Planning and Control.* Homewood, Ill.: Richard D. Irwin, 1968.

Eilon, S. *Elements of Production Planning and Control.* New York: Macmillan Publishing Company, 1962.

Fetter, R.B., and Dalleck, W.C. *Decision Models for Inventory Management.* Homewood, Ill.: Richard D. Irwin, 1961.

Fisherman, A. For optimum inventory: go back to basics. *Hospital Purchasing Management* 2 (September 1977):6-9.

Giroux, F. Security in stores. *Dimensions in Health Service* 54 (October 1977):20-22.

Hadley, G., and Whitin, T.M. *Analysis of Inventory Systems.* Englewood Cliffs, N.J.: Prentice-Hall, 1963.

Hanssmann, F. *Operations Research in Production and Inventory Control.* New York: John Wiley and Sons, 1962.

Hospitals have inventory ranging from $50 per bed to $1,000 per bed. Why the large variance? *Hospital Forum* (California) 19 (January 1977): 16-17.

Housley, C. What is your inventory and other good questions. *Dimensions in Health Service* 54 (December 1977):37-39.

Schlag, D.W., Jr. Hospitals need proper accounting of inventories. *Federation of American Hospitals Review* 10 (August 1977):46.

Schrock, R.D. Cart exchange system aids financial control. *Hospital Financial Management* 31 (May 1977):50.

Stafford, D. Monitoring materials flow through inventory control. *Hospitals, JAHA* 51 (June 1978):99-101.

Stewart, C.E., Jr. A manual system for storage and inventory control of laboratory supplies. *American Journal of Medical Technology* 43 (September 1977):864-869.

Uneven inventory performance reflects poor organization. *Hospital Purchasing Management* 3 (January 1978):7-9.


**Supplies and Equipment**

Alexander, M. Accountability in selection and use of products in the operating room. *AORN (Association of Operating Room Nurses)* 25 (February 1977):230-232.

Banasik, R.C. Hospital purchasing: developing and measuring performance standards. *Purchasing Administration* 1 (November-December 1977): 16, 18-19, 22.

Begole, C. Analysis of telephone costs, ownership. *Hospitals, JAHA* 51 (April 1977):110-111.

Blessing, J.A. Management considerations in medical equipment acquisition. *Medical Instrumentation* 11 (January-February 1977):35-36.

Boudreau, E.M. Rhode Island Hospital: Regulate capital equipment budget, role played by purchasing grows more important. *Hospital Purchasing Management* 2 (March 1977):11-13.

Buyers guide surveys. *Medical Electronics* 8 (December 1977):71-85.

Disposables vs. reusables: A special report. *Hospital Purchasing Management* 2 (February 1977):7-13.

Harris, J.L. Is your standardization committee really doing its job? *Hospital Purchasing Management* 2 (October 1977):18-19.

Housley, C. Product standardization—a team effort. *Dimensions in Health Service* (Canada) 54 (June 1977):8.

HSA's making hospitals more cautious in buying new imaging equipment. *Modern Healthcare* 7 (August 1977):36.

Kohn, J. Hartford. Consortium Shares Scanner. *Modern Healthcare.* 7 (February 1977):24-25.

Krumrey, N.A. Equipping a new hospital. Bringing method to the madness. *Hospitals, JAHA* 51 (June 1977):109.

Laufman, H. Classification of medical devices and priorities in standards-setting in the United States. *Medical Instrumentation* 11 (May-June 1977):180-182.

Lloyd, R.S. Ohio hospital packs up wasted dollars. *Executive Housekeeper* 24 (March 1977):41.

Medical equipment. *Surgical Business* 40 (December 1977):33-35.

New Medicare law pushes durable equipment buying. *Medical Products Salesman* 8 (December 1977):1, 11.

Nichols, R. Telephones: What to do when you have outgrown or worn out your system. *Hospital Engineering* 22 (July-August 1977):8-9.

Price monitor—disposable syringes: Low-volume users sometimes pay lower prices. *Hospital Purchasing Management* 3 (January 1978):5-6

Schropp, M.L. VA expands testing of medical products. *Medical Products Salesman* 8 (March 1977):28-29.

Simple form brings order to equpment, supply loans. *Hospitals, JAHA* 51 (October 1977:14, 16.

Smith, M. A rational approach for making major equipment purchases. *Hospitals, JAHA* 51 (December 1977):16, 78-79, 82.

Steps taken to reduce cost of medical/surgical supplies. *Hospital Central Service* 11 (July-August 1977):3-4.

Ten tests of capital equipment purchasing effectiveness. *Hospital Purchasing Management* 2 (March 1977):9.

Veterans Administration expands product evaluation program. *Hospital Purchasing Management* 2 (October 1977):9-12.

Wallgren, L.R. How to make your standardization committee more effective. *Hospital Purchasing Management* 2 (October 1977):13-15.

X-ray film prices: The small hospitals sometime do better than the large ones. *Hospital Purchasing Management* 2 (July 1977):4-6.

# Appendix A:
# Glossary of Terms

**ABC analysis.** Breakdown of inventory items into three categories as follows:

A items: The 10-20 percent of items that account for 70-80 percent of the dollar value.

B items: The 30-40 percent of items that account for 15-20 percent of the dollar value.

C items: The 40-50 percent of items that account for 5-10 percent of the dollar value.

**ABC analysis report.** A report showing all inventoried items in descending order of annual dollar volume of usage.

**ABC inventory control.** An inventory-classification system that recognizes that, given any inventory, a small percentage of the number of the components will make up a large percentage of the annual dollar value; and a large percentage of the components will make up a small percentage of the annual dollar value.

**Absorption.** One carrier assumes the charges of another without any increase in charges to the shipper.

**Absorption costing.** A type of product costing that assigns fixed manufacturing overhead to the units produced as a part of product cost.

**Abstract symbol.** A symbol whose form does not suggest its meaning and use. Such symbols must be defined for each specific application.

**Accelerated depreciation.** Depreciation methods that write off the cost of an asset at a faster rate than the writeoff under the straight-line method. The three principal methods of accelerated depreciation are: sum-of-years'-digits, double declining balance, and units of production.

**Acceptable quality level (AQL).** This is a standard for the buyer to use in accepting material that does not, in its entirety, meet specifications. For example, an AQL of 0.98 indicates that the buyer is willing to accept shipments that have 2 percent of the items out of specification or more characteristic properties.

**Acceptance.** A promise to pay by the debtor against whom a draft or bill of exchange has been drawn, usually evidenced by signing the draft or bill and writing "accepted" on its face.

**Access mode.** In COBOL, a technique that is used to obtain a specific logical record from, or to place a specific logical record into, a file assigned to a mass-storage device.

**Access time.** In computer applications, the time interval between the instant at which the data are called for from a storage device and the instant delivery begins.

**Accessorial notice.** A service in addition to the line-haul service, usually at an added cost, consisting of heating, packing, loading, storage, and so on.

**Account number.** The code to which the vendor charges any sales, credits, or adjustments for any items with the purchases.

**Accumulation bin.** Where a product is assembled, this is usually a physical location used to accumulate all the components that go into the assembly before sending the assembly order out to the floor.

**Active inventory.** Covers raw material, work-in-process, and finished products that will be used or sold within the budgeted period without extra cost or loss.

**Activities.** In PERT and CPM, the specific jobs or tasks that are the components of a particular project.

**Activity ratio.** The ratio of the number of records in a file that have activity to the total number of records in the file.

**Add-in memory.** A method of increasing computer memory by adding new circuitry to existing memory. This is distinguished from *add-on* memory, which involves increasing memory by adding additional peripheral devices.

**Address.** The location of an area where data or instructions can be stored in computer-related equipment, such as the main memory unit of the central processing unit or direct-access devices like magnetic disk and magnetic drum. The address is stated as a number. Persons working with higher-level programming languages seldom if ever directly use the storage address. It is maintained within the computer system.

**Administered vertical marketing systems.** The necessary coordination of production and marketing activities achieved essentially through the domination of one powerful channel member.

**Adoption notice.** One carrier lawfully takes over another carrier's operations and obligations.

**ADP system (automatic data-processing system).** Data processing performed by a system of electronic or electrical machines so interconnected and interacting as to reduce to a minimum the need for human assistance or intervention. Synonymous with EDP (electronic data processing).

**Advertising.** Communications about a product or service that are nonpersonal, paid for, identified with the firm, and intended to encourage consumer purchase.

**Advice notice.** The usual document used when goods are sent any appreciable distance. The note is posted in advance to warn the customer that the goods are on the way.

**Agent wholesaler.** Middleman who does not take title to the goods he handles.

**Aggregate inventory.** The sum of the inventory levels for individual items. For example, the aggregate finished-goods inventory would be made up of one-half the sum of all the lot sizes plus the sum of all the safety stocks plus any anticipation or seasonal inventory.

**Aggregate-inventory management.** Specifically, planning the overall levels of inventory that will be required and making sure that the individual reordering techniques execute this overall policy.

**Aging schedule.** A report showing how long accounts receivable have been outstanding. It gives the percentage of receivables now past due and the percentage past due by, for example, one month, two months, or other periods.

**ALGOL (ALGOrithmic Language).** An international language to represent and communicate information using algebraic symbols.

**Algorithm.** A prescribed set of well-defined rules or processes for the solution of a problem in a finite number of steps. The algorithmic approach is in contrast with the heuristic approach.

**Allocation.** Assigning one or more items of cost or revenue to one or more segments of an organization according to benefits received, responsibilities, or other logical measures of use.

**Alphanumeric.** A contraction of alphabet-numeric, the system of communication employing letters of the alphabet, numerals, and other symbols such as punctuation or mathematical symbols.

**Alphanumeric data.** The set of data that includes the letters A-Z, the numbers 0-9 and special symbols like $+$, $-$, \$, #, *, ., and so on.

**Amortize.** To liquidate on an installment basis; an amortized loan is one in which the principal amount of the loan is repaid in installments during the life of the loan.

**Amount to reorder.** A predetermined amount of material to be ordered, usually calculated by same decision rule, such as the economic lot size.

**Analog.** The representation of numerical quantities, generally by means of continuously variable physical quantities. Contrast with digital (computer).

**Analog plotter.** A type of printer (device) that takes digital or discrete entities as generated by a digital computer and plots them out in a continuous fashion.

**Analytical model.** An operational representation of a given problem in terms of mathematical, graphical, or verbal symbols.

**Annual-usage value.** The number of units forecasted or used over a year multiplied by the item's unit cost.

**Annuity.** A series of payments of a fixed amount for a specified number of years.

**Anticipation.** An amount taken off a bill when an invoice is paid in advance of the discount or net due date. This is granted in addition to any discounts and is calculated at a stated percentage rate for the number of days between that of actual payment and the due date.

**Anticipation inventories.** Additional inventory above basic pipeline stock to cover projected trends of increasing sales, planned sales, promotion programs, seasonal fluctuations, plant shutdowns, and vacations.

**Application** (computers). The use of computer-based routines for specific purposes such as accounts-receivable maintenance, inventory control, or new-product selection; software or computer programs that process data and provide output for the stated purpose.

**Appropriation.** An authorization to spend up to a specified dollar amount.

**Arbitrage.** Buying in one market and selling simultaneously in another in order to profit from price variances.

**Architecture** (computers). Refers to the design of a system. It can be the way the hardware, software, or network manipulate data. *Topology* is another term for network architecture. It describes a network by its geometric form.

**Arithmetic, decimal.** Addition, subtraction, multiplication, and division of decimal quantities.

**Arithmetic and logic unit.** The unit of the central processor of a computer that performs the mathematical operations as well as the so-called logical operations, such as branching and decision operations, which means making choices between alternative sets of instructions.

**ASCII.** American Standard Code for Information Interchange.

**Asepsis.** The methods of making or keeping free from pathogenic microorganisms.

**Assembler.** A computer program that translates symbolic operation codes into instruction in machine language, one for one, which the machine can understand and perform. The assembler provides computer-operating instructions; assigns locations in computer storage for successive instructions; and computes locations for the data, instructions, and successive results of computer operations.

**Assembly.** A group of subassemblies and/or parts that are put together; the total unit constitutes a major subdivision of the final product.

**Assembly bill-of-materials form.** Copies of a bill of material or parts list, which are used as requisitions for issuing balanced groups of materials and parts for assembly orders.

**Assembly parts list.** A list of all parts (may include subassemblies) making up a particular assembly, as used in the manufacturing process.

**Assignment problem.** A special type of problem involving, for example, the assignment of jobs to machines, workers to tasks, and so on, such that one job or worker is assigned to one and only one machine or task. The objective is usually expressed in terms of finding the assignment that minimizes costs, minimizes time, maximizes profits, and so on.

**Attributes of information.** Characteristics of information that make the information useful to the receiver, such as accuracy, timeliness, reliability, and origin.

**Audio-response unit.** A device that generates output from computer systems in the form of spoken words; words stored on a magnetic medium for use in output.

**Audit trail.** A technique that makes it possible to retrace processing of data in order to change, add, or delete records in a file; or to locate the origin of a transactions generation.

**Automatic stocking.** A predetermined quantity of one or more line items routinely issued at a specified time.

**Auxiliary storage.** Storage that supplements the main memory section of the central processing unit. Auxiliary storage may be on-line or off-line.

**Availability.** A term usually interpreted to mean "material available for planning" and thus including not only the on-hand inventory, but also inventory on order.

**Available stock.** Stock on hand plus stock on order less any unfilled customer demand.

**Available time.** Used in stock control to mean the interval between the earliest time at which a specific requirement of an item can be calculated and the time at which it is required.

**Available work.** Work that is actually ready to be worked on, as opposed to scheduled work that may not yet be on hand.

**Average costing.** Inventory-valuation method where a weighted average unit cost is computed, that is:

$$\frac{\text{Total goods available for sale (cost)}}{\text{Total goods available for sale (units)}} = \text{Average cost/unit for the period}$$

**Average inventory.** In a simple inventory system, this is the sum of one-half the lot sizes plus the reserve stock.

**Backhaul allowance-pickup allowance.** Price difference when the buyer does the transportation.

**Backlog of orders.** The sum of all the unfilled orders waiting to be filled or processed.

**Backorder.** The receipt of a demand for a product when there are no units on hand in inventory. These backorders become shortages, which are eventually satisfied when a new supply of the product becomes available.

**Backspace.** In computer input, to backspace is to move back the reading or display position according to a prescribed format.

**Backup.** Standby, substitute, or alternate components in a computer processing system that can be used in case of failure or damage to the primary component, for example, backup copies of data or programs or backup equipment and facilities that can be used in the event of hardware failure or emergencies.

**Backward scheduling.** A scheduling technique where the schedule is computed, starting with the due date for the order and working backward to determine the required starting date.

**Balanced loading.** Loading a starting department with a product mix that should not overload or underload subsequent departments.

**Balance-of-stores record.** A double-entry record system that shows at all times the balances of material on order and "available" for future orders.

**Balance out.** At the end of a model year, or in anticipation of an engineering or design change, the stocks of all subordinate items can be reduced in a balanced way. Items that can be carried over to the next model are stocked somewhat below forecast requirements. Items that can be carried over can be stocked to a level somewhat above forecast.

**Band.** A group of circular recording tracks on storage devices such as drums or discs.

**Bank.** A quantity of materials that is awaiting further processing.

**Base index.** One way of expressing a seasonal profile is by a set of base-index numbers, one for each forecast period of the year. Usually the values express the expected ratio of demand in that period to the demand in an average period. Sometimes base-index numbers represent differences. The whole pattern is also called a "profile." If the index numbers are cumulated, they may be expressed as a "percentage done," meaning the cumulative percentage of the total season sales done by any period within the season.

**Base inventory level.** The normal inventory level made up of the lot-size inventory plus the safety-stock inventory.

**Base pipeline stock.** Inventory in transit to fill the many stocking points in the distribution system.

**Base series.** A standard series of demand-over-time observations used in forecasting seasonable items. This series is usually based on the relative level of demand during the corresponding period of previous years.

**Base stock.** A minimum quantity of inventory that can be identified as necessary in certain types of operations to maintain a continuing service or production.

**Base stock system.** A method of inventory control that issues replenishment orders whenever an order is received for an item. Base-stock orders are also used to adjust the level of the base stock for each item.

**Basic producer.** The manufacturer that uses material resources to produce materials for other manufacturing.

**Basic stock.** The desired level of the average inventory.

**Batch.** The material and/or information required or used in one production or processing cycle.

**Batch processing.** A mode of computer operation in which transactions are accumulatd over a period of time and then processed in the computer at the same pass-through or as a batch. It is the most common form of computer processing. Batch processing is distinguished from *real-time* processing, in which transactions are processed as they are generated.

**Batch production.** A type of production in which work is processed in batches, each of which has its own sequence of operations.

**Baud** (communications). A unit of signaling speed equal to twice the number of Morse code dots continuously sent per second. In terms of binary signals, one baud is one bit per second.

**Behavior segmentation.** Identification of a target market according to common needs, characteristics, or consumption patterns.

**Benchmark.** An approach of testing the computer software or hardware with an actual application to demonstrate that it works.

**Benefit segmentation.** Identification of a target market group in terms of the benefits its members want from a product or service.

**BID.** (a) A price offer by a prospective purchaser. (b) A quotation given, usually in competition with other vendors, in response to an intending buyer's request.

**Bill of lading.** Document issued by common carrier inventorying the containers that are shipped.

**Bill of landing.** An order-negotiable or straight nonnegotiable document that is a contract for transportation between the shipper and the carrier.

**Bill of materials.** A listing of all the subassemblies, parts, and materials that go into an assembled product, showing the quantity of each required to make one assembly.

**Bill of sale.** A written agreement transferring ownership of a property from one party to another.

**Binary.** A numbering system consisting of only two digits or states, that is "on" = "1" and "off" = "0", or "bit" and "no-bit." If zero (0) and one (1) are used as the only digits, the decimal number 13 is represented as 1101.

**Bin cards.** Cards bearing records of receipts, issues, and stock balances, held in the stores in which the items are stocked although not necessarily in the bins. The essential difference between a bin card and a stock card is that the primary purpose of the stock card is to provide information as a basis for placing replenishment orders. A bin card is merely a local record of what is currently in store, and may also carry its location. Bin cards and allocation cards can be combined.

**Bin-location file.** A listing that specifically identifies the physical location of each item stored in inventory.

**Bin tag.** A type of perpetual inventory maintained at the storage area for each inventory item.

**Bin trips.** The number of times (per year) that an item is ordered by separate customer transactions, regardless of the number of units ordered.

**Bit.** Abbreviation of BInary digiT. A single character in a binary number (that is, 0 or 1).

**Blanket order.** A purchase order issued by a buyer to a vendor for a year's requirements of a particular item. The items are shipped against the blanket order when the vendor receives a release from the buyer. Generally, the release is made for relatively small quantities to replenish in-house inventories.

**Block.** A group of computer words handled as a unit because they are stored in successive memory locations.

**Block control.** Control of the production-process groups or "blocks" of shop orders for products undergoing the same basic processes.

**Block diagram.** A diagram of a system or a computer in which the principal parts are represented by suitably associated geometrical figures. A diagram shows both the basic functions and the functional relationships among the parts.

**Block scheduling.** This is a detailed scheduling technique where each operation is allowed a fairly long period or block of time, such as a week.

**Book inventory.** A definition of inventory units or value obtained from perpetual-inventory records rather than by actual count.

**Book value.** The accounting value of an asset. Normally it is the original acquisition cost less all depreciation taken.

**Boundary.** The separation between two elements, systems, or processes; often an imaginary line of demarcation that separates and distinguishes two or more different entities for purposes of analysis.

**Branch.** In programming, a branch is a set of instructions that are executed between two successive decision instructions.

**Branch warehouse.** A separate stocking location removed from the main manufacturing plant.

**Break.** In computer usage, to halt the execution of a routine. A routine in this mode may be restarted from the break point, or terminated.

**Break-even analysis.** An analytical technique for studying the relationships among fixed costs, variable costs, and profits. A break-even chart graphically depicts the nature of break-even analysis. The break-even analysis. The break-even point represents the volume of sales at which total costs equal revenues (that is, profits equal zero).

**Break-even point.** The level of production or the volume of sales at which operations are neither profitable nor unprofitable.

**Bridging run.** The quantity ordered when tooling is to be changed or when the unit cost of the materials is to be changed. The quantity ordered will last longer than usual and will bridge over the period when the source cannot supply more, because the plant is being re-tooled.

**Budget.** A plan that includes an estimate of future costs and revenues related to expected activities.

**Budget variance.** The difference between the actual amounts incurred and the budget figure.

**Buffer.** A storage area or storage device that is used to assemble input and output for processing. Buffers help to compensate for speed differences between the central processing unit and various input-output devices.

**Buffer stock.** A stock allowance to cover errors in forecasts of demand during the procurement period or to cover for a production-facility maintenance shutdown.

**Bug.** A mistake in a computer program or an equipment malfunction.

**Build schedule.** The master plan that states the number of units of the product to be assembled during each period. The build schedule may identify only the generic product line. Specific configurations may be specified later as customer orders are received.

**Bulk breaking.** Breaking a large-quantity order into smaller units for resale.

**Bulk-order quantity.** A quantity larger than the EOQ, which may be ordered in order to get a lower unit price.

**Bunching.** The accumulation and tender of railroad cars en route, resulting in deliveries that differ from normal schedules.

**Burst.** To separate continuous-form paper (computer printouts) into discrete sheets.

**Business analysis.** A stage in new product or service development in which detailed forecasts of probable sales, income, and expenses are prepared.

**Business cycle.** A seemingly recurring change in general business activity going from a low point (depression) to a high point (prosperity); important for forecasting.

**Business risk.** The basic risk inherent in a firm's operations. Business risk plus financial risk resulting from the use of debt equals total corporate risk.

**Buyer's market.** A market condition favorable to purchasers existing when the forces of supply and demand keep prices relatively low.

**Buyer's risk.** The possibility that a sample will contain fewer defects than the rest of the lot.

**Buying.** The function of finding sources of supply, obtaining quotations, and placing purchase orders. Issuing delivery schedules to suppliers and progressing the supply of goods are often included in the buying function.

**Buying center.** The organizational members actually involved in purchase decisions. This could include users, buyers, influencers, and decision makers.

**Byte.** A data-storage unit made up of six or eight bits. A bit is the smallest unit of storage and is filled with either a 1 or a 0. A series of bits produces the binominal equivalent of the data.

**Calendar time.** Refers to the passage of days or weeks, as in the definition of lead time or scheduling rules, in contrast to running time.

**Call-off quantity.** On a delivery schedule sent to a supplier, the quantity specified to be delivered at one time (and paid for) against a covering order for a larger quantity.

**Call reports.** Reports prepared by salespersons after calling on prospective customers.

**Capacity.** The highest sustainable output rate that can be achieved with the current product specifications, product mix, worker effort, plant, and equipment.

**Capacity planning.** The management task of deciding what alterations are to be made to manufacturing capacity and by what time they are to be completed. This should be carried out as part of a routine procedure that culminates in periodic issue of a sales program and a production-capacity program.

**Capital asset.** An asset with a life of more than one year that is not bought and sold in the ordinary course of business.

**Capital budgeting.** The process of planning expenditures on assets whose returns are expected to extend beyond one year.

**Capital costs.** Cost of monies tied up. If average inventories increase, then the capital invested in inventory increases proportionately. In general, the appropriate rate to use should reflect the alternative opportunities for investment of comparable funds. The cost of borrowed funds would represent the lower limit.

**Capitalization rate.** A discount rate used to find the present value of a series of future cash receipts; sometimes called discount rate.

**Card.** A machine-processable card of eighty numbered columns that can be keypunched according to column numbers.

**Card column.**  On a data-processing card, a column is a single line of punch positions parallel to the short edge of a 3¼" × 7" punched card.

**Card hopper.**  The portion of a card-processing machine that holds the cards to be processed and makes them available to a card-feed mechanism.

**Card row.**  On a data-processing card, a row is a single line of punch positions parallel to the long edge of a 3¼" × 7" punched card.

**Card stacker.**  The portion of a card-processing machine that receives processed cards.

**Carrier.**  Any individual, company, or corporation engaged in transporting goods.

**Carry-back; carry-forward.**  For income-tax purposes, losses that can be carried backward or forward to reduce federal income taxes.

**Carrying cost.**  The cost of carrying inventory, consisting of cost of capital invested, taxes, and insurance, obsolescence and spoilage, and space costs.

**Cartage.**  Intracity hauling.

**Cascaded systems.**  Multistorage operations where the input to each stage is the output of a preceding stage.

**Cash budget.**  A schedule showing cash flows (receipts, disbursements, and net cash) for a firm or institutional unit, such as a pharmacy, over a specified period.

**Cash cycle.**  The length of time between the purchase of raw materials and the collection of accounts receivable generated in the sale of the final product.

**Cash discounts.**  Cash discounts are awarded for prompt payment of bills. A policy such as "2/10 net 30" means the purchaser can deduct 2 percent of the list price if he pays for the order within the first ten days of the month following receipt of the bill. Payment is expected within thirty days, even if the discount is not utilized. Vendors offer cash discounts to improve their cash-flow positions and thus to reduce the need for borrowing money to pay their bills on time.

**Cash flow.**  Movement of money in and out of business.

**Cash-receipt journal.**  Journal designed to record all cash receipts.

**Catalog number.**  An assigned number (typically five to eight digits) used as an identifying and locating factor for the institution and its computer service.

**Cathode-ray tube (CRT).**  A vacuum tube containing a screen on which information may be shown electronically.

**Central control unit.**  The part of the central processor that (1) receives and interprets instructions and (2) sends appropriate signals to the executing hardware.

**Centralized dispatching.** Organization of the dispatching function into one central location.

**Centralized system.** A set of functions or programs processed by or in a single center and servicing several locations.

**Central processing unit (CPU).** The main work of the computer system where all control and processing work is based. The unit of the computer that controls all processing of data, movement of data, and execution of instructions. Sets of circuits that together make up the control unit, the arithmetic/logic unit, and the main-memory unit. Also called the CPU or the mainframe.

**Central processor.** *See* Central processing unit.

**Certificate of compliance.** A supplier's written assurance to the effect that the supplies or services delivered fulfill specified requirements.

**Chain of distribution.** The path of an item from producer to final user.

**Change order.** A formal notification that an order must be changed in some form. This may result from a changed date or specification by the customer, an engineering or design change, a change in inventory requirement date, or some other change.

**Changeover cost.** Setup cost and tear-down cost.

**Channel** (physical goods). The route goods or services travel to get from producers to consumers. It can be direct or indirect (through wholesalers and/or retailers).

**Channel** (Information). The path along which information in general, or a series of digits or characters in particular, may flow, such as input channel or output channel.

**Channel functions.** The tasks that must be performed for goods to move from producers to consumers: promotion, transportation, storage, financing, risk bearing, marketing information.

**Character.** A digit, letter, or other symbol that is used as part of the organization, control, or representation of data.

**Character data.** Letters and symbols (e.g., +, −, *, /, and so on) that can be processed as data in a computer system.

**Chip.** Integrated-circuit module of varying sizes, complexities, and functions, such as a memory chip or a processor chip.

**Christmas tree.** A bill of material in the form of graphic product-structure chart showing how the assembly is made up of subassemblies, the subassemblies made up of lower-level components, and so on.

**Classification-of-goods theory.** A breakdown of goods and services based on product or service characteristics and consumer purchasing behavior; the three general categories are convenience, shopping, and specialty goods.

**Clerical system.** A system where work is performed according to fixed, standardized procedures that have been developed as a result of the frequent recurrence of the work. Computer-based clerical systems are those manual systems of a routine type that have merely been automated. Clerical systems are not considered decision-oriented procedures.

**Closed-loop system.** A system in which the computer directly controls an external process without human intervention. In a closed-loop process-control system, for example, the computer may be connected directly to instrumentation through a digital-to-analog converter. The computer can then apply control action directly to the process by actuating valves, setting controls, and so forth.

**Closed shop.** Pertaining to the operation of a computer facility in which most productive problem programming is performed by a group of programming specialists rather than by the problem originators. The use of the computer itself may also be described as a closed shop if full-time trained operators rather than user programmers serve as the operators.

**Closed short.** An order is closed short when less than the quantity order will be delivered to stock. This may be the result of scrap losses or unavailability from the vendor.

**COBOL** (COmmon Business Oriented Language). A business-data-processing language.

**Code.** A verb denoting the assignment of a number or letter to identify and designate a specific character or group of characters.

**Codec.** An acronym for a coder-decoder device. It is used to regroup multiplexed data. It is often used with a *modem*, which transforms digital signals to analog signals so that information can be sent over telephone lines.

**Cognitive dissonance.** Tendency of consumers to have doubts after purchases.

**Collate.** To combine parts or all of two or more ordered sets (files) of information in any way so that a similar sequence is observed in the combined set.

**Collateral.** Assets that are used to secure a loan.

**Commercialization.** The final stage of new product development, that is, full-scale introduction and marketing.

**Commissary.** Large facility with sophisticated, automated equipment.

**Commitment fee.** The fee paid to a lender for a formal line of credit.

**Commitments.** Orders that have been accepted but not yet filled, including backorders.

**Commodity records.** Extensive card indexes of where to buy goods and materials.

**Common carrier.** A transportation company operating under a Certificate of Convenience and Necessity, which provides service to the general public at published rates.

**Common parts.** Those elemental parts that are used in two or more products.

**Common system.** The use of the same computer programs at separate locations. For example, facilities having their own computer systems may each process materials-transaction data but both use the same programs.

**Communication Access Method (CAM).** Hybrid software or microcode hardware used to gain efficiency. It implements a systems-hardware interface and protocol. *Protocol* is a software package that allows incompatible computers in a network to communicate.

**Compatibility.** Capacity of interchangeability among products, programs, and media.

**Compensating balance.** A required minimum checking-account balance that an institution must maintain with a commercial bank. The required balance is generally equal to 15 to 20 percent of the amount of loans outstanding. Compensating balances can raise the effective rate of interest on bank loans.

**Compile.** To produce a machine-language computer program from a series of symbolic operation codes or statements. A special compiler program is used to perform the translation from nonmachine to machine language.

**Compiler.** A type of translator that converts computer programs written in higher-level programming languages into signals that can be interpreted and executed by the CPU.

**Complementary product.** When demand for one product increases with demand for another, they are complementary.

**Component.** An inclusive term used to describe a subassembly or part that goes into higher-level assemblies.

**Component parts.** An inventory grouping that comprises items that are either purchased or manufactured from raw material and stored for use in assemblies or for sale to customers as repair or replacement parts. (Parts may be held in component-parts stores and still require further processing or finishing at final assembly.)

**Composite cost of capital.** A weighted average of the component costs of various debts and, in proprietary institutions, of preferred stock and common equity. Also called the weighted average cost of capital, it usually reflects the cost of each additional dollar raised, not the average cost of all capital the institution has raised throughout its history.

**Computer.** A device capable of solving problems by accepting data, performing prescribed operations on the data, and supplying the results.

**Computer-controlled exchange (CBS).** A digital or analog private-branch exchange (PBX) that is automatically controlled. The CBX is also referred to as a multichanneled switching node. The PBX is a system for rerouting voice or data communications.

**Computer program.** A set of instructions or commands that guide the processing of data in a computer system.

**Computer programmers.** Those who translate an analyzed problem solution into a set of computer instructions (programs) in a language that the computer understands and can process.

**Concurrent processing.** A method of processing in which two or more jobs *appear* to be getting processed at the same time. The instructions of each job are processed one at a time, but alternate in such a fashion as to make the most-efficient use of the system.

**Condition sales contract.** A contract for the financing of new equipment that calls for paying off the loan in installments over a one- to five-year period. The seller retains title to the equipment until payment has been completed.

**Consignment goods.** Goods held for sale but not owned by the holders. These goods would not be considered part of the consignee's inventory.

**Console** (computer). That part of a computer used for communication between the operator and the computer.

**Constant demand rate.** An assumption of many inventory decision models, which states that the same number of units are taken from inventory in each period of time.

**Constant supply rate.** The situation in which the inventory is built up at a constant rate over a period of time. This assumption is used in many production and economic-lot-size models.

**Constraint.** The limitations placed on the maximization or minimization of an objective function, as in mathematical programming.

**Constraints.** Restrictions or limitations imposed on a particular problem situation.

**Consumer information-retrieval system.** An innovative method whereby consumers can get information and assistance over the phone.

**Consumerism.** A general term referring to identification and resolution of problems that consumers experience.

**Consumer-product-safety commission.** A federal regulatory agency charged with identifying and investigating products that may harm consumers.

**Containerized freight.** Shipments packaged in standard-size and -shape containers for transportation by truck, train, or ship.

**Continuous budget.** A budget that perpetually adds a month or quarter into the future as the month or quarter just ended is dropped.

**Continuous production.** Production method that is performed on an ongoing basis. Examples are refineries, chemical plants, and so on.

**Contract carrier.** A motor carrier, other than a common carrier, hauling under contracts in accordance with a permit issued by a government regulatory body.

**Contract market.** The "nonpublic" market composed of governmental, institutional, or commercial buyers who purchase goods and services on behalf of the final market.

**Contractual vertical-marketing systems.** Independent institutions—producers, wholesalers, jobbers, retailers—are banded together by contracts to achieve the necessary economic size and coordination of effort.

**Contracyclical buying.** Buying goods during the "off" season for a particular industry. The incentives for the buyer are usually major price concessions.

**Contribution.** In marginal analysis, the difference between price per unit and variable cost per unit. It is the amount left over to cover fixed costs and provide a profit.

**Control board.** A visual means of showing machine loading or project planning. Usually a variation of the basic Gantt chart.

**Convenience goods.** A classification of consumer goods. These are generally inexpensive items for which substitutes are available.

**Conversational mode.** A procedure for communication between a terminal and the computer in which each entry from the terminal elicits a response from the computer, with the response governing or affecting the next action to be taken by the terminal operator.

**Conversion cost.** The cost of converting prime goods to finished goods. These costs include overhead and indirect labor.

**Converter.** A manufacturer who changes the products of a basic producer into a variety of industrial, institutional, and/or consumer products.

**Conveying equipment.** Equipment used to transport solids, such as belt conveyers, vibrating conveyers, skip hoists, elevators, and trucks.

**Coordinated orders.** A family of items obtained from the same source. A single order is placed at one time for a list of items. Some of the items are ordered in sufficient quantities when they are needed, so that they do not need to be included on every order.

**Coordination models.** A class of analytical models involving the relationship between starting times of the component tasks of a project and the completion date of the project.

**Core storage.** A storage device in which binary data are represented by the direction of magnetization in units of doughnut-shaped magnetic materials. Synonymous with Magnetic core storage, Magnetic storage.

**Corporate vertical marketing.** A situation in which all facilities from production through sales are owned by one company.

**Corrective action.** Action that must be taken to get actual inventories or production back on plan, such as expediting.

**Correlation coefficient.** A measure of the degree of relationship between two variables.

**Cost accounting.** A quantitative method that accumulates, classifies, summarizes, and interprets information for three major purposes: (1) operational planning and control, (2) special decisions, and (3) product costing.

**Cost-benefit analysis.** A technique of assessing the impact of projects, new systems, procedures, products, and/or information systems in organizations by identifying the costs and benefits of acquisition.

**Cost center.** A subdivision of the institution established for the purpose of assigning or allocating costs.

**Cost center code.** Typically a two- to five-digit numeric code used to disburse the cost of operating an overhead account.

**Cost effectiveness.** The relationship between cost measured in terms of dollars and cents (foregone opportunities, and so on) on the one hand, and effectiveness measured in terms of specified performance characteristics on the other. Cost can be held constant and effectiveness varied, or effectiveness held constant and cost varied in order to arrive at a specified cost-effectiveness relationship. *Similar to* Cost-benefit.

**Cost factors.** The units of input that represent costs to the materials management system, such as labor hours and purchased material.

**Cost of capital.** The discount rate that should be used in capital budgeting and/or establishing the cost of holding inventory.

**Cost of goods sold.** The cost of merchandise sold. This includes direct materials, direct labor, and overhead costs.

**Cost of holding inventories.** The cost incurred over time because the inventory exists. *See* Holding costs.

**Cost plus.** A pricing method allowing the vendor to charge his costs plus a fixed percentage of those costs.

**Coupler.** A piece of equipment into which the user places a telephone receiver to establish telephone communications between the computer and a terminal.

**Coupon system.** A control method for issuing materials. This system requires that an identifying coupon be attached to each container for each lot or shipment. The identifying coupons should indicate the time when the goods were received. Thus each container can be identified by lot; typically the oldest lot is used first.

**Covenant.** A protective clause typically contained in loan agreements. Covenants are designed to protect the lender and include such items as limits on total indebtedness, restrictions on dividends, and minimum current ratio.

**CPM (Critical-path method).** Method outlining the expected times of completion of each part as well as of the total system project. A critical path is the longest path (time) through the network.

**CPU.** The central processing unit of a computer.

**Crashing**. In CPM, the process of reducing an activity time by adding resources and hence usually costs.

**Creeping inventories**. The gradual increase in inventories often owing to suppliers shipping ahead of schedule and/or users hoarding.

**Critical-path scheduling**. A technique that is intended for project planning and control. It is a variation of the Gantt chart. *See* CPM.

**Critical rate**. A priority factor for workshop scheduling, which measures the ratio of the proportion of stock on hand relative to the order point to the proportion of time remaining relative to the total lead time.

**CRT (Cathode-ray tube)**. An electronic display device used to input information and/or request information from the computer. (The CRT resembles a television picture tube placed on top of a typewriter.)

**Culture**. One of the external environments marketers must understand and deal with; the social heritage of a society, including living habits, arts, aspirations, and the distinctive "style" of an aggregate of people.

**Cumulative scheduling**. Scheduling production on an aggregate basis to achieve economical run lengths.

**Current purchase-unit price**. The current purchase price of a single item or unit of issue of that item. Used as an input in choosing the quantity to be purchased and in evaluating vendors.

**Customer order**. A customer order is an offer to buy received from a prospective customer of the organization. It can be prepared by customers such as hospitals contracting to buy certain goods or services from local or regional cooperative or sharing organizations. Information contained on customer orders is basically the same as that found on purchase orders.

**Customer-service costs**. These include cancelled or lost orders, both current and future; expediting costs; extra freight; more-expensive substitutes; and special-handling charges.

**Cycle**. The time interval during which a system returns to similar initial conditions, for example, the length of time between replenishment shipments.

**Cycle stock**. Stock that depletes gradually and is replenished cyclically as orders are received.

**Cycle time**. The length of time between cycles, for example, between placing two consecutive orders.

**Cyclical-inventory count**. A physical-inventory-taking technique whereby inventory is counted continuously rather than once a year.

**Cycling**. Creation, deletion, or modification of file records according to a predetermined fixed schedule.

**Damages**. Money demanded by the buyer as compensation for a late delivery.

**Data.** Facts, ideas, or concepts that can be collected, communicated, or processed. The representation of facts, ideas, or concepts electronically in digital form. Contrast with information.

**Data administrator.** Person (or group) responsible for control and integrity of a set of files.

**Data bank.** A series of easily accessed integrated master files (usually magnetic tapes or discs) eliminating record duplication.

**Data base.** A collection of interrelated data stored together with controlled redundancy to serve one or more applications; the data are stored so that they are independent of programs that use the data.

**Data-base management system (DBMS).** A software system that allows access to stored data by providing an interface between users or programs and the stored data.

**Data dictionary.** A documentation of the data items included in a data base together with their relationships with other data and programs or routines that use them.

**Data flow chart.** A flow chart representing the path of data from collection through processing. It defines the major phases of the processing as well as the various data media used.

**Data packing.** A method of sending data by holding the data at the sending location or node until a channel clears to send it.

**Data phone.** Any of a family of devices used to permit the transmission of data over telephone channels.

**Data processing.** The preparation of data or basic elements of information, and their handling, according to precise rules of procedure to accomplish such operations as classifying, sorting, calculating, summarizing, and recording. *Synonymous with* Data handling.

**Data reduction.** The process of transforming masses of raw test or experimentally obtained data, usually gathered by automatic-recording equipment, into useful, condensed, or simplified intelligence.

**Data switching.** A method of data transmission where the data is broken down into words and sent over any number of channels. The words are reassembled by a codec when transmission is received.

**Dead load.** The orders ahead of any manufacturing facility that have not yet been released. Usually used in dispatching to indicate the orders on hand for which work has not yet been received.

**Debug.** To detect, locate, and remove mistakes from a program system or procedure and/or malfunction from a computer or other hardware.

**Decentralized dispatching.** The organization of the dispatching function into individual departmental dispatchers.

**Decision table.** A tabular chart showing the logic relating various combinations of conditions to a set of actions. The decision table is extremely useful whenever a choice must be made between several feasible alternatives.

**Decision tree.**  A branching chart showing the actions that follow from various combinations of conditions. The concept of decision trees has been used extensively in formalizing administrative and diagnostic decisions.

**Deck.**  A collection of cards, commonly a complete set of cards that have been punched for a definite service or purpose.

**Decode.**  Interpretation of bits of data into alphanumeric symbols.

**Decoupling inventory.**  Inventory maintained between two operations in order to control them independently.

**Decrement.**  The quantity of inventory reduction. Example: Internal medicine requisitions two pens. Upon computer processing, these pens are immediately recorded as a reduction of inventory and charged to that department. This reduction of inventory is called a decrement.

**Dedicated.**  Pertaining to a mode of operation in which a procedure requires all the resources of the system.

**Delay report.**  A regular report issued from the production floor, usually by the dispatcher, showing which jobs are behind schedule and why.

**Deliver to.**  Denotes the final destination of materials shipped or distributed.

**Delivery date.**  Date on which a shipment is expected to arrive.

**Delivery lead time.**  The elapsed time between the placement of an order and the time of receipt by the order-placing agency.

**Delivery period.**  The time from receipt of a customer's order to dispatch of the goods.

**Demand.**  (1) The requirement rate of any item in terms of quantity per unit of time. (2) The interactive-processing mode usually to and from the computer and remote terminals. (3) The desire to purchase a commodity, accompanied by the means of payment.

**Demand distribution.**  A relative arrangement of a set of demand data.

**Demand during a lead time.**  The expected demand over the lead-time period.

**Demand filter.**  As total demand is posted during a forecast-review period, it is compared with the most recent forecast for that period. If the difference is large compared to the standard deviation, the demand filter creates an exception report, in case something is wrong with the value being posted. The objective is to catch very serious errors in entry or in coding special orders as normal.

**Demarketing.**  A firm's attempt to discourage consumption for a product or service, particularly when shortages of necessary resources occur.

**Demodulation.**  The process of reconstituting digital signals from a modulated transmission circuit. Modulation and demodulation equipment is needed to make communication signals compatible with business-machine codes.

**Demographics.** A set of objective data about a group of people. Generally the data include such factors as age, sex, marital status, mobility, income.

**Demurrage.** Charges assessed by the carrier against the shipper or consignee for delay of a car, vessel, or vehicle beyond a specified time allowed for unloading or loading and releasing the equipment to the carrier.

**Departmental stock.** An informal system of holding stock in a production or service department.

**Dependent demand.** Demand (typically for components) that is dependent on requirements generated by higher-level subassemblies and assemblies.

**Depreciation.** Decrease in value of a capital asset because of use, deterioration, inadequacy, obsolescence, and/or applicable tax laws.

**Descriptive text.** A complete description of a single line item. Typically, an eighty-alphanumeric-character statement used to print the storeroom catalog and produce some inventory listings and/or MMS reports.

**Design modification.** An alteration, specified by the design function, to a product specification already issued to the production department.

**Detailed scheduling.** Scheduling items only after an order for them is received.

**Detail persons.** Salespersons who do not attempt to make immediate sales, but who foster "goodwill," make informal presentations, and/or leave samples.

**Detention.** Penalty against shipper or receiver for delaying beyond the allowed time in the trucking industry.

**Deterioration.** Product spoilage, damage to package, and so forth.

**Deterministic model.** An adequate and appropriate representation of phenomena, repeated observations of which warrant the assumption that the statistical fluctuations are small enough to be ignored. *Contrast with* Probabilistic model.

**Diagnostic routine.** A routine used to locate a malfunction in a computer or to aid in locating mistakes in a computer program; thus, in general, any routine specifically designed to aid in debugging or trouble shooting.

**Dictionary.** A list of codes or references intended to facilitate managerial access to the data base. The dictionary may be tailored to the needs and vocabularies of individual managers; it may be maintained externally in the form of a user's handbook or stored within the system itself as a specialized kind of index.

**Digital computer.** A computer that processes information represented by combinations of discrete or discontinuous data as compared with an analog computer with continuous data. Sequences of arithmetic and logical operations are performed not only on data but on its own program, which can be stored as well.

**Direct access.**   Refers to the process of obtaining data from, or placing data into, storage where the time required for such access is independent of the location of the data most recently obtained or placed into storage.

**Direct-access index.**   A list of storage locations and contents by means of which data can be directly located and taken from, or placed into, secondary storages.

**Direct channel.**   Goods or services that move directly from a manufacturer to ultimate consumers with no wholesale or retail intermediaries.

**Direct competition.**   Organizations in the external environment that offer similar products or services.

**Direct cost.**   Cost that can be directly attributed to a particular job or operation.

**Direct costing.**   The type of product costing that charges fixed manufacturing overhead immediately against the revenue of the period in which it was incurred, without assigning it to specific units produced.

**Direct labor.**   Labor that is specifically applied to the product being manufactured.

**Direct materials.**   Raw materials and components that become a part of the final product in measurable quantities.

**Direct ordering.**   One of the basic methods of ordering an item in which the item is ordered only when it is known to be required for a firm customer's order and then only in the quantity needed to execute that order.

**Direct pickup.**   Method of dispatching materials from stores to the requisitioner or user in which the person or department requisitioning the material either waits for the requested material or arranges to pick up the material as soon as it is ready.

**Disbursement.**   The issuance of raw material or components from a storeroom.

**Disc.**   A portion of the computer that stores data, sometimes referred to as the working file. It retains information on inventory levels, vendor's addresses, descriptive text, and so on.

**Discontinue date.**   The date after which no further demand is to be served, for example, after an engineering or design change, the end of the season, or the last recorded demand. Controlled by both the planning and the forecast horizons.

**Discounted cash-flow techniques.**   Methods of ranking investment proposals. Included are the rate-of-return method, the net-present-value method, the equivalent-annual-cost method, and the profitability-index or benefit-cost ratio.

**Discounting.**   The process of finding the present value of a series of future cash flows. Discounting is the reverse of compounding.

**Discounting of accounts receivable.**   Short-term financing whereby accounts receivable are used to secure the loan. The lender does not buy the accounts receivable but simply uses them as collateral for the loan. Also called assigning accounts receivable.

**Discount order quantity.**   The order quantity based on a discount that the vendor will give if a fairly large quantity is ordered.

**Discounts.**   List-price deductions offered to final consumers and/or middlemen who perform some service or marketing function for the manufacturer.

**Disk-drive storage device.**   Computer peripheral equipment that stores data for ready access by a sequential, indexed, or random method.

**Dispatching.**   The function of assigning jobs to the appropriate work centers and/or workers.

**Display.**   In computer terminology, a visual presentation of data.

**Distributed computing.**   A system-design philosophy in which computational capability is distributed among two or more processing facilities rather than centralized at a single site. Typically, these facilities are linked by a communication network and often exhibit functional specialization. Not all facilities in a distributed network need to have equipment of the same size and configuration.

**Distributed data processing (DDP).**   The term used to describe all computer networks. *Clustered network* refers to any number of "dumb" terminals connected to one processor.

**Distribution.**   The assignment of costs or revenue to the various accounts affected.

**Distribution channel.**   A system through which material is transported from its source to its destination.

**Distribution system.**   An organization of administrative procedures, transport facilities and warehousing or storage facilities used to move materials.

**Distributor.**   A business that purchases and resells its products, usually maintaining a finished-goods inventory.

**Diversion.**   A change in routing of a shipment.

**Document.**   Any drawing, parts list, or product specification used to define a product.

**Documentation.**   The process of recording in unambiguous and operationally meaningful ways every step in a process, procedure, or system, so that it can be completely replicated or understood in the future if need be.

**Double-bin system.**   A control method for issuing materials in which the area or bin space allocated to an item is approximately twice the amount required for a standard lot or shipment. As each new lot is received, it is placed in the empty space and not used until the older items have been used.

**Downtime.**   Time when needed equipment is unavailable for use for any reason.

**Drayage.**   Charge made for local hauling by dray or truck; usually refers to the segments where the back of the truck is placed on a rail car.

**Drop shipper.**   A middleman who holds title to goods in transit but who does not handle the goods.

**Drop time.**   Amount of time needed to unload a vehicle and take goods into the receiving dock.

**Due date.**   The calendar date at which an operation or order is to be completed.

**Dumb terminals.**   Computer input-output stations that have no processing abilities and must be connected to the main processor at all times. *Smart terminals* are able to do some data-processing chores.

**Dump.**   A transfer of the contents of a storage device to other media, such as punched cards or printout. Frequently used in debugging when the contents of internal storage need to be listed for visual examination.

**Dunnage.**   Lumber or material used to brace materials in carriers' equipment.

**Dynamic memory.**   A memory device that must be instantly reminded of the data it stores by maintaining an electric current through it. *Static memory* is a device that will maintain its data even if the computer system shuts down.

**Earmarked material.**   Reserved material on hand that is physically identified rather than reserved in a record.

**Echelon.**   Any stage in the physical distribution system, such as a vendor, the manufacturing plant, finished goods at a master warehouse, regional warehouses, or local stocking outlets.

**Economic order quantity (EOQ).**   The amount to be purchased or manufactured in one lot in order to minimize the cost of carrying inventory and of ordering and/or of setup for manufacturing.

**Economic run length.**   The equivalent of EOQ when the material ordered is produced in house.

**Economic time cycle.**   The number of periods of demand that corresponds to the economic batch quantity over the planning horizon.

**Edit.**   To rearrange data or information. Editing may involve purging unwanted data, selecting pertinent data, applying format techniques, inserting symbols such as page numbers and typewriter characters, applying standard processes such as zero suppression, and testing data for reasonableness.

**Effectivity date.**  The date when demand is expected to start being recorded, as when the item is released for sale to customers or when it appears in the bill of materials of some parent item.

**Efficiency.**  The relationship between the planned labor requirements for a task and the actual labor time charged to the task.

**Eighty-twenty rule.**  This rule of thumb states that about 80 percent of the institution's total demand or usage is accounted for by 20 percent of the items.

**Elasticity.**  (1) An indication of the ability of a material to adapt to different circumstances. (2) The idea that when unit prices drop, revenue increases (more units are sold at lower prices).

**Electronic data processing.**  A term used to identify both the industry associated with the manufacture and use of computing equipment and the function of processing and/or manipulating data by electronic means.

**Elemental parts.**  Those parts that require no assembly in their manufacture or generation, such as nuts, bolts, and so on.

**Emergency orders.**  Some companies provide different services and different payment terms for "emergency" orders from customers, such as to repair a machine that is out of operation, in contrast to stock orders, which may take longer to fill but have more attractive payment terms.

**Empirical distribution.**  A probability distribution based on direct observation of data, rather than on some mathematical formula to describe the essential nature of the distribution.

**Encode.**  Translation of information or data into machine-readable format.

**End item.**  A product sold as a completed item or repair part.

**Engineering change.**  A revision to a parts list, bill of materials, or drawing made and authorized by the engineering department and usually identified by a control number.

**Engineering drawing.**  A blueprint that visually represents the dimensional characteristics of a part or assembly.

**Environment.**  That which makes up the physical surroundings of a material, usually referring to requirements for proper storage or use.

**Erase.**  To obliterate information from a computer storage medium.

**Esteem value.**  A monetary measure of the properties that contribute to the product's acceptability or desirability.

**Exception reports.**  Reports that list or flag only those items that deviate from plan or fall above or below some prescribed standards or criteria.

**Excess-material requisition.**  A requisition to authorize withdrawal from stores of material, or parts for assembly, in excess of the planned quantity.

**Exchange value.**  A monetary measure of the qualities and properties of an item that enables it to be exchanged for something else.

**Exclusive distribution.**   A pattern usually used for specialty goods, which are made available by only a few outlets, or possibly only one, in a given area.

**Ex-dock.**   Buyer takes titles to goods after they are unloaded from a ship.

**Execute.**   To interpret a machine instruction and perform the indicated operation(s) on the operand(s) specified. An operand is that which is operated on.

**Expected demand.**   An estimate of the average demand that should occur during some future period of time.

**Expediting.**   The function of searching out and correcting conditions accounting for discrepancies between planned and actual performance.

**Expendable item.**   An item that is consumed in use, losing its original identity, or the cost of which does not warrant approval by some higher body such as the equipment committee.

**Explosion.**   An expansion of a bill of materials into the total of each of the components required to manufacture an assembly or subassembly quantity.

**Exponential decay.**   A fixed fraction of stock on hand that is lost at the end of each period.

**Exponential smoothing.**   A technique of forecasting sales or demand that uses a smoothing factor in adjusting the difference between the last period's actual sales and the forecast.

**External funds.**   Funds acquired through borrowing or by selling new common or preferred stock.

**External storage.**   Storage facilities that are removable from the computer itself but that hold information in a form acceptable to the computer (magnetic tape, punched cards, and so on).

**Fabrication.**   A term used to distinguish manufacturing operations for components as opposed to assembly operations.

**Factor.**   An agent for the sale of merchandise who may hold possession of the goods in his own name or that of his principal. He is permitted to sell and to receive payment for the goods.

**Factory loading.**   Conversion of a sales forecast or order book into load on production departments and comparison with their capacity as part of the function of capacity planning.

**Factory-owned retail outlet.**   A direct channel in which a company's goods or services are offered only through retail outlets established and operated by the producer.

**Failure rate.**   Number of items failing a test, divided by the number tested.

**Feedback.**   The flow of information back into the control system so that actual performance can be compared to planned performance.

**Feeder ships**.  Ships that supply goods for use in later stages of production. This relates mostly to the manufacture of components and fabricated subassemblies for subsequent assembly.

**Field**.  (1) A set of one or more bits or characters treated as a unit of information. Commonly used synonym for *data element*. (2) An assigned area in a record to be marked with information.

**Field warehousing**.  A method of maintaining inventories in a "warehouse" at or close to the buyer organizations.

**FIFO (First-in, first-out)**.  (1) A method of inventory valuation which assumes that the oldest units in are the first units out. (2) A policy for scheduling work.

**File**.  A collection of related records that are stored together. The records are organized or ordered on the basis of some common factor called a key. Records may be of fixed or varying length and can be stored on different devices and storage media.

**File maintenance**.  Adding, deleting, or changing the contents of records in a file. Reorganizing the structure of a file to improve access to records or to change the storage space required.

**File management**.  A term that includes the functions of creation, insertion, deletion, or updating of stored files and records in files—the operations that are performed on files.

**File organization**.  A method for ordering data records stored as a file and providing a way to access the stored records. Examples: sequential, indexed, list, and random.

**Final assembly**.  The highest-level assembled product.

**Final market**.  Consumers who purchase goods or services for final use.

**Financial Accounting Standards Board (FASB)**.  A private (nongovernment) agency that functions as an accounting-standards-setting body.

**Financial lease**.  A lease that does not provide for maintenance services, is not cancellable, and is fully amortized over its lifetime.

**Financial structure**.  The entire right-hand side of the balance sheet; the way in which a firm is financed.

**Finished goods**.  Complete units and assemblies carried in stock ready for delivery to customers or for transfer to other plants. Generally, they are items that have been produced by a company or institution, although they may include complete items purchased for resale.

**Finished-goods inventory**.  The cost of a manufacturer's completed product that is being held for sale.

**Finished product**.  The end result of a process. Note: The finished product may be sold as is for consumption or may be the raw materials for another process.

**Firm program procedure**.  A procedure to permit orderly manufacture and maximum possible output, particularly when the production facilities as a whole are overcommitted. Its essential feature is that for a time ahead, which has to be decided, the production program is held firm. The latest priorities can be reflected in the orders that are included in the firm program, but the priorities of orders that have been included in the firm program cannot be changed.

**Firmware.**   Electronic circuitry built into a computer to replace common software functions.

**First-in, first-out.**   *See* FIFO.

**First-off inspection.**   Inspection of the first parts produced after a machine has been set up, prior to proceeding with the whole batch.

**Fixed charges.**   Costs that do not vary with the level of output, especially fixed financial costs such as interest, lease payments, and sinking-fund payments.

**Fixed cost.**   Costs that are not related to volume.

**Fixed-interval-reorder system.**   A periodic-reordering system in which the time interval between the orders is fixed but the size of the order may vary according to usage.

**Fixed-length record.**   A record that always contains the same number of data items and the same number of characters in a particular data item. Contrast with variable-length record.

**Fixed order cycle.**   Any system of stock control in which an order can be placed only at fixed review times.

**Fixed-order system.**   An inventory-control system in which the size of the order is fixed but the time interval between orders depends on actual demand.

**Fixed-period control system.**   The time between orders is kept fixed in this system. At each ordering time, an amount is ordered to bring the stock on hand and on order up to the estimated maximum required over the replenishment lead time.

**Flexible budget.**   A budget, usually referring to overhead costs only, that is prepared for a range, rather than for a single level of activity; one that can automatically be adjusted to changes in the level of volume.

**Flip-flop.**   A circuit or device containing active elements capable of assuming either one of two stable states at a given time.

**Floating order point.**   An order point that is responsive to changes in demand and/or lead time.

**Floor stocks.**   Stocks of inexpensive production parts held in the production facility from which production workers can draw without requisition.

**Floppy disc.**   Magnetic storage device; usually used on smaller computer systems.

**Flow chart.** A pictorial representation of processes and procedures for operation on data. A diagram that describes documents, procedures, processes, and equipment used in processing data in a specific application.

**Flow-process chart.** A graphic presentation of the sequence of operations, transportation, delays, and storages occurring during a process.

**Flow production.** A type of production in which all the batches of work follow the same sequence of operations, or predominantly so. Production processes that satisfy the criterion of flow production are sometimes erroneously classified as batch production merely because work is processed in batches. To discourage this mistake, the term *batched-flow production* is sometimes used.

**Flow racks.** Slides or conveyors on which gravity feeds items forward to the picker.

**Flow shop.** A shop in which machines and operators handle a standard, usually uninterrupted material flow, performing the same operations for each production run.

**FOB (Free on board).** A pricing strategy in which the seller bears all costs up to the point of placing the product on board a carrier at the point of the product's origin.

**FOB destination.** The seller assumes the cost of freight and title passes to the buyer at the destination.

**FOB point.** The location from which the consignee has title to the goods and is responsible for their continued distribution.

**Follow-up.** Monitoring of job progress to see that operations are performed on schedule or that purchased material or products will be received on schedule.

**Forcing orders.** Starting jobs ahead of their planned release time in order to level the work load.

**Forecast.** An objective projection into the future of historical data and/or a subjective estimate reflecting management's anticipation of changes or new factors influencing demand.

**Forecast error.** The difference between actual and forecast demand.

**Forecast interval.** The length of time into the future for which the forecast is computed.

**Forecasting.** The mechanism of arriving at measures for planning the future. This covers such things as product demand, supply, cost, prices, and lead times.

**Format.** The arrangement of data for computer input or output and/or the arrangement of any information as in a report.

**FORTRAN (FORmula TRANslating system).** A programming language for problems that can be expressed in algebraic notation.

**Forward load.** That part of the future load on a work center which is not yet available to run because previous operations have not been completed or materials or tools are not available.

**Free stock.** Physical stock less requirements allocated, usually used as part of a shortage-control procedure.

**Freeze period.** The number of planning periods within which the quantity and possibly schedule dates for open replenishment orders are not to be changed automatically by the system. Net requirements stated by the user are transferred from the supplier's inventory account into the user's inventory account under a dual accounting system, one freeze period after they are computed.

**Frozen order.** An order due within the freeze period which is not to be changed automatically by the system.

**Gantt chart.** The earliest and best-known type of control chart, especially designed to show graphically the relationship between planned performance and actual performance.

**Generator.** As in *program generator*, a program that permits the computer to write other programs automatically.

**GFE.** Government-furnished equipment.

**Going-rate pricing.** Used with homogeneous products, where prices tend to be the same for all products.

**Goods-in-process inventory.** Goods (or work) in the process of being manufactured, which when complete will be finished-goods inventory.

**Goods-received note.** A document used to record particulars of a consignment of goods when it arrives.

**Goods receiving.** The operations of receiving goods as they arrive in a factory, comprising checking the quantity against the order and/or advice note, recording details of the consignment on a goods-received note, and releasing the goods for storage or production. Goods inwards inspection, in which the quality is also checked, may be included.

**Goodwill cost.** A cost associated with a backorder, a lost sale, or any form of stockout or unsatisfied demand. This cost may be used to reflect the loss of future revenues because a customer experienced an unsatisfied demand.

**Grades.** Government-specified labels that reflect quality standards of certain goods.

**Graphics.** Output displays embodying graphs or other pictorial symbols, as contrasted with output of information in strictly digital form.

**Gravity feed.** This system requires special equipment such as either gravity-feed storage bins or double-access bins. In either case, incoming material is sequenced behind the old stock. Thus the old stock is removed first either from the front of the bin or from the lower end of the rack or incline.

**Gross requirements.** The total requirements for a particular component, not taking into account any inventory of that component which is currently on hand.

**Grouping orders.** Combining orders for several items from one vendor to take advantage of cost reduction.

**Group technology.** A technique for securing to a large extent the advantages of flow production where otherwise batch production would have to be used. Its basis is to split a large part of the output of the shop into families of sufficiently similar components to enable a flow line to be set up to manufacture each family.

**Handleability.** An indication of the ease of manipulating, directing, controlling, or transporting a material.

**Handling.** All movements of goods and materials in or about the undertaking.

**Handling and storage costs.** Some incremental costs vary directly with the size of inventories. There are handling costs when materials must be placed in inventory or issued from inventory. Included also are costs associated with storage, such as rent or prorated space costs, insurance, taxes (in proprietary institutions), obsolescence, spoilage, and capital costs. If average inventories increase, these costs will also increase and vice versa. *See* Holding costs.

**Hard copy.** A printed copy of system output in a form readable by human beings.

**Hardware.** A term used to describe the physical units and capabilities of a computer. This includes the central processing unit as well as the peripherals such as the encoders or input devices such as teletypes, printers, CRTs, and so on. *Contrast with* software.

**Hash total.** A control total, accumulated manually from a batch of input documents, that helps ensure that entry of data into the computer system is correct and documents are not lost. Hash totals can be kept on quantities, part numbers, invoice numbers, and so on.

**Head.** A device that reads, records, or erases information in a storage medium.

**Hedging.** A practice of selling for future delivery utilized by dealers or processors to protect themselves against loss. Any profit owing to subsequent price increases is also sacrificed.

**Heuristic.** Pertaining to exploratory methods of problem solving in which solutions are discovered by evaluation of the progress made toward the final result. *Contrast with* algorithm.

**Hidden quality.** Product or service characteristics that are not immediately obvious to potential purchasers but that may differentiate the item from competitors sufficiently to encourage purchase.

**High-level language.**   User-oriented symbolic programming language with high degree of readability, hence maintainability, such as COBOL, FORTRAN, and Pl1.

**Holding or carrying cost.**   All costs associated with maintaining an inventory, including the cost of the capital invested in the inventory, insurance, taxes, warehouse overhead, and so on. This cost is often stated as a percentage of the cost of the units stored in inventory.

**Hold order.**   A written order directing that certain operations or work be interrupted or terminated, pending a change in design or other disposition of the material.

**Hold points.**   Stock points for semifinished inventory.

**Horizontal marketing.**   An organization concentrated on one level of the distribution channel.

**House accounts.**   Customers who are called on by upper-level sales executives rather than by field representatives.

**Idea generation.**   The first stage in new product or service development, which involves gathering all possible concepts from a variety of internal and external sources.

**Ideal capacity.**   The absolute maximum number of units that could be produced in a given operating situation, with no allowances for work stoppages and repairs.

**Idle time.**   Time when operators or machines are not producing product because of setup, maintenance, lack of material, tooling.

**Illegal character.**   A character (symbol) or combination of characters that is not valid according to some criterion.

**Immediate access.**   Retrieval of a piece of data from a data store faster than it is possible to read through the whole data store searching for the piece of data, or to sort the data store.

**Impact.**   An acronym for Inventory Management Program and Control Technique. This term refers to an application developed by IBM Corporation for determining when to order and how much to order.

**Impact printer.**   A printer device in which the printing mechanism physically touches the page.

**Impulse goods.**   Goods or services that consumers tend to purchase impulsively, with little planning or consideration.

**Inactive inventory.**   Designates the stocks that are in excess of the contemplated or actual consumption within the budgeted period.

**Increment.**   The quantity of addition to inventory. Example: One hundred boxes or units of issue of tongue depressors are checked in by the receiving department. When the one hundred boxes are entered into the computer inventory, this action is called an increment.

**Incremental cost of capital.** The average cost of the increment of capital raised during a given year.

**Independent demand.** Demand that is directly related to customer demand and as such must be forecast. (The demand for finished-goods inventories is typically an independent demand, whereas the demand for components is dependent and may be calculated.)

**Independent-demand items.** Distribution inventory from which any buyer may order.

**Index.** A computer-stored table containing the addresses of records in a data base. There may, for example, be a part-number index used to refer to a file of inventory records. Also referred to as a *list*.

**Indexed sequential.** A method of data retrieval where information is acquired based on some group of unique identifying characters on the input record matching a similar field on the stored record.

**Indirect channel.** A route for goods and services from producers to consumers that includes wholesale or retail intermediaries.

**Indirect cost.** Cost that is not directly incurred by a particular job or operation, such as heating costs.

**Indirect materials.** Raw materials that become part of the final product but in such small quantities that their cost is not applied directly to the product. Instead their costs become part of the overhead associated with producing goods or services.

**Inelasticity.** If lower prices do not result in increased total dollar sales, the product or service is price inelastic.

**Information.** Data that have been processed into a meaningful form. It adds to a representation and tells the recipient something that was not known before. What is information for one person may not be information for another. Information should be timely, accurate, and complete. Information reduces uncertainty. *Contrast with* Data.

**Information flow.** Describes flow of information from one institution to another.

**Information retrieval.** The techniques for optimally storing large amounts of data for easy and economic access or for future references.

**Information system.** A computer-based system that processes data into a meaningful form that can be used by the recipient for decision-making purposes.

**Initialize.** To set various counters, switches, and addresses to zero or other starting values at the beginning of or at the prescribed points in a computer routine. Initialization is used as an aid to recovery and restart during a long computer run.

**In-process inventory.** Unfinished goods awaiting completion.

**Input.** Information or data transferred from an external storage medium into the internal storage of the computer; the device or collective set of devices necessary for input; the coded instructions arranged in proper sequence to direct the transfer of data or information.

**Input-output devices.** Devices used to enter data into a system or to record results from the computer.

**Input validation.** Performing tests and checks on input to ensure that the input operation is legal and the input itself is correct. Pertaining to a wide variety of tests that can be applied to ensure the correctness of data being input to a computer system.

**Inquiry.** A request for information from storage, for example, a request for a display of the number of available airline seats or the year-to-date usage of a product.

**Insistence.** The final level of consumer brand acceptance—the consumer has become so loyal to the brand that he will not accept any substitute.

**Inspection order.** An authorization to an inspection department or group to perform an inspection operation.

**Instruction.** A set of characters that defines an operation together with one or more addresses, and that, as a unit, causes the computer to perform the operation on the indicated quantities.

**Integrated data processing.** Data moves automatically from operation to operation by means of a job-control program.

**Integrated system.** The system characteristic in which input data can be directed to service all required users with minimal duplication of process.

**Intelligent terminal.** A computer-oriented terminal that has built-in data-checking capabilities and a small memory. Special functions may also be built into the terminal to perform certain checks on the data or to handle certain kinds of transactions (for example, bank deposit and withdrawal transactions).

**Intensive distribution.** Placing goods or services in multiple outlets; mainly used for impulse or convenience goods.

**Interactive computing.** The type of computer processing in which the user of the system communicates directly with the system to input data and instructions and receive output. *See also* On-line.

**Interactive mode.** A mode of operation in which information is entered, acted on by the computer, and then responded to by the computer.

**Interface.** (1) The hardware and programs that permit exchange of information between computer systems or among devices. (2) The facility to allow information to pass from one application to another. (3) A shared boundary between two systems.

**Intermediaries.** Various types of institutions, middlemen, or agents serving in various capacities in the distribution channel.

**Intermediate clause**.  A clause in tariffs providing for the application of rates from or to points not listed that are the same as those published from or to more distant points via the same route.

**Intermediate market**.  The market composed of industrial, governmental, and institutional buyers, who purchase goods or services for resale or for their own operation.

**Internal storage**.  Addressable storage directly controlled by the central processing unit of a digital computer.

**Interval time**.  A term sometimes used in shop loading for the interval of time to be allowed from the completion of processing on one operation to the start of processing on the next operation on a batch of work. It comprises transit time and queueing time.

**Intrinsic forecast**.  A forecast based on past history, such as a forecast made from a moving average.

**Inventory**.  Stock-keeping items that are held in a stock point and that serve to decouple successive operations in the process of manufacturing a product and distributing it to the customer. Inventories may consist of finished goods ready for sale or use, of parts or intermediate products, or of raw materials. Inventory is also frequently used to mean the investment in inventoried stock.

**Inventory analysis**.  Determination of the levels of investment in inventory that are necessary to support various commercial, institutional, and production policies on delivery periods, service levels, plant utilization, and the extent to which the output required from the production facility is to be allowed to fluctuate.

**Inventory-carrying costs**.  One type of cost involved in planning and controlling inventory. Factors included in inventory-carrying costs are cost of money invested, obsolescence, deterioration, shrinkage or loss, taxes, insurance, space charges, and handling costs. *See* Holding costs.

**Inventory control**.  The control of inventory, and particularly tradeoffs between the various associated costs on the one hand, and the service level or stockout rate on the other.

**Inventory-cost method**.  To apportion the cost of goods available for sale or use between the cost of goods sold or used and ending inventory.

**Inventory cost of capital**.  The inventory dollar value times the current rate of interest on borrowed money.

**Inventory data base**.  A record of all the information relevant to each item carried in stock.

**Inventory file**.  A record containing the net quantity of all parts and subassemblies normally maintained in inventory.

**Inventory investment**.  The number of dollars that are tied up in inventory.

**Inventory models**.  Models relating to inventory management that answer the questions "How much?" and "When?" They permit the manager to determine the point at which orders should be placed for repeat goods, and the quantity of each order.

**Inventory policy.** A definite statement of the philosophy of management on inventories.

**Inventory shorts list.** A listing of all items that are low or out of stock.

**Inventory shrinkage.** Losses resulting from scrap, deterioration, breakage, pilferage, and so on.

**Inventory simulation.** The use of simulation to determine how different inventory-control techniques will work.

**Inventory standard.** A standard level, expressed in monetary value, for any class of inventory (material, parts, work in process, and so on) calculated realistically to take account of operating policy and decision rules to be used in stock control and operation scheduling.

**Inventory team.** Team for taking physical inventory, consisting of one or two counters, a checker, and a writer.

**Inventory turnover.** The number of times that an inventory cycles during the year. The inventory turnover is arrived at by dividing the average inventory level into the annual sales or usage.

**Inventory usage.** The value or the number of units of an inventory item consumed over a period of time.

**Inventory value.** The sum of the number of units of each item on hand or in storage in the storerooms and elsewhere of each line item times its current purchase unit price or market value.

**Invoice.** An invoice is a notice from a seller to a buyer that goods ordered have been delivered or shipped and that appropriate payment is expected. It indicates the purchaser, seller, amount to be paid, discounts, and other terms of payment.

**I/O.** Input-output.

**JCL (Job-control language).** (1) Specific directions used in computer processing to direct the input and output and to mark the beginning and end of a job. (2) A set of statements that are used to describe a job (program) and its requirements to the operating system. The language makes it possible to identify such requirements as amount of processing time, memory space, translators, and files used in executing a job.

**Job-order costing.** A system of applying manufacturing costs to specific jobs or batches of specialized or unique production in proportion to the amounts of materials, attention, and effort used to produce each unit or group of units.

**Job scheduling.** Provides each major department or assembly foreman with a schedule or orders to be completed by a specific date.

**Job-shop operation.** A functional organization centered around particular types of equipment or operations.

**Job status.** A periodic report showing the plan for completing a job; usually the requirements and completion date, and the progress of the job against that plan.

**Jobber.** A dealer who purchases goods or commodities from manufacturers or importers for resale to retailers.

**Jobbing production.** Production of products designed to meet individual customers' requirements, usually in small quantities.

**Journey time.** Loading time plus travel time plus drop time.

**Judgment items.** Those inventory items that cannot be effectively controlled by mechanical means because of age (new or obsolete product) or management decision (promotional product).

**Key.** A data element (or group of data elements) used to find or identify a record.

**Keypunch.** Process of punching a hole into a card to denote a specific unit of data for feeding into the computer.

**Keypunch machine.** A device that is activated by depressing a key on a typewriterlike keyboard to punch holes in a card. The punched holes represent data.

**Knocked down.** Articles that are taken apart for shipping purposes so as to reduce the cubic-foot displacement.

**Labor claim.** A production worker's regular report detailing the jobs he or she has worked on; the number of pieces, number of hours, and so on; and often the amount of money to which he or she is entitled.

**Labor ticket.** A form used to record the application of labor to specific jobs or production operations.

**Landed price.** Vendor's price, which includes the cost of the goods, transportation, and other costs relating to delivery to the location specified by the purchaser.

**Language.** A set of representations, conventions, and rules used to convey information into and out of computers.

**Last-in-first-out (LIFO) inventory accounting.** (1) Valuation of inventory by assuming that the items most recently received are used first. (2) Policy for scheduling work.

**Layout.** The kits of components ahead of the assembly department waiting to be put together.

**LCL.** Less-than-carload quantity.

**Lead time.** The time interval needed to complete a portion or all of the activities in a replenishing cycle. It includes the time needed to identify a replenishment requirement, process the order, and receive the item in stock ready for use.

**Lead-time demand.** The number of units demanded and removed from inventory during the lead-time period.

**Lead-time-demand distribution.** In probabilistic inventory models, this is the probability distribution that describes the possible number of units demanded during the lead-time period.

**Lead-time offset.** A term used in time-series planning where a requirement in one time period will require release of an order in some earlier time period based on the lead time for an item.

**Leading indicators.** Specific business-activity indexes that are useful to the forecaster since any trends in these indicators will later reflect on the forecast. For example, number of housing starts is a leading indicator for the industry that supplies builders' hardware.

**Learning curve.** A job takes longer to perform at first than after a similar job has been repeated several times. The time per job frequently is reduced by the same percentage every time the total number of jobs completed has doubled. Hence at the beginning of a new production run there will be some loss in efficiency compared with a standard based on long runs.

**Letter of intent.** An order for equipment that may be used to reserve a delivery position or tentative delivery date at some future time.

**Level.** Each agent or institution in the distribution channel, beginning with the producer, that takes title ownership or selling responsibility constitutes a channel level; for example, two level—producer to consumer; three level—producer to retailer to consumer; four level—producer to wholesaler to retailer to consumer; five level—producer to wholesaler to jobber to retailer to consumer. Also used to denote the structure of a product. Level 0, for example, would be the final assembled product. Level 1 would include all the subassemblies that go into the final assembly. Level 2 would be all the components that go into the level-1 subassemblies.

**Level-by-level planning.** A term used in materials planning to describe a technique that involves the determination of gross requirements at the highest level and the comparison of this gross requirement with available inventory, which then determines the net requirements at that level. The net requirements at that level are the gross requirements for the next level of inventory down. Level-by-level planning takes into account available inventory of components at all levels.

**Library routine.** A proven set of coded instructions arranged in proper sequence, which is maintained in a collection of computer programs.

**Lien.** A lender's claim on assets that are pledged for a loan.

**Life-cycle status.** The stage of an individual product on the "normal" continuum progressing from product birth to death; a useful concept for final market segmentation.

**LIFO (last-in, first-out).** In cost determination, a pricing technique used in the issuance of materials that requires the cost of materials last acquired to be recorded first for current issues. Also, a policy for scheduling work.

**Light pen.** A device available with certain visual-display units that enables the operator to change the information displayed by pointing the light pen at the screen.

**Limiting operation.** In a series of operations with no alternative routings, the capacity of the total system can be no greater than the operation with the least capacity. As long as this limiting condition exists, the total system can be effectively scheduled by simply scheduling the limiting operation.

**Line balancing.** An assembly-line process can be divided into elemental tasks, each with a specified time requirement per unit of product and a sequence relationship with the other tasks. Line balancing is the assignment of these tasks to work stations so as to minimize the total amount of unassigned time at all stations.

**Line management.** Those managers in an organization whose duties are concerned with direct executive control of the institution's main operations. *Contrast to* staff functions.

**Line of credit.** An arrangement whereby a financial institution (bank or insurance company) commits itself to lend up to a specified maximum amount of funds during a specified period.

**Line printer.** A device capable of printing one line of characters across a page simultaneously as the paper advances continuously over a type cylinder containing all characters in all positions.

**Linear programming.** A mathematical approach to a group of management problems that contain many interacting variables expressed as linear inequalities and that basically combine limited resources to maximize profits or minimize costs.

**Liquidated damages.** A sum agreed on between the parties to a contract as damages for breach of contract, to be paid by the breacher or nonperformer.

**List price.** The basic price the manufacturer asks final consumers to pay for a product or service.

**Live load.** This is the load of manufacturing orders against a manufacturing facility that are actually available to be worked on.

**Load.** This is the amount of scheduled work ahead of a manufacturing facility, department, or section, usually expressed in terms of hours of work.

**Load leveling**. Spreading orders out in time so that the amount of work that falls in the time periods tends to be distributed evenly.

**Loading**. Comparing the hours required for each operation with the hours available in each work center in the time period scheduled.

**Loading time**. Amount of time needed to load goods onto the delivery vehicle.

**Locator file**. A file used in the stockroom where each item does not have a specific location. The locator file records where the product has been stored.

**Logistics management**. A segment of materials management concerned with getting the material to the right place at the right time. The basic problem in logistics management is to determine optimum investment and location of materials.

**Lot size**. The amount of a particular product that is normally ordered either from the plant or vendor. *See* Order quantity.

**LTL**. Less-than-truckload quantity.

**Machine address**. Synonymous with *absolute address*. An absolute, direct identification represented by a name, label, or number for a register or location in the device. A machine address refers to a unique location consisting of electronic, electrostatic, electrical, hardware, or other elements into which data may be entered and from which data may be obtained as desired.

**Machine center**. A group of similar machines that can all be considered together for purposes of loading.

**Machine language**. Synonymous with machine-oriented language, a system for representing and communicating information or data that the machine can interpret and use without translation.

**Machine sensible**. Information or data represented in a form that can be read by the machine in question.

**Machine utilization**. The percentage of time that a machine is running or producing as opposed to idle time.

**Macroinstruction**. A statement to the compiler or assembler written in the same general manner as source instructions. It tells the computer both to insert a specially coded subroutine and to modify that subroutine in accordance with the additional information given as part of the statement. Many compilers allow the programmer to define his own macroinstructions.

**Mad (mean absolute deviation)**. Calculation used in measuring and updating forecast error.

**Magnetic-ink-character reader**. An input device that can recognize and accept input data that are recorded on documents in magnetic ink.

**Magnetic tape.** A device used to record and store the information extracted from the disc and used in producing reports and listings.

**Main frame.** The central processing element of a computer, containing the main memory, arithmetic units, and registers.

**Main memory.** Usually the fastest storage device of a computer and the one from which instructions are executed. *Contrast with* Auxiliary storage.

**Makespan.** *See* production cycle.

**Make to order.** Manufacture only to customer orders.

**Make to stock.** Manufacture and carry in a finished-goods inventory for sale "off the shelf."

**Management by exception.** The practice of focusing attention mainly on significant deviations from expected results.

**Management information system (MIS).** A system designed to provide the information that management needs to make decisions.

**Manifest.** A statement listing the particulars of all shipments loaded in a car, ship, truck, and so on. Usually refers to the ship's manifest.

**Manufacturer's agent.** Wholesalers whose main function is selling the goods they carry.

**Manufacturer's brand.** Identifies a product with the name of a manufacturer.

**Manufacturing forecast.** The sales forecast translated into meaningful terms for the manufacturing departments. A sales forecast might show total units, whereas the manufacturing forecast might be broken down into total hours by significant machine center.

**Manufacturing order.** A document conveying authority for the manufacture of specified parts or products in specified quantities. The manufacturing order sometimes also shows the date by which the job must be completed and due dates for individual operations that have been assigned by the scheduler.

**Manufacturing process.** The series of activities performed on material to convert it from the raw or semifinished state to a state of further completion and a greater value.

**Margin** (profit on sales). The profit margin is the percentage of after-tax profit to sales.

**Marginal cost.** The cost of an additional unit. The marginal cost of capital is the cost of an additional dollar of new funds.

**Marginal revenue.** The additional gross revenue produced by selling one additional unit of output.

**Markdown pricing.** A pricing strategy design to "move out" excess inventory by cutting product price.

**Market.** A group of buyers with significant buying potential and with unfilled needs or desires, who have the means to purchase, and whom a marketer can profitably serve.

**Market classification.** The process of separating potential customers into two broadly defined groups—the intermediate and the final markets.

**Market segmentation.** The process of identifying market "groups" with common needs, consumption patterns, and so on.

**Market share.** The percentage of a given market controlled by an individual seller; obtaining a specific share of the market is a standard pricing objective.

**Market stability.** A basic marketing strategy in which a firm tries to maintain a less-competitive, steadier price structure, in times of high and low demand.

**Market testing.** A stage in new-product or -service development during which the idea is actually tried out in a small number of authentic sales situations.

**Marketing.** The business function concerned with directing goods and services from the producers to the consumers, including: finding out what people need, helping them to develop need satisfiers, informing and persuading, moving properly priced goods and services to consumers, and keeping consumers satisfied.

**Marketing concept.** A business philosophy that accepts as its basic premise that firms must first begin to understand their consumers.

**Marketing cycle.** The idea that marketing is a continuing process that begins with understanding consumers and continues over a period of time as consumers purchase products.

**Marketing information system (MIS).** A structured flow of data that is collected, analyzed, and distributed to marketing executives on a continuing basis, designed to evaluate and improve marketing decisions and programs.

**Marketing mix.** The set of "competitive tools" available for marketing managers—marketing research, product or service development, pricing, promotion, and distribution.

**Marketing plan.** A written statement of objectives and of how marketing management will utilize the controllable tools (product, price, promotion, channels) to accomplish them.

**Marketing research.** Systematic gathering, recording, and analyzing of data related to marketing.

**Marshaling.** The preparation of kits of parts and/or subassemblies ready for assembly.

**Marshaling list.** A list of items to be marshaled for an assembly batch.

**Master file.** A permanent file of data pertaining to the history or current status of a factor or entity of interest to an organization. A master file is periodically updated to maintain its usefulness. *Contrast with* Transaction file.

**Master procurement plan.** A schedule of those items that must be purchased in future time periods.

**Master production schedule.** A forecast of what items must be produced in future time periods.

**Master tariff.** A tariff with the Interstate Commerce Commission applying to a large number of applicable tariffs. Used mainly to publish general rate increases.

**Master warehouse.** Safety stock to cover all regions of the country is carried in a master warehouse. Satellite or field warehouses fill orders from customers in their territories. The master-warehouse location can coincide with a satellite, in which case the inventory balances are merely a bookkeeping convenience and there is not necessarily any physical segregation. In general, a given product has only one master warehouse, but for different products the master warehouse can be at different sites.

**Material.** Any commodity used directly or indirectly in producing a product, raw materials, component parts, subassemblies, and supplies.

**Material control.** This term is sometimes used synonymously with stock control and sometimes to cover one or more of the following: calculation of requirements, ordering and stock control, store keeping, goods receiving, and possibly buying.

**Material-flow-process chart.** A graphic representation of the sequence of operations, transports, delays, and storages occurring during a process. The material-flow-process chart presents the process in terms of the events which occur to the material such as distances moved and the time required to move it.

**Material hold tag.** Form used to identify and hold certain materials in store for specific orders.

**Material obsolescence report.** A report showing slow-moving and inactive items prone to obsolescence.

**Material-requirement plan.** A schedule that outlines the time-phased priority plan for assemblies, necessary to support the master schedule.

**Material requisition.** A document issued by an authorized person instructing a store keeper to issue certain items from stock.

**Material transfer.** Document used to effect the transfer of material between stock rooms and/or divisions of the institution or company.

**Materials control.** The function of maintaining a constantly available supply of raw materials, purchased parts, and supplies that are required for the manufacture of products or for the performance of a service. Functional responsibilities include the requisitioning of materials for purchase in economic quantities at the proper time, and their receipt, storage, and protection; the issuing of materials or use upon authorized request; and the maintenance and verification of inventory records.

**Materials management.** A term used to describe the grouping of management functions related to the complete cycle of material flow, from the requisitioning, purchase, and internal control of materials; to the planning and control of work in process; to the warehousing, shipping, distribution, and/or disposal after use of a product.

**Materials-management information system (MMIS).** The combination of human and computer-based resources that results in the collection, storage, retrieval, communication, and use of data for the purpose of cost-effective management of materials and for planning of materials-related operations.

**Materials-ordering system.** System used in the development and monitoring of ordering quantities to optimize inventory-related costs and service levels.

**Materials planning.** In manufacturing, the planning of requirements for components based on requirements for higher-level assemblies. The production schedule is exploded or extended through the use of the bill of materials, and the results are netted against inventory.

**Materials schedule.** A listing of the specifications, quantities, and deliveries of the materials to be purchased during the next period.

**Matrix.** A rectangular arrangement of elements in rows and columns.

**Matrix bill of material.** Bills of material for groups of products in families having common components that are arranged in a matrix so that all requirements for common components can be readily totalled.

**Max-min.** *See* Min-max system.

**Maximum level.** The largest amount of stock permitted to be on hand for an item at any one time.

**Mean time to failure.** Expected average interval between periods of equipment inoperability.

**Media.** Newspapers, television, radio, and magazines in which advertising is placed in order to reach potential customers.

**Median.** A measure of the center of a set of numbers such that half the observations are larger and half are smaller than the median. *See* Probability distribution.

**Memory.** An organization of storage elements, primarily for the retrieval of information; examples are semiconductor memory, magnetic-core memory, magnetic-disk memory. The rapid-access storage elements from which program instructions are executed and data operated on are referred to as *main memory.*

**Merchandise inventory.** Goods held for resale, acquired through purchase without further processing.

**Merchant wholesaler.** A middleman who buys, pays for, and takes title to goods.

**Merge.**   To combine into a single set two or more sets of information without altering the order of the items.

**MICR (magnetic in-character recognition).**   A device that detects the presence or absence of a photosensitive mark.

**Microinstruction.**   An instruction consisting of a small, single, short command, such as add, shift, or delete.

**Microprogramming.**   The use of a certain special set of characters that defines an operation together with one or more addresses, or no address, and that, as a unit, causes the computer to perform the operation on the indicated quantities. The set consists of only basic elemental operations that the programmer may combine into higher-level instructions, which he or she may then program using the higher-level instructions only.

**Middleman.**   Wholesalers and/or retailers who assist manufacturers in moving goods to consumers.

**Min-max system.**   In inventory control, usually a fixed-interval-reorder system, which consists of reviewing stocks at regular intervals but placing a replenishment order only when stocks on hand plus stocks on order have fallen to (or below) some specified order point (minimum). When this occurs, an order is placed to bring the amount on hand plus that on order up to a specified ceiling level (maximum).

**Minicomputer.**   Small, compact, relatively inexpensive, and easy-to-install computer equipment.

**Minimum stock.**   This term is sometimes used variously to mean the alarm level, the reorder level, or the buffer stock of an item.

**Mix control.**   The control of the individual products going through the plant.

**Mnemonic.**   A technique used to assist human memory. A mnemonic represents and resembles the original word by using several letters of the original word in sequence; for example, "mlpy" for "multiply."

**Mode.**   An established method of operation, such as batch-processing mode, on-line mode, foreground mode.

**Model.**   An approximate representation of a process or system that attempts to relate the most important variables in the system in such a way that an increased understanding of the system is attained.

**Modular bill of materials.**   Capital products have a large variety of options and accessories and are usually assembled to order. Each of the stockable subassemblies can be forecast and planned, so that there are reasonable stocks available to meet customer requirements. In that case, the end product is made up from modular bills of materials; and the particular mix of features is specified as firm orders are received from customers.

**Modularity.** A consideration in the design of systems and programs. A system has modularity when its constituent parts can be readily identified, altered, or augmented.

**Modulation.** The process by which business-machine codes are made compatible with communication-carrier transmission facilities.

**Money market.** Financial market in which funds are borrowed or lent for short periods (less than one year). The money market is distinguished from the capital market, which is the market for long-term funds.

**Monitoring report.** A non-decision-oriented report that summarizes or describes events that have taken place.

**Monte Carlo.** A method to derive statistically valid conclusions about the entire span of outcome of a process, one or more of whose components are characterized by numbers that can only be specified within limits. The method consists of selecting, repeatedly and separately, collections of numbers that represent the individual characterizations of one or more components such that, together, these selections duplicate the essence of the process as a whole.

**Motivation research.** Attempts to demonstrate, using analytical techniques from psychiatry, the true reasons for consumer behavior.

**Move order.** The authorization to move a particular item from one location to another.

**Move ticket.** A card used in dispatching to authorize movement of a job from one work center to another, and report the progress of the job toward completion.

**Move time.** The actual time that a job spends in transit from one operation to another in the shop.

**Movement inventory.** A type of in-process inventory that arises because of the time required to move goods from one place to another.

**Moving annual total.** Total inventory throughout for the last twelve months.

**Moving weighted average.** The average cost of all inventory in stock is charged as the cost of each unit out.

**MRP (Materials-requirements planning).** Refers to systems that keep track of requirements and plan production in discrete time intervals. Usually the term includes explosion of net requirements from a parent schedule to dependent requirements on subordinate items.

**Multilevel bill of materials.** A bill of materials that shows all the components going into the assembly at the various assembly levels.

**Multiplexing.** The process of transferring data from several devices operating at relatively low-transfer rates to one storage device operating at a higher-transfer rate in such a manner that the high-speed device is not obliged to wait for the low-speed devices.

**Multiprocessing.** Cooperating computer processors working together on the same task.

**Multiprogramming.** The more efficient use of computer hardware resources for simultaneous processing of two or more jobs.

**Nanosecond.** One-billionth of a second.

**Need date.** The date at which net requirements become positive; there is not sufficient stock on hand and on order to cover gross requirements. *Contrast* Schedule date.

**Needs.** A psychological or physiological necessity; everyone has basic needs that, when stimulated, provoke action.

**Net change.** A materials-planning system in which the materials plan is not recalculated periodically but instead is updated as each requirement change occurs.

**Net requirement.** The actual manufacturing or purchasing requirements for a particular component. The net requirements are calculated by deducting the available inventory from the gross requirements.

**Net-requirements schedule.** The outstanding manufacturing or purchasing requirements for an item, taking account of all existing stock and orders in process.

**Network.** A complex of data terminals all eventually able to communicate with a central computer(s) across data lines, telephone lines, telecommunication lines, or other lines.

**Network-analysis techniques.** A collection of techniques well suited to the planning and progress control of one-of-a-kind projects. *See* PERT or CPM.

**Network-description table (NDT).** Specifies the topology of the entire network. The *nodal-route vector (NRV)* is part of the NDT in that it describes modal addresses and routing specifications and eliminates the need for programmers to adjust for different routing procedures.

**Network planning.** This is a broad generic term for techniques that are used to plan complex projects. Two of the most important network-planning techniques are CPM and PERT.

**Node.** Any station in a telecommunications network. Can be used for transmission, reception, or switching.

**Noise.** Distortions in data as they are communicated to a receiver or user. The distortions may block the data to make them useless.

**Noise level.** A general term in communications theory, which relates to extraneous messages that interfere with the intended message.

**Nominal interest rate.** The contracted or stated interest rate, undeflated for price-level changes.

**Non-patient-charge item.** An item charged to a department overhead account and not directly to a patient, for example, pencils, batteries, tongue depressors.

**Nonsignificant part numbers.** Part numbers that are assigned to each part but do not convey any information about the part.

**Nonlinear programming.** The maximization or minimization of the value of a linear expression of variables that are subject to increasing or decreasing returns to scale. The "nonlinear" nature comes from the fact that a doubling, say, of the inputs of one variable would not double the output, but instead would more than double or less than double it, depending on the increasing or decreasing returns to scale.

**Normal probability distribution.** A symmetrical, bell-shaped probability function.

**Normalize.** To adjust the representation of a quantity so that the representation lies in a prescribed range.

**Numeric data.** Data consisting of the numbers 0-9 on which arithmetic operations are performed.

**Numerical analysis.** The construction of effective methods to calculate quantitative solutions to mathematical problems that may or may not have analytic solutions, and the specification of the errors and the ranges of errors in obtaining such solutions.

**Object program.** Synonymous with *target program* and *object routine*. The complete sequence of machine instructions and routines necessary to solve a problem, usually coded in machine language as the output of an automatic coding system. *Contrast with* Source program, written in symbolic or algebraic language.

**Objective probability distribution.** Probability distributions determined by statistical procedures.

**Obsolescence.** Loss of product value resulting from a model or style change or technological development.

**Off line.** The condition of not being in direct communication with the computer, machines, or devices that are under the control of the central processing unit.

**On hand.** The balance shown in perpetual-inventory records as being present at the stocking location.

**On line.** (1) Characterization of a system and of the peripheral devices in a system in which the operation of the peripheral equipment is under the control of the central processing unit. Information of the current activity is introduced into the data-processing system as soon as it occurs. *Contrast with* Off line. (2) The condition of being in direct communication with the computer, machines, or devices that are under the direct control of the central processing unit. Airline-reservations systems are the best known on-line systems. This is distinguished from batch-processing.

**On order.** The stock on order is the quantity represented by the total of all outstanding replenishment orders.

**Open-account purchase.** A purchase made by a buyer who has established credit with the seller. The transaction is charged to the purchaser's account, payment for which is to be made at some future date agreed on by buyer and seller.

**Open insurance policy.** A type of insurance covering shipments for a designated time or a stated value and not limited to a single shipment.

**Open item.** A system in which the computer does not directly control a process but instead displays or prints out information to assist the operator in determining and taking appropriate action. Management information systems are open-loop systems.

**Open-purchase-order report.** A listing of all open orders currently in the system.

**Open shop.** Pertaining to the operation of a computer facility in which most productive problem programming is performed by the problem originator rather than by a group of programming specialists. The use of the computer itself may also be described as open shop if the user/programmer also serves as the operator.

**Open to buy.** (1) A retailer's term referring to the largest total value or or volume of an item available for purchase. (2) The volume or total value of goods remaining to be purchased against a specific requisition.

**Operating level.** The maximum level of stock in a min-max system. The order quantity is the difference between the operating level and the available stock when a replenishment order is triggered.

**Operation card.** A document printed for each operation to be done. It shows some or all of the following: product, part or assembly number, operation number, work center, tool number, standard times, batch quantity, and start and completion date for the operation.

**Operation layout.** A list of production operations in the order in which they are to be carried out in the manufacture of an item.

**Operation scheduling.** Specifying by a routine procedure the planned start and/or finish dates for each operation.

**Operations research.** A profession or discipline devoted to the application of science-based methods to solving problems in which there is a choice of a number of cost-effective or optimum solutions.

**Operations sequence.** The sequential steps which manufacturing engineering recommends that a given assembly or part follow in its flow through the plant.

**Opportunity cost.** The return on capital that could have resulted had the capital been used for some other purpose.

**Optical scan.** Equipment that recognizes characters by their visual images acceptable as input into computer.

**Optimal.** Giving rise to the best combination of values for all the variables involved. Computer processes are optimized by rearranging the instructions or data in storage in such a way that the program can be run with a minimum number of time-consuming jumps or transfers.

**Optimization.** The process of determining those values for the variables in a system that will give the best or most-desired values for the output variables.

**Order.** A request from a customer for goods to be delivered or services to be performed.

**Order backlog.** Orders that have been received for which goods are not yet available.

**Order control.** Control of the progress of each customer order or stock order through the successive operations in its production cycle.

**Order cost.** Procurement costs originate from the expanse of issuing an order to an outside supplier or from internal-production setup costs. Order costs include the fixed cost of maintaining an order department and the variable costs of preparing and executing purchase requisitions. Even when orders are delivered from other parts of the same institution, order costs still apply. The same purchasing routine of checking inventory levels, issuing orders, follow-up, inspection, and updating inventory records pertains to internal procurement.

**Order-intake control.** The function of ensuring that completion dates agreed to between the production and sales departments on customers' orders are realistic in that they do not exceed available or planned capacity.

**Order number.** A number assigned by production control to a given order in the manufacturing facility.

**Order point.** The level of total stock on hand and on order at which action is taken to replenish the stock.

**Order quantity.** The quantity ordered. The term is frequently used to mean batch quantity.

**Ordering.** The function of specifying what shall be made or bought, in what quantity, and by what date it is to be available.

**Ordering cost.** The fixed cost (salaries, paper, transaction, and so on) associated with placing an order for an item.

**Original-equipment manufacturer (OEM).** Seller's classification of a buyer whose purchases are incorporated into a product he manufactures, usually without changing the item he acquires.

**Outgoing materials systems.**  A system used in the receipt and control of the finished product from production, the warehousing of the product, and shipment of the finished product to the customers. This might run the whole gamut from the proper recording and handling of a single item of a finished product to be shipped against a specific customer order, to a whole elaborate system of branch warehouses located in various geographical locations, with inventories to support orders of various finished products for many customers.

**Out-of-pocket costs.**  The net additional costs incurred when some change is made in business operations.

**Output.**  Data that have been processed; the device or collective set of devices used for taking data out of a device; the information transferred from the internal storage of a computer to a secondary or external storage, or to any device outside the computer.

**Output control.**  This includes dispatching, expediting, and any other follow-up to get the right work out of a vendor or manufacturing facility.

**Output data.**  Data to be delivered from a device or program, usually after some processing has taken place.

**Overhead.**  Costs or expenses that are not directly identifiable with or chargeable to the manufacture of a particular part or product.

**Overhead account.**  Fixed expenses required to operate a department.

**Overlapped schedule.**  The "overlapping" of successive operations, whereby the completed portion of a job lot at one work center is processed at succeeding work centers before the pieces left behind are finished.

**Overrun.**  The quantity received from manufacturing in excess of quantity ordered.

**Overtime.**  Work beyond normal established working hours, which usually requires that a premium be paid to the workers.

**Ownership of materials.**  The person with title to the goods and therefore the responsibilities that go along with ownership (profits, losses, accountability).

**Partial order.**  Any shipment received or shipped that is less than the amount ordered.

**Pass.**  One cycle of processing a body of data.

**Passage of title.**  Title to goods passed when the goods reach the point designated by seller as the FOB destination or shipping point.

**Past due.**  An order that has not been completed on time.

**Patient-charge item.**  A specific item used for one patient and one patient only, such as a heart valve or an elbow prosthesis.

**Payback period.**  The length of time required for the net revenues of an investment to return the cost of the investment.

**Payment flow.**   Describes flow of cash payment from one institution to another.

**Penetration pricing.**   A new product or service pricing strategy in which a product or service is deliberately priced low to assure wide penetration of the market and wide consumer acceptance; once these objectives have been met, the seller may raise the initial penetration price.

**Percent of fill.**   A measure of the effectiveness with which the inventory-management system responds to actual demand. The percentage of customer orders filled off the shelf can be measured in either units or dollars.

**Periodic inventory.**   Accounting method to determine inventory by (1) periodically taking a physical count of merchandise on hand and (2) valuing the inventory by multiplying the quantity by the appropriate price and costs of shipment.

**Periodic-inventory system.**   No detailed record of inventory is maintained. However, at the end of a period a physical count is made to determine the amount and cost of the goods sold.

**Peripheral function.**   Secondary or lower-priority activity that can be performed in a different environment of time and of processing constraints.

**Perpetual inventory.**   Usually used to describe an inventory record-keeping system in which each transaction in and out is recorded and a new balance is computed.

**Perpetual-inventory record.**   A record of specific items, containing an updated history of all inventory transactions, including receipts and issues of some specific items.

**Perpetual-inventory system.**   For each type of goods stocked, a detailed record is maintained that shows (1) units and cost of each purchase, (2) units and cost of the goods for each sale, and (3) the units and amount on hand at any point in time.

**Perpetual stockchecking.**   A method of checking recorded stock balances against a count of the physical stock which is operated continuously, a proportion of the balances being checked each week.

**PERT (Program Evaluation and Review Technique).**   A network of activities showing their precedence and time relationships. It is used to plan and control work on large, complex, one-of-a-kind projects. *See also* CPM.

**Physical distribution.**   The combination of activities associated with the movement of products from the manufacturer to the user.

**Physical file.**   The data contained in or on one storage device like a magnetic tape or magnetic disk.

**Physical flow.**   Actual movement of material.

**Physical inventory.** The determination of inventory on hand by actual count.

**Picking list.** An order bill of materials, used as the basis for the stockroom to actually select and withdraw from the shelves or bins the components to make up a product or the finished goods to ship to a customer.

**Picking sheet.** List of items to be packed and shipped on one order to one destination.

**Piece parts.** Consists of individual items in inventory at the simplest level in manufacturing.

**Pipeline.** A system of pipes, valves, pumps, or compressors for transporting gasses or liquids. Also used in describing the entire physical distribution system (trucks, railroad cars, storage in transshipment points, and so on) of rigid materials.

**Planning.** A statement of goals and of means for reaching them.

**Planning horizon.** The period of future time for which plans are formulated.

**Pledging of accounts receivable.** Short-term borrowing from financial institutions where the loan is secured by accounts receivable. The lender may physically take the accounts receivable but typically has recourse to the borrower; also called discounting of accounts receivable.

**Plotter.** A visual-display board on which output is graphed by an automatically controlled pen or pencil.

**Plug-compatible unit.** A piece of computer hardware manufactured by one company but capable of operating in a functionally compatible manner with hardware manufactured by another company.

**Plugged level.** When a new product is to be released, the forecast model can be set up initially on the basis of a rate of demand specified by a product planner or marketing manager. That level is "plugged" into the record, as distinguished from an average that later can be estimated from actual demand.

**Positioning.** Determining the placement of a product or service item in terms of existing competitive offerings.

**Postinventory review.** A procedure used to recount the mistakes so that they can be documented and avoided the next time in order to improve inventory-taking quality.

**Preference.** The second level of consumer brand acceptance; consumers prefer a brand, but will accept substitutes if necessary.

**Prepaid expenses.** Expenses entered in the accounts for benefits not yet received.

**Preproduction planning.** This term is used to mean collectively the planning activities that precede production. It may refer to various combinations of the following activities: capacity planning, establishment of production-stage charts, product specification, process planning, stock control and ordering, shop loading, and operation scheduling.

**Prescheduling.** A scheduling technique used for repetitive products. The amount of time to be allowed for each operation is calculated once; then, as each order is received or as the due date or start date changes, the schedule can be recalculated without having to refer to the scheduling rules.

**Present value (PV).** The value today of a future payment or stream of payments discounted at the appropriate discount rate.

**Price.** The dollars-and-cents amount charged by a seller for a product or service.

**Price breaks.** Changes in the unit price of a purchased item as the order quantity or batch quantity is increased.

**Price lining.** A pricing strategy in which certain classes or lines of merchandise are sold at a limited number of price levels.

**Price maintenance.** A price established by a manufacturer or wholesaler below which the product will not be allowed to be sold.

**Price prevailing at the date of shipment.** An agreement between purchaser and vendor that the selling price may be modified by the vendor between the order and delivery dates.

**Price protection.** An agreement between purchaser and vendor granting purchaser any discount established by the vendor, generally prior to shipping date.

**Price variance.** The difference between the actual price and the standard price, multiplied by the total number of items acquired.

**Primary file.** The main file from which a program first reads records. In multifile processing, it is used to determine the order in which records are selected for processing.

**Prime cost.** The sum of direct material and direct labor costs.

**Prime operations.** Critical or most significant operations whose production rates must be planned.

**Prime rate.** The lowest rate of interest commercial banks charge very large, strong corporations.

**Priority list.** A list of tasks arranged with the most urgent at the top. Priorities can be assigned by latest start date, slack time, critical ratio, or any of several other techniques.

**Priority rules.** Rules that are given to the dispatcher so that he can decide which job to do next.

**Pro forma invoice.** An invoice received before a sale is consummated, informing the buyer of the terms of sale.

**Probabilistic demand.** Situations in which demand for the inventory item is not known exactly and probabilities must be used to describe the demand alternatives for the product.

**Probabilistic model.** The representation of a process, event, or relationship in terms of relative frequency of occurrences (logical relations between statements instead of events, degree of one's belief in the outcomes, and/or abstract characteristics associated with groups of entities). The distinguishing feature in all these representations is that the outcome at any time period is not known, but only a group of possible outcomes, any one of which may materialize.

**Probability distribution.** The distribution of chances of an observation taking on any value within the possible range. The form of the distribution could be normal, log normal, uniform, exponential, and so on if the variable can take on a continuous range of values. If the variable is inherently discrete (integer) valued, then the distribution forms might include Poisson and binomial. (There are a great many other forms.)

**Procedure-oriented language.** A higher-level language that is used to formulate computer programs by specifying the procedures or algorithms that are to be executed.

**Process average.** Average percentage of defective units present in the shipment.

**Process control.** Automatic control of continuous manufacturing operations by means of computers.

**Process costing.** Employed when manufacturing involves many units of a single product over a long period of time, (for example, manufacturing concrete).

**Process industry.** An industry such as food processing, in which work flows through a fixed continuous manufacturing process as opposed to an intermittent type of industry.

**Process planning.** Specification of the sequence of processes or operations and the machines, tools, and miscellaneous equipment to be used in producing a particular part, subassembly, or product.

**Process time.** That part of the throughput time of a batch during which operations are being carried out on the batch.

**Processing.** The operation in which a computer works on or manipulates data.

**Processing, asynchronous.** Computer processing involving simultaneously two or more independent operations that have no time relationship to each other or are "asynchronous," such as transferring data from a communication line while performing an arithmetic operation. *Contrast with* synchronous processing.

**Processing, background.** A type of multiprogrammed computer operations on data and programs coded and collected in advance in batches. This operation can be set aside temporarily to accept and process on-line inputs as priority tasks. *Contrast with* Foreground processing.

**Processing center.**   Location on the production floor where work is done directly on the goods being produced.

**Processing, foreground.**   A type of multiprogrammed computer operations on on-line inputs as priority tasks, which set aside temporarily the operation of data and programs coded and collected in advance in batches. *Contrast with* Processing, background.

**Processing, parallel.**   A form of multiprocessing whereby two or more operations are handled simultaneously on two or more central processing units. Parallel processing and multiprogramming are the two ways to accomplish multiprocessing.

**Processing, synchronous.**   Computer processing during which two or more operations are controlled by common timing signals, such as data transfer from arithmetic register to memory.

**Processor.**   The main frames or central logic unit of a computer to which peripheral input-output units are attached.

**Procurement time.**   The time from the decision to place an order until the goods are available for use.

**Product.**   A tangible want-satisfying unit, with a definable lifetime, which can be stored, transported, and resold; something someone makes for someone.

**Product acquisition.**   Purchase of new or existing product or service items or lines.

**Product life cycle.**   The idea that product or service items, like people, are mortal; they are born, grow, and decline.

**Product-line breadth.**   The number of different lines of products or services offered.

**Product-line depth.**   The variety of product or service items offered.

**Product management.**   An organizational design based on specific products or product lines.

**Product manager.**   An individual who is assigned complete responsibility for marketing a product or service line, or even a single item.

**Product orientation.**   A view of business that holds that "the firm knows what customers want," and that views the role of marketing as being limited to selling.

**Product/service deletion.**   The process whereby weak product or service items are eliminated from the firm's or institution's product or service mix.

**Product/service-development system.**   A structured set of activities for developing, analyzing, screening, and ultimately producing new products and services.

**Product/service item.**   A single product or service.

**Product/service line.**   A group of related products or services, distinguished by features and prices.

**Product/service mix.**   The total array of products and services offered for sale by a firm.

**Product/service policies.**   Concise written guidelines governing the type of product or service items a firm will offer, defined by "the business the firm is in."

**Product specification.**   A document or documents that completely define the content and form of a product and its components and specify all the quality standards to be met.

**Product structure.**   A bill-of-materials format that lists the components required to make a product and indicates the levels at which they are assembled, such as an indented bill of materials.

**Production-capacity program.**   One of the end products of the capacity-planning function, a document that specifies, against a time scale, the capacity of all kinds that the production department is to provide.

**Production control.**   The function of directing or regulating the orderly movement of goods through the entire manufacturing cycle from the requisitioning of raw materials to the delivery of the final product to meet the objectives of customer service, minimum inventory investment, and maximum manufacturing efficiency.

**Production costs.**   The unit personnel, materials energy, and prorated overhead costs attributable to production of goods used in providing care. In addition, there are some other production costs that can have a direct bearing on inventory models. These include overtime premiums and the incremental costs of changing production levels, such as hiring, training, and separation costs.

**Production cycle.**   The overal time required from the start of manufacture or from an earlier stage to completion of the product. Thus the production cycle may include the time required for specification of a customer's product, ordering, and procurement of special items. *Synonymous with* Makespan.

**Production-load program.**   A statement of the load on the production departments corresponding to the company's commitments.

**Production order.**   A production order instructs a "production" facility to produce something. It will indicate what is to be manufactured or otherwise produced, how much to make, and when the production should be completed.

**Production planning.**   The function of setting the limits or levels of manufacturing operations in the future, consideration being given to sales or usage forecasts and the requirements and availability of workers, machines, material, and money. The production plan is usually in fairly broad terms and does not specify in detail each of the individual products to be made, but usually specifies the amount of capacity that will be required.

**Production program**.   This term is used in a variety of ways, but the most common meaning is a document showing the products and the quantities of each that are to be produced in a given period of time; it tends to relate to output of finished products from the entire production facility or factory rather than output of partly finished items from individal departments.

**Production-rate-change costs**.   These comprise overtime, hiring, laying off, training, extra outside-material procurement, temporary labor premiums, and increased scrap and rework costs.

**Production schedule**.   A document that relates to a period of time, most commonly a week or a month, and that specifies the items that are to be made in that period and in what quantities. It usually relates to a manufacturing department or section, and as such is a collective shop order for a number of items; but it sometimes relates to the whole production facility.

**Production-stage chart**.   A chart that shows against a time scale the sequence of activities by which finished products are made. Although it is called a production-stage chart, the activities are not usually all production activities but may also include design activities, preparation of programs or schedules, data processing, ordering, procurement of purchased items, and anything else that is relevant.

**Production stores**.   Stores for direct material at all stages of manufacture other than finished goods.

**Productivity**.   Refers to a relative measure of output per labor or machine hour.

**Profit center**.   A unit of a large, decentralized firm that has its own investments and for which a rate of return on investment can be calculated.

**Program**.   (1) A sequence of instructions used in a computer to solve a problem or to perform a function. (2) A series of actions proposed in order to achieve a certain result.

**Program, general-purpose**.   A program having wide application, written by the vendor and designed to be used as a library routine.

**Program, special-purpose**.   A program written by a user organization to accomplish a specified task. A special-purpose program usually has less usage than function-specific programs, and may only be run once.

**Programmed decision**.   A frequently recurring decision that is well understood and well structured, resulting from routines developed to state how the decision should be made.

**Programming**.   A management task by which the sales program and production-capacity programs are compiled, authorized, and issued at regular intervals.

**Progress record.** A document for each shop order, which shows all the operations to be performed and on which the release and completion of each operation is recorded.

**Progress section.** The individual or group of individuals in a manufacturing shop who are responsible for progress control and usually carry out the functions of shop loading, shortage control, operation scheduling, work sequencing, anticipation of potential delays, and recording progress on all shop orders.

**Promotion.** Communications designed to present a company and its products to prospective customers, in order to make known need-satisfying attributes of products and to encourage purchase.

**Promotional mix.** The blend of advertising, personal selling, and sales promotion designed to accomplish a firm's promotion objectives.

**Protection time.** A number of days used as a safety buffer between the date on which demands are due and that on which supply orders are to be completed.

**Protocol.** Usually line protocol. The interactive code by which the computer and the terminal device are able physically to send data to each other.

**Provisioning.** The act of providing and particularly the steps taken beforehand to lay in provisions.

**Publicity.** Communiations about a firm or product not generated by the firm or not specifically designated to promote the firm or product.

**Pull and push systems.** If replenishment of stocks in one location can be determined without reference to the stock status elsewhere, that is essentially a pull system of field replenishment. In a push system the total stock status is taken into account in computing fair shares for all locations from the stock of a given product.

**Pull strategy.** A promotional strategy intended to develop consumer demand for a product or service and thus to "pull" it through the channel.

**Pulse-code modulation (PCM) and delta modulation.** Methods for converting analog signals to digital signals.

**Punch card.** A card for computer use that may be punched with holes to represent letters, digits, or characters.

**Purchase journal.** Used to accommodate the entry of all purchases made on credit.

**Purchase order.** (1) A purchaser's formal written offer to a vendor containing all terms and conditions of a proposed transaction. (2) An offer to buy goods and services. A purchase order is prepared by an authorized agent, buyer, or other person to obligate the institution to pay for the merchandise ordered. Prepared in response to an approved purchase requisition, purchase orders contain much the same information as that found on the requisition.

**Purchase requisition.** A purchase requisition is prepared by a department or employee of an organization to indicate that goods or services should be purchased. Usually, the preparer does not have the authority to order the merchandise directly from the vendor, hence the term "requisition." Purchase requisitions normally indicate a suggested vendor, the amount of goods required, estimated price, and shipping instructions.

**Purchasing specifications.**   Documents giving quality standards required in purchased materials, laid down as part of the function of product specification.

**Push strategy.**   A promotional strategy intended to encourage middlemen to stock and sell a product, rather than to rely on consumer demand.

**Qualitative standards.**   Standards such as personableness, responsibility, and cooperativeness that are difficult to measure but that should be considered in evaluating a salesperson's performance.

**Quality control.**   A continuous managerial system to ensure the quality of a material by a critical study or test of that material or product.

**Quantitative standards.**   Standards such as total sales volume and revenue per sales call that can be used to evaluate the performance of a salesperson.

**Quantity discounts.**   Discounts or lower unit costs offered by a manufacturer whenever a customer purchases larger quantities of the product.

**Quarterly-ordering system.**   A periodic-inventory-replenishment system whereby all requirements are reviewed and replenishment orders placed four times a year.

**Queue.**   (1) A sequence of elements, one waiting behind the other. (2) A waiting line of jobs available to go through an operation in the shop or service facility.

**Queueing time.**   The time after a batch is available for an operation during which it waits for a machine or an operator to become available.

**Quick-deck explosion.**   Method whereby quantities of components at all levels are simply ordered to meet assembly-quantity requirements.

**Quotation.**   A statement of price, terms of sale, and description of goods or services offered by a vendor to a prospective purchaser; a bid.

**Rack jobber.**   A jobber who stocks and maintains his own rack in a large retail outlet.

**Random.**   A method of data retrieval whereby information is acquired in any order that may be required.

**Random access.**   The process of obtaining data from, or placing data into, storage in which the time required to obtain or place any one element is the same as for any other, being independent of the particular location in storage.

**Random- or direct-access devices**. A device in which access to a stored record is not dependent on the position of that record within the file.

**Random-use item**. Any item the usage of which does not conform to an average quantity.

**Random variable**. A variable for which the occurrence of any one value within the specific range is as likely as any other.

**Range of items stocked**. The list of items carried in a particular location without regard to the quantity of each actually in or planned to be in stock.

**Rate of return**. The internal rate of return on an investment, calculated by finding the discount rate that equates the present value of future cash flows to the cost of the investment.

**Raw materials**. Items that are purchased and converted by processing into finished or component parts.

**Raw-materials inventory**. Items acquired through purchase, extraction of natural resources, or growth, (for example, food items) for the purpose of processing into finished goods.

**Reaction time**. The period of time from the moment at which a decision is made to do something, until that act can actually be accomplished.

**Read**. Transfer information from a source, such as punched-card storage, to a part of the computer; for example, to transfer the information contained in the holes of the punched card into electrical or electronic impulses for the magnetic storage. The process of reading may include translation.

**Real time**. A computer system in which the computer receives data processes it, and returns results sufficiently quickly that they can affect the functioning of the actual or real-world system at that time.

**Real-time processing**. (1) The processing of data simultaneously with the related physical process so that the results of the processing can be used to guide the physical process. (2) Pertaining to the processing of a request in an on-line system and making the results available to the user in a rapid-enough time frame to control or affect the activity in which the user is involved.

**Receiving**. This function is generally responsible for the following activities: physical report of incoming materials, inspection of shipment, identification and delivery to destination, and preparation of a receiving report.

**Receiving record**. A receiving record or receiving report is prepared when goods are received from a vendor. A receiving clerk uses it to list the items received, their quantities, and their condition. It is then sent to other parts of the organization requiring this information.

**Reconciling inventory**. Comparing the physical-inventory figures with the perpetual-inventory record and correcting the record.

**Reconsignment.** A change of consignee for a particular shipment.

**Record.** An organized collection of information (elements) about a single subject, treated as a unit. Two or more records form a file.

**Record key.** A field in a record that identifies the record in a file.

**Rectification.** Work done to correct defective items or to comply with design modifications.

**Register.** A hardware device used for temporarily storing data or instructions in the algorithm or logic unit of the central processor.

**Regression analysis.** A statistical procedure for predicting the value of one variable (dependent variable) on the basis of knowledge about one or more other variables (independent variables).

**Regulatory power.** The power of federal agencies to influence or control business or institutional activities.

**Reinvestment rate.** The rate of return at which cash flows from an investment are reinvested. The reinvestment rate may or may not be constant from year to year.

**Reject note.** A document raised by inspectors or quality-control staff to say that certain items fall short of specifications and are not to be used.

**Release.** The authorization to produce or ship material that has already been ordered.

**Release date.** The date on which new items are released for sale to customers.

**Reliability.** The consistency with which a material or data will be within certain quality parameters.

**Remittance advice.** A document prepared by the purchaser and enclosed with his check to describe the invoices being paid. It generally shows invoice numbers, invoice amounts, and discounts taken.

**Remote access.** Pertaining to communication with a data-processing facility by one or more stations that are distant from that facility.

**Remote batch processing.** A data-processing mode combining the features of on-line communications and batch processing. Batches of data are entered into a system from a remote terminal, then communicated to a central computer for subsequent processing.

**Reorder point.** The inventory level at which a new order should be placed. *Also* Reorder-point level.

**Reorder quantity.** In a fixed-order system of inventory control, the fixed quantity that should be ordered each time the available stock falls below the order point.

**Reorder report.** A listing of all items that are being reordered because the stock level is below the reorder level.

**Repair parts.** Parts required for maintenance of an assembled product, generally ordered and supplied at a date after the shipment of the product.

**Replacement-cost accounting.** A requirement under SEC Release no. 190 (1976) that large companies disclose the replacement costs of inventory items and depreciable plant.

**Replacement order.** A manufacturing order for the replacement of material that has been scrapped during a production cycle.

**Replenishment lead time.** The total period of time that elapses from the moment it is determined that a product is to be reordered until the product is back on the shelf available for use.

**Requirements.** Those raw materials, parts, or assemblies necessary to finish a given order or series of orders or forecast.

**Requirements scheduling.** Calculation of gross and net requirements. The task includes summarizing, that is, combining individual requirements of the same item for different products or customers' orders.

**Research and development.** A functional area in business which conducts ongoing research designed to develop and improve a firm's product or service offerings.

**Reserved material.** Material on hand or on order that is assigned to specific future production orders.

**Response.** System acknowledgment of a terminal input. Such a response might consist of a light display, a printout, or merely a carriage return.

**Response time.** The amount of time that elapses between a request for data or for processing and the receipt of the data or processing results.

**Retailers.** Outlets where consumer goods are sold.

**Retrieve.** To find and select specific information, especially a record or group of records from a data base.

**Returns.** Items that are sent back to the vendor and for which credit is given.

**Review interval.** The time period between successive inventory checks.

**Review period.** In a fixed-order-cycle system of stock control, the interval of time between reviews at which replenishment orders may be placed.

**Rework order.** A manufacturing order to rework and salvage defective parts or products.

**Risk premium.** The difference between the required rate of return on a particular risky asset and the rate of return on a riskless asset with the same expected life.

**Rolling forecast.** A forecast that is recalculated periodically and extended one period further into the future.

**Route sheet.** A document specifying the operations on a part and the sequence of these operations, with alternate operations and routings wherever feasible. *Also* Route card.

**Routine.** In computer terms, a set of coded instructions arranged in proper sequence to direct the computer to perform a desired operation or sequence of operations. A subdivision of a program consisting of two or more instructions that are functionally related—therefore, a program. *Also* Subroutine.

**Running parallel.** The running of a newly developed system in a data-processing area in conjunction with the continued operation of the current system; or the final step in the debugging of a system. This step follows a system test.

**Running time.** The time during which a machine is actually producing a product.

**Rush order.** An order that for some reason must be filled in less than normal lead time.

**Safety stock.** The buffer or cushion of stock kept on hand to protect against stockouts caused by uncertainty of future demands or lead time.

**Safety time.** In a time-series planning system, material is frequently ordered to arrive ahead of the forecast requirement date to protect against forecast error. The difference between the forecast requirement date and the planned in-stock date is safety time.

**Sale and leaseback.** An operation whereby a firm sells land, buildings, or equipment to a financial institution and simultaneously executes an agreement to lease the property back for a specified period under specific terms.

**Sales forecast.** An estimate of future sales and income to be derived from the sale of a product or service or line of products or services; the sales forecast is the heart of the marketing plan.

**Sales journal.** Journal for posting all sales.

**Sales program.** An instruction to the sales department which shows against a time scale of completion dates the volume and mix of the company's products for which they are to obtain customer's orders.

**Sales promotion.** Promotional activities designed to support advertising and personal selling; includes offers of free samples, premiums, and so on.

**Salvage.** Material that cannot be used for its original purpose, some part of which can be reconditioned or reused.

**Salvage and supplies disposal.** Arrangements for the disposal or reuse of supplies, redundant waste, obsolete materials, or plant and equipment.

**Salvage value.** The value of a capital asset at the end of some specified period. It is the current market price of an asset being considered for replacement in capital-budgeting problems.

**Sample.**   A small portion of goods taken as a specimen of quality.

**Samples (sampling).**   A sales-promotion technique whereby free samples of goods are given to consumers; in market research, "samples" of target markets are selected as representatives of the total market's characteristics and are surveyed or observed.

**Sampling.**   Selection of a proportion or sample of a total number of items, called the population, in such a way that the sample can be considered as representative of the population.

**Satiety.**   Availability of as much of the product as can be used.

**Sawtooth diagram.**   A quantity versus time graphic representation of the order-point-order-quantity inventory system showing inventory being received and then used up and reordered.

**Schedule.**   A listing of jobs to be processed by a work center, department, or plant; their respective start dates; and other related information.

**Schedule date.**   The date when a production lot is due to be completed. It may be the same as the need date, or earlier if lots are released early to stabilize production, or later if there are limitations on material or capacity.

**Scheduled delivery.**   Method of dispatching materials in which the storeroom provides regularly scheduled deliveries throughout the plant.

**Scheduling.**   The process of setting operation-start dates for jobs to allow them to be completed by their due dates.

**Schema.**   A description of a data base, including a statement of the characteristics of the data and the relationship between different data elements. *Contrast with* subschema.

**Scientific inventory control.**   The use of statistical techniques to determine proper reserve-stock levels.

**Scrap.**   Material that is of no further use to the institution or company and that should be sold for whatever price can be obtained for it.

**Scrap allowance.**   An allowance of additional items or material over and above the quantity theoretically required, to cover, to a predetermined extent, the likelihood of scrap being produced.

**Scrap note.**   A document that authorizes disposal of goods as scrap.

**Scrap rate.**   The ratio of the difference between the amount or number of units of product started in a manufacturing process and that amount or number of units that are completed at an acceptable quality level, divided by the latter.

**Screening.**   The first filtrating stage in product or service development, during which new ideas are analyzed in reference to a firm's product or service policies.

**Sealed-bid pricing.**   Competitive pricing where suppliers compete for jobs on the basis of bids.

**Seasonal.** Daily, weekly, or monthly sales data that show a repetitive pattern from year to year with some periods considerably higher than others.

**Seasonal inventory.** Inventory built up in anticipation of a peak season in order to maintain production level.

**Secured account.** An account on which the purchaser assumes liability for the debt incurred by a purchase transaction by signing a negotiable instrument at the time the transaction is settled or at the time of delivery.

**Securities and Exchange Commission (SEC).** The federal agency that supervises the operation of securities exchanges and related aspects of the securities business and with which a registration statement must be filed on new issues of securities.

**Selective distribution.** Placing goods or services in a number of retail outlets, but not in all within a given area; appropriate for shopping goods.

**Seller's market.** A market condition favorable to vendors, which exists when the forces of supply and demand keep prices at a relatively high level.

**Seller's option.** Seller's privilege to require the buyer to purchase at an agreed price and within a given period of time.

**Seller's risk.** The possibility that a sample will contain more defects than the rest of the lot.

**Selling agent.** A wholesaler responsible for selling a company's entire line of goods.

**Selling on consignment.** An arrangement whereby the seller takes possession of the goods from the producer but does not take title to them. Ownership passes directly from producer to buyer.

**Semiconventional system.** One in which certain components of a conventional system have been changed.

**Semifinished goods.** Products that have been stored uncompleted awaiting final operations that adapt them to different customer specifications.

**Sequence number.** The identification of the sequence of steps in the manufacturing process.

**Sequencing.** Determining the order in which a manufacturing facility is to process a number of different jobs in order to achieve certain objectives.

**Sequential access.** A condition where the first unit of data is read through the record and so on until the operation is complete.

**Sequential control.** A process implying an ordered control over the steps of an operation.

**Service.** An intangible want-satisfying unit, which has a short life and cannot be transported, stored, or resold; something someone does for someone.

**Service level.**   The proportion of total demand of an item that is met from stock. It is sometimes expressed as the proportion of total demand *value* that is met from stock.

**Service-parts-transfer order.**   Form used to transfer parts from parts stores for resale to individual customers.

**Service time.**   The time required to serve the customer after he places a demand on an inventoried item.

**Setback time.**   The expected lead-time requirements that are deducted from the required finish date to set the start date.

**Setup.**   Preparing a machine or workplace for the performance of an operation on a batch. It usually includes production of the first few items and may include procurement of signature for first-off inspection.

**Setup costs.**   Setup costs account for the physical work incurred in preparing for a production run (setting up equipment and adusting machines) and include the clerical costs of shop orders, scheduling, and expediting. External orders, internal procurement, and setup costs remain relatively constant regardless of the order size.

**Setup time.**   Time required to adjust a work station or a machine and/or to attach the proper tooling to make a particular product.

**Shared file.**   Data storage available to several computers.

**Shelf life.**   The length of time a material may be stored without affecting the usability or salability of the material.

**Shipping.**   This activity normally is concerned with outgoing shipment of parts, products, and/or components, including packaging, marking, weighing, and loading for shipment.

**Shipping authorization.**   Form used to release stores materials for shipping to outside vendors for processing and fabrication.

**Shipping order.**   Shipping orders are instructions to a shipping department to package and ship merchandise or other goods from one place to another. The document indicates what and how much is to be shipped, to whom it is to be sent, and when and how it is to be sent.

**Shop.**   A manufacturing department or section.

**Shop-load summary.**   A document showing the analyzed load by work centers compared with available capacity.

**Shop loading.**   Analysis of the future load arising from shop orders on hand and as yet uncompleted and its comparison with available capacity. The anlaysis usually has to be by work center and by operation schedule date, with subdivision of the future load on each work center into live and forward load.

**Shop order.**   An instruction issued by the ordering function to a shop to produce a specified quantity of an item by a specified date.

**Shop order documents.**   A set of documents produced to facilitate control of production. It frequently includes a progress report, a material requisition, a route card, and operation cards.

**Shop planning**.   The coordination of material handling, material availability, setup, and tooling availability so that a job can be done on a particular machine.

**Shopping goods**.   Goods that are not frequently purchased, that are relatively expensive and durable, and that consumers take time and care in purchasing.

**Shortage**.   The quantity of an item that is shown to be required, beyond what is available.

**Shortage control**.   The process of checking, either clerically or physically, the availability of materials a few hours, days, or weeks before they are due to be issued from stores. When the goods are received, the proccess ensures that shortages are cleared before the goods are put into storage.

**Shortage costs**.   Costs incurred when stockouts occur, such as the incremental cost of more expensive items used as substitutes, (for example, a larger-than-necessary X-ray film). A part shortage can also be the cause of idle "labor" in a radiology department and of incremental labor cost to perform operations out of sequence. The magnitude of the opportunity cost incurred when patients are referred out for some service because of stock shortages. Shortage costs also include emergency measures to expedite a rush delivery. This cost is easily identified as the difference between the usual cost of procurement and the extra cost for accelerated service. When emergency procedures cannot provide a wanted item, the client is left unsatisfied. The only apparent costs are billings lost from the potential service. The reaction of a dissatisfied patient in terms of future "business" is a cost that can only be estimated.

**Shortage note**.   A document sent to all concerned to notify them of the existence of a shortage.

**Short date**.   A replenishment order that is scheduled for the end of the freeze period but is needed earlier.

**Short sale**.   A sale of a commodity for future delivery that is not owned by the seller who expects to buy it at a lower rate before the delivery date.

**Shrinkage**.   Loss of materials due to theft.

**Significant part numbers**.   Part numbers that are intended to convey certain information such as the source of the part, the material in the part, or the shape of the part.

**Simulation**.   Generally a computer-based imitation of the operation of an actual or real-world system, so that one may study its behavior and its reaction to specific changes.

**SKU (Stock-keeping unit)**.   A particular part number at a particular location.

**Slack time**.   The time allowance for contingencies in excess of the time usually required to carry out a process.

**Slanted chart.** A record with one column for each month. A new line is posted whenever the forecast or the production plan is revised so that forecasts, production, and planned-inventory budgets can be compared from month to month as they are revised.

**Small Business Administration (SBA).** A government agency organized to aid small firms with their financing and other problems.

**Smoothing constant.** In exponential smoothing, the fraction of the difference between the actual result and forecasted result that is added to the previous smoothed value to arrive at a new smoothed value.

**Sociographics.** Social or group influences on consumer behavior.

**Software.** (1) The totality of programs and routines associated with a computer, such as compilers, assemblers, narrators, and routines. (2) Sometimes, the documentation of procedures, programs, or hardware.

**Sort file.** A temporary file used for sequencing or placing data into order in a transaction or master file.

**Source document.** The original record of a transaction.

**Source program.** A program written in other than machine language that must be translated into machine language before use.

**Spare parts.** Extra parts supplied with an assembled product for maintenance purposes.

**Special.** Refers to a part or group of parts that are unique to a particular order.

**Special delivery.** Unscheduled delivery of materials direct to the requisitioner to meet emergency demands for materials and supplies, or to deliver material to areas not normally serviced by a scheduled delivery plan.

**Special use.** Procedure in which material may be issued and dispatched to persons authorized to approve the requisitioning of material.

**Specific identification.** Inventory-valuation method where each good purchased is identified. When a sale is made, the cost of that unit is identified and recorded.

**Specifications.** Comprehensive and accurate statements of the technical requirements descriptive of a good or service, and of the procedure to be followed to ascertain that the requirements are met.

**Split lots.** A replenishment order initially issued under one reference number may be split into smaller pieces to get some material through a bottleneck quickly or to allow for better materials handling in the shop.

**Spoilage.** Products lost due to defects in workmanship or in the material.

**(S.s) inventory policy.** A two-level control system in which a replenishment order is issued if the available stock is equal to or less than the order point $s$, (the lower level), and in which the amount ordered is equal to $S$ (the upper level) minus the available stock.

**Staff functions.** Those activities that are not a part of line management but which assist line management by providing specialized advice or services.

**Staging.** Pulling of the material requirements for an order from inventory before the material is required.

**Standard.** A quantitative target that is expected to be achieved or surpassed by a predetermined margin.

**Standard cost.** The cost of an operation, process, or product, including labor, material, and factory overhead, calculated on the basis of standard performance and prices.

**Standard deviation.** A statistical measurement of the variability of a set of observations from the mean of the distribution.

**Standard hour.** A unit of work used to express the work content of an operation or the load on a shop or section. It is the amount of work that will be completed in one hour at a standard rate of working.

**Standard purchase order.** A purchase order tailored to the kinds and types of materials and services being purchased by a specific company or institution.

**Standard-purchase unit price.** Set pricing for a fixed period of time until a total issue unit-price revision is instituted.

**Standard times.** The total time in which a job would be completed at a standard rate of working.

**Start date.** The date that an order should be placed into the shop based on some form of scheduling rules.

**State-preference model.** A framework in which decisions are based on probabilities of payoffs under alternative scenarios or "states of the world."

**Statement.** A document periodically sent by the vendor to the customer (frequently at the month's end) that shows the total amount owed to the vendor on unpaid bills.

**Step.** One operation in a computer routine.

**Stochastic process.** Used synonymously with *random process*, and applied to diverse phenomena such as coin tossing, time-series analysis, and fluctuations of demand. Generally involves time.

**Stock.** Stored goods, products, or service parts ready for sale or use.

**Stock card.** A document showing all transactions that affect the balance of physical stock. Also, computer punch cards identifying a particular stock item by catalog number and other pertinent data.

**Stock check.** A reconciliation of a stock balance on record with counted physical stock.

**Stock control.** A means of deciding when an item should be ordered, made, or bought and in what quantity. The alternative to direct ordering. Also, the clerical control of movement of goods into and out of stores and the level of stocks at all times.

**Stockout.** Lack of materials or products that are normally expected to be on hand in stores or stock.

**Stockout costs.** All costs associated with a stockout, such as goodwill cost and reorder costs. *See* Shortage costs.

**Stock records.** Stock records are maintained for items of inventory and indicate the amount on hand, the quantity level at which more of the item should be ordered, the vendor or supplier, receipts of stock, and issues of stock. When used, they serve as perpetual-inventory records that indicate the amount of the item on hand at any one time.

**Stock status.** A periodic report showing the inventory on hand and usually showing the inventory on order and some sales or usage history for the products that are covered.

**Stocked item.** An item ordered on the basis of stock control.

**Stocking location.** Any warehouse that carries a particular item in its range of products. Distinguished from *bin location*, which is the place within a warehouse where the item is stored.

**Stockyard.** Outdoor storage facility.

**Storage bins.** Storage facilities generally used for solids.

**Storage, buffer.** An element between two devices, for example, external and internal, that temporarily compensates for the difference in their respective rates of throughput.

**Storage, bulk.** Storage for larger amounts of programs or data. The contents of the bulk storage first must be transferred to the main storage before they can be processed on a computer.

**Storage cost.** The cost of facilities, personnel, taxes, and so on to provide physically for the storage of inventory. *See* Holding cost.

**Storage, refresher.** Storage to rewrite (refresh) continually the image (data) "written" on the face of a cathode-ray tube.

**Storage tanks.** Storage facilities generally used for liquids and gases.

**Store.** A place where objects are kept and protected against unauthorized removal.

**Storeroom.** Any area where an inventory is maintained.

**Stores.** Stored materials used in making a product.

**Storing.** The supervision, identification, and storage of materials and goods in sound condition for safety and readiness for use when needed.

**Strategy.** A method or plan of action designed to accomplish objectives.

**String.** A linear sequence of entities such as characters or physical elements.

**Subassembly.** An assembly that is used at a higher level to make up another assembly.

**Subjective probability distributions.** Probability distributions determined through subjective procedures.

**Suboptimization.** (1) The achievement of the best combination of values for only a part of the total number of variables involved in the system.

(2) Optimization of one subsystem at the expense of another, for example, optimizing production costs at the expense of inventory costs.

**Subroutine.** A subunit of a routine. The smallest unit of a program that can be named and run apart from another subroutine.

**Substitute products.** Products whose demand decreases as demand for another product increases.

**Substoreroom.** A secondary storage area where a portion of the total inventory is maintained.

**Supplies.** Materials used in providing higher-order services or in production of other products. Supplies are not readily charged to the client or to finished production (for example, tongue depressors, lubricating oils, repair parts).

**System.** (1) An assemblage of parts into a meaningful whole. (2) A set of resources—personnel, materials, facilities, cash, time, and/or information—organized to perform designated functions, in order to achieve desired results. (3) EDP systems are of two kinds: units of equipment or hardware called *computer systems* and units of programs called *computer-applications systems* or software.

**System engineers.** For the purposes of this book, this is the job title of those engaged in the anlaysis, design, programming, and implementation of materials and/or information systems.

**System test.** (1) The running of the whole system against test data. (2) A complete simulation of the actual running system for purposes of testing. (3) A test of an entire interconnected set of components for the purpose of determining proper functioning and interconnection.

**Tactics.** The specific means used for accomplishing objectives, as opposed to strategy.

**Tangible assets.** Physical assets, as opposed to intangible assets such as goodwill or the stated value of patents or copyrights.

**Tape drive.** Sequential-access storage device used to read a magnetic tape.

**Target-inventory level.** The target inventory is equal to the order point plus the order quantity. It is often used in a periodic-review system.

**Taxonomy.** The systematic distinguishing and naming of types or categories that group similar objects or ideas.

**Technical development.** The stage in new-product or -service development during which actual prototypes, or scale models, of the product or service item are developed to test out its technical feasibility.

**Teleprocessing.** The use of communication equipment to transmit data automatically to remote locations.

**Teletypewriter.** A term used by the Bell System to refer specifically to teleprinter equipment.

**Telpak.** A service offered by communications common carriers for the leasing of wideband channels between two or more points.

**Term discount.** Synonym for cash discount.

**Term loan.** A loan with a maturity greater than one year, generally obtained from a bank or an insurance company. Term loans are usually amortized.

**Terminal.** A device capable of transmitting input to and obtaining output from the system of which it is a part.

**Test marketing.** Marketing research designed to try out a new product in actual situations.

**Throughput.** The flow of materials, people, and/or information through a system. Also a term describing the total elapsed time in the performance of a computer job.

**Through rate.** A rate that applies from origin to destination.

**Time clerk.** An employee whose principal job is to record or supervise the recording of operators' attendance and/or start and finish times on operations for the purposes of wage, bonus, and/or cost determination.

**Time-division multiplex.** A method of breaking data down to individual bits and sending it over a single line in any order that corresponds to available channel space. Reframe time is the time required to reassemble the data in the correct form after time-division multiplexing.

**Time-series planning.** A materials-planning technique whereby demand is expressed by specific time periods out into the future and order-release dates are planned based on the anticipated inventory that will be on hand in future time periods.

**Time sharing.** The use of a device such as a computer for two or more purposes, such as different computations, during the same time span; accomplished by arranging parts of one sequence of events or relations in such a way that they can alternate with parts of other sequences without losing their identity.

**Time standard.** The predetermined labor times allowed for the performance of a specific job. The standard will often consist of two parts, that for setup and that for actual running.

**Time ticket.** A labor claim entered by an operator, frequently in the form of a handwritten report or punched card.

**Title.** That document that evidences ownership (car title, purchase order, cancelled check, receipt).

**Title flow.** Describes actual passage of title (of ownership) from one institution to another.

**Tool order.** A document authorizing withdrawal or issue of specific tools from the tool crib or other storage.

**Top-down development.** A development strategy whereby the executive control modules of a system are coded and tested first, to form a "skeleton" version of the system; when the sysem interfaces have been proven to work, the lower-level modules are coded and tested.

**Total cover.** The total of the stock and outstanding-order balances.

**Total-inventory report.** A listing of all items in inventory with quantity, price, and lead-time information.

**Total system.** A general term relating to an information system addressed to a broad range of user information requirements.

**Toughness/fragility.** An indication of how much abuse or rough handling a material can be subjected to before damage will result.

**TPOP (Time-Phase Order Point).** A technique to determine when to order independent demand items and when to reschedule to adjust to changes in demand.

**Trade credit.** Interfirm debt arising through credit sales and recorded as an account receivable by the seller and as an account payable by the buyer.

**Trade discount.** Deductions from list or catalog price offered to channel members for performing certain marketing functions for the manufacturer.

**Trademark.** A brand that has been registered with the U.S. Patent Office and has legal protection against use by someone else.

**Traffic.** An organizational unit charged with responsibility of arranging the most economical classification and method of distribution or shipment for both incoming and outgoing materials and products.

**Traffic control.** Supervision of a firm's or institution's use of transportation facilities in order to obtain their optimum use.

**Transaction.** An event that involves or affects a business or organization. Events taking place during the course of routine business activities (for example, user's replenishing of stocks or central ordering materials from a supplier).

**Transaction control block (TCB).** Acts as a memory buffer in a virtual-access system. It keeps the local sequence number (LSN) or modal address of the master program while one node is waiting a reply from another.

**Transaction file.** A file containing relatively transient data that, for a given application, is processed together with the appropriate master file.

**Transfer price.** The price charge by one segment of an organization for a product or service that it supplies to another segment of the same organization.

**Transit time.** The time required to move a batch from the completion of one operation to its availability for the next.

**Translator.** A software program that operates on or uses as data other computer programs to translate higher-level instructions into machine-executable instructions.

**Transportation costs.** These costs are primarily a function of four basic elements: the distance a shipment must travel, the weight of the shipment, the nature or type of product, and the mode of transportation utilized.

**Transportation inventories.** Inventories that exist because materials must be moved.

**Transportation problem.** A special type of problem usually involving the determination of how many units should be shipped from each of several supply locations to each of several demand locations so that all demands are satisfied and transportation costs are minimized.

**Transshipment.** Shipment of material to an intermediate location from which it is then shipped to its ultimate destination on another vehicle or carrier.

**Traveling requisition.** A purchase requisition that is made up once and then used each time the raw material or product is reordered.

**Traveler.** A copy of the manufacturing order that actually moves with the work through the shop.

**Truncate.** To terminate a computational process in accordance with some rule.

**Turnaround time.** The elapsed time between generation of input by a user entering it into some process and the receipt of the results of that processing by the user.

**Turnover.** The number of times inventory is replaced during a time period.

**Two-bin system.** A type of fixed-order system in which inventory is carried in two real or imaginary bins. A replenishment quantity is ordered when the first bin is empty.

**Two-level reorder system.** A system of ordering in which the major volume of demand is supplied by a low-cost and low-speed system. A second system is made available for high-speed (quick-response) ordering and thereby reduces the required safety-stock needs.

**Ultimate consumer.** The buyer who is the last user of a good or service.

**Unbundling.** User of computer hardware pays a separate price for use of vendor's licensed systems software on already-installed hardware.

**Uniform delivered price.** A pricing strategy in which delivery price charged to all buyers, regardless of location, is the same. The delivery charge is included in the net price of the product.

**Unit load.** A number of items or bulk material arranged and restrained so that the combination can be picked up and moved as a single object too large for manual handling.

**Unit of issue.** The unit in which the inventory is maintained and the charge to a department is determined.

**Unit of purchase.** The packaging routinely supplied by the vendor (case, box, carton, and so on).

**Unplanned-production orders.** Orders for small quantities and unplanned operations in which material requirements are not preplanned or when no production-control system exists.

**Update.** To modify a file or report with current information according to a specified procedure.

**Usage.** The number of units of an inventory item consumed over a period of time.

**Usage-value classification.** Division of the stocked items into categories according to the value of an average period's consumption or usage of each so that appropriate stock-control procedures can be devised for each category.

**Use value.** A monetary measure of the qualities of an item that contribute to its performance.

**Utility routine.** A standard subprogram provided by the vendor to assist in the preparation of user programs, such as a conversion routine or sorting routine.

**Utilization factor.** In waiting-line systems, the ratio of the mean arrival rate to the mean service rate. It indicates the proportion of the time the service facilities are in use.

**Values.** Criteria by which people evaluate and/or conduct their own and others' behavior.

**Variable.** A quantity that can assume any of a given set of values.

**Variable costs.** Expenses like labor, raw materials, and packaging, which vary depending on the number of units being produced or sold.

**Variable-length record** A record that can contain a varying number of characters or data items. *Contrast with* fixed-length record.

**Variance.** The difference, positive or negative, between actual performance and a preset standard, budget, or target.

**Vendor file.** A file including complete addresses of all specific vendors to which requests for bids and/or purchase orders are submitted.

**Versatility.** An indication of the number of different applications for which a material can be used.

**Vertical distribution (marketing).** An organization set up in sections such that one section's finished product becomes the next section's raw material.

**Virtual access.** A data-access method used when data is stored at a specific address. The system must execute a search routine for that address each time it is used if no TCB (task-control block) is used.

**Visual-review system.** A simple inventory-control system whereby the the inventory reordering is based on actually looking at the inventory on hand.

**Volatile storage.** A storage device in which stored data are lost when electrical power is removed.

**Volatility/stability.** An indication of the ease and/or speed at which a material may change states.

**Voucher.** An authorization to pay. For example, a purchasing agent who has ordered merchandise receives an invoice from the vendor that indicates the terms of payment for the merchandise and a receiving report from the receiving department, which indicates that the merchandise has been delivered according to the order. The purchasing agent, not having authority to write and sign checks against the institution's checking account, prepares a voucher authorizing the accounting department or other organizational section to prepare and deliver a check to the vendor in payment for the merchandise. The vouchers will show, usually, the vendor to whom payment is to be sent, the purchase order (by number) that has been filled, the vendor's invoice number, and the amount to be paid.

**Wait time.** The time a job spends waiting to be moved or waiting to be worked on in the shop; the time during which an operator is not usefully employed.

**Wall-to-wall inventory.** Raw materials, parts, or assemblies that may enter the plant at one end and are processed through the plant into end products without ever having entered a formal stock area.

**Warehouse.** Indoor storage facility.

**Waybill.** A transportation-line record issued for each shipment, showing all details and with copies sent to all interested agents.

**Week supply.** Amount of inventory on hand divided by the weekly usage rate.

**Weighted cost of capital.** A weighted average of the component costs of debt and/or preferred stock and of common equity. Also called the composite cost of capital.

**Where used.** A method of retrieving all "parents" that show a given material in their product structures, used for engineering or technical changes and for coping with shortages and substitution.

**Wholesaler.** An intermediary between the producer and the retailer.

**Wide-area telephone service (WATS).** A service provided by telephone companies that permits a customer, by use of an access line, to make calls to telephones in a specific zone on a dial basis for a flat monthly charge.

**Won (impact printer).** A printer device utilizing lasers, or other technology, to transfer an image to paper. It does not require a printer device to touch the page.

**Word.**  A sequence of characters treated as a unit and capable of being sorted in a single computer location.

**Work center.**  A subunit of a production or service department to indicate either a group of people or of specific machines that are more or less interchangeable.

**Work in process.**  Product in various stages of completion throughout the production facility or factory. *Also* Work in progress.

**Work-in-process inventory.**  The cost of uncompleted goods still on the production line.

**Work measurement.**  The establishment of the work content of an operation, expressed in standard minutes or standard hours, by time study, work sampling, or use of synthetic data.

**Work order.**  A document sent by the sales department to the production department specifying that a product or batch of products shall be made. It may correspond with a customer's order or may be for finished-stock replenishment.

**Work sampling.**  The use of a large number of random-sampled observations to determine the frequency with which certain activities are formed.

**Work sequencing.**  Ensuring, by a routine procedure, that work is fed to the production resources in the best sequence.

**Work station.**  The assigned location where a worker performs his or her job. Its object is to enable best use of material, human, and plant resources.

**Working capital.**  The part of the capital of a company that is used to pay for materials, wages, and services and is being continually recovered in the selling price of the product. It represents all the capital of the company other than that which is invested in fixed assets.

**Working stock.**  That element of the stock of an item which fluctuates between zero and the batch quantity, the other element being buffer stock.

**Write.**  To record data in a storage device or a data medium. The recording need not be permanent (for example, the writing on a CRT display device).

**Yield.**  The rate of return on an investment; the internal rate of return.

**Yield factor.**  The ratio of the average good quantity at the end of the production process to the quantity originally scheduled.

**Zoning.**  Division of warehouse stock into zones to ease order picking.

# Appendix B: Recommended Materials-Processing Procedures and Equipment

The central processing department can and should be designed to combat and control cross-contamination. "Clean" and "soiled" areas should be separated by physical barriers such as masonry walls, and materials flow patterns should preclude mixing of clean with soiled materials. Department layout, personnel duties and procedures, and system equipment should be designed to preclude transmission of contamination from one area to another.

## Decontamination Area

This is the area to which using units send soiled materials for processing and/or disposal.

Soiled materials for processing consist of the following:

1. Heat- and moisture-stable items.
2. Heat- and/or moisture-sensitive items.
3. Infectious items (for special handling).
4. Medical equipment.
5. Distribution vehicles.

### Heat- and Moisture-Stable Items

Heat- and moisture-stable items include all those that may be subjected to steam decontamination at 285°F. Mechanical washing followed by steam decontamination is required to control infection within both the department and the hospital. Items for processing should be unloaded from the distribution vehicles for racking.

Rapid racking is essentially to system operation to preclude congestion of carts, especially at peak periods, and to maintain continuous washer-sterilizer operation. Equipment such as the rotary holding table (a circular rotating table top on a fixed base) and the racking station (a counter-type unit that hold sthe washer-sterilizer loading racks) provide highly efficient facilities for rapid racking of heat- and moisture-stable items. Both

The author is grateful to the American Sterilizer Co. for supplying the information contained in this appendix.

items are available from American Sterilizer Company, Erie, Pennsylvania, and from other suppliers.

When the solid items are unloaded from modules, the rack-loading personnel place them into the proper rack on the racking station. If the racking station does not have the proper rack on it at that time, the item is placed onto the rotary holding table. When a rackload accumulates on the table, the proper rack is selected to fill a vacancy on the racking station, and the items are transferred to this rack.

A rack loader need not leave his station to perform these duties. The rotating table top increases efficiency by bringing all items within easy reach of the rack loader at the racking station. Productivity is increased by the use of this labor-saving specialized equipment. Larger volumes may be easily and efficiently handled by a minimum of personnel; smaller volumes are racked in shorter times, thereby releasing the personnel for other processing functions in the same area.

Mechanically powered roller-type units that transport filled racks from the racking station to automated washer-sterilizers are also available from various sources. They can be electrically and mechanically interfaced with the washer-sterilizers to (1) advance the queue of racks on the units as racks are accepted by the washer-sterilizers and (2) advance racks onto the washer-sterilizer loading units as vacancies occur.

Their length (queue of racks in linear feet) can be determined to provide adequate queueing for maximum numbers of racks at peak periods while occupying minimum floor space.

*Loading racks* are available in various configurations to ensure proper processing of different types of materials.

*General-purpose racks* have single compartments to hold instrument trays or individual items. Hold-down screens are used to retain smaller items during processing.

*Tray racks* accommodate 16″ × 22″ or 11½″ × 15″ shallow trays. Spacers hold the trays upright and separated.

*Basin racks* have sets of spacers, each set supporting and separating basins and bowls.

*Bedpan racks* also have sets of spacers, each set holding a bedpan or fracture pan upright for drainage. These rack compartments have spray nozzles connected to common manifolds especially designed to fit valves in the chamber of the companion washer-sterilizer.

*Glassware racks* have sets of spacers, each designed to support an inverted flask, beaker, bottle, jar, or urinal. These racks also have spray nozzles.

Prefabricated structures (modular-wall assemblies), which have front-curtain wall with openings through which one or more washer-sterilizers can be installed, are also available commercially.

Double-door, through-the-wall types of washer-sterilizer equipment can be commercially obtained. (The Amscomatic Washer-Sterilizers are produced and marketed by American Sterilizer Company.) Such units provide mechanical washing, rinsing, and steam decontamination of heat- and moisture-stable items such as utensils, glassware, and surgical instruments. As previously stated, each washer-sterilizer can be interconnected with the horizontal rack transporters so that racks automatically advance to and into the machines as vacancies occur. When a rack enters the chamber and the door closes, the cycle begins automatically. At its conclusion, the items are decontaminated and are completely safe for handling in the "clean" area.

*Heat- and/or Moisture-Sensitive Items*

Heat- and/or moisture-sensitive items (excluding medical equipment) are those which, by their nature, cannot be subjected to a sterilizing temperature or to the moisture inherent in steam decontamination. These items are processed manually according to specific procedures and techniques and, if required, by gaseous decontamination.

Commercially available *portable sonic cleaners* provide a means for effective cleaning of small items with sonic vibrations passed through detergent-laden wash water. Such units are used for processing heat-sensitive items; delicate or multiple-jointed cutting instruments, such as eye knives; items that are not easily cleaned by manual or mechanical methods; delicate or non-heat-resistant glassware; and plastic components of aspirators and other equipment.

Following ultrasonic cleaning, the items are rinsed and then transferred to a *cleaning counter* for chemical disinfection (or they are otherwise decontaminated for further processing).

The cleaning counter is a specially designed work station for manually cleaning and chemically disinfecting or decontaminating certain items that cannot be processed in washer-sterilizers. Such units may include sinks with hot- and cold-tap-water faucets for cleaning, and wells for short-term and long-term soaking of items as well as distilled-water and compressed-air outlets.

The heat- and/or moisture-sensitive items may next be sent to the "clean" preparation and packaging area via a pass-through window. Depending on the technique used, the items processed at the cleaning counter may require ethylene-oxide-gas decontamination. For many years, certain heat- and/or moisture-sensitive items could only be cleaned and disinfected by manual methods. Recent development of a safe sterilant consisting of 12 percent ethylene-oxide gas and 88 percent dichloro-difluoromethane combined with specialized sterilizing equipment provides a means for total decontamination of supplies and equipment such as the following:

*Telescopic instruments:*
Bronchoscopes
Cyctoscopes
Electrotomes
Endoscopes
Esophagoscopes
Opthalmoscopes
Ostoscopes
Pharyngoscopes
Proctoscopes
Resectoscopes
Sigmoidoscopes
Thoracoscopes
Urethroscopes

*Plastic goods:*
Catheters
Nebulizers
Vials
Syringes
Gloves
Test tubes
Petri dishes
IV sets
Infant incubators
Heart-lung machines
Heart pacemakers
Artificial-kidncy machincs

*Rubber goods:*
Tubing
Surgical gloves
Catheters
Drain-and-feed sets
Sheeting

*Instruments and equipment:*
Cautery sets
Eye knives
Lamps
Needles

Neurosurgical instruments
Scalpel blades
Speculae
Syringes
Dental instruments
Oxygen tents

*Miscellaneous:*
Dilators
Electric cords
Hair clippers
Miller-Abbott tubes
Pump motors
Books
Toys
Pottery
Blankets
Sheets
Furniture
Sealed ampules
Sutures
Medicine droppers

Ethylene-oxide-gas sterilizers are available in double-door units so that they can be loaded or unloaded from either the decontamination or the preparation and packaging area. The use of sterilizers in the preparation and packaging area will be discussed later. Their use in the decontamination area is for gaseous sterilization of heat- and/or moisture-sensitive items and bagged infectious items from isolation or other areas.

Some of these units are automated to the extent that, once they are loaded, the operator merely selects the proper programming cycle, temperature, and exposure time and presses a "start" button. No further attention is necessary until the cycle is completed. Labor-saving devices are also available for loading and unloading of the gas sterilizers.

### Infectious Items

Infectious items from isolation and other areas normally are bagged and either tagged or color coded for easy identification by processing personnel. These bags are not opened until they have been decontaminated in one of the previously discussed sterilizers, depending on the nature of the items. Following decontamination the bags can be opened and the articles either racked or taken to the cleaning counter.

General-purpose sterilizers are available in double-door units for steam sterilization of bagged heat- and/or moisture-stable infectious items from isolation or other areas, and also for general steam sterilization, for emergency sterilization, and for small loads. Flasked solutions may be processed in units such as those discussed in the section concerned with the preparation and packaging area. Automatic controls allow the operator to select the proper programming cycle (for wrapped goods, unwrapped goods, or liquids) by pressing the appropriate button on the main control panel. After programming the processing temperature and exposure time, no further attention is necessary until completion of the cycle on this unit. Both ethylene-oxide-gas sterilizers and general-purpose sterilizers can be recessed in masonry walls.

### Medical Equipment

Medical equipment is a term encompassing a broad spectrum of items and devices used directly and indirectly in the care and treatment of patients. Some items require sanitization; some, disinfection; and others, decontamination. The nature and size of the items determines the processing methods. The following are some typical medical-equipment items:

| | |
|---|---|
| Air kems | Morch respirator |
| Air mattress | Ostoscope |
| Bed board | Oxygen gauge |
| Bed cradle | Oxygen regulator |
| Bennett respirator | Oxygen tent |
| Blood pump | Pacemaker |
| Cast cutter | Restraints |
| Chaffin Pratt machine | Rotating tourniquet |
| Cosmo cautery unit | Rubber ring |
| Croupette canopy | Sand bag |
| Croupette | Steam inhalator |
| Crutches | Suction machine |
| Food pump | Tapewriter |
| Hot-water bottle | Traction accessories |
| Humidifier | Traction cart |
| Hydrocollator | Wangensteen |
| Ice bag | Wire cutter |
| Ice collar | Vital-capacity apparatus |
| Isolation cart | |

The decontamination area includes the means to process such equipment properly. Provisions are included for washing, rinsing, soaking, treated-water rinsing, sanitization with flowing-detergent steam, and rinsing with clean steam and/or water. Items requiring steam or ethylene-oxide-gas decontamination are processed in the equipment previously described. Small windows can be used as a convenient pass-through opening for small items that require only manual cleaning before being stored or returned to the using units.

Equipment-assembly and -inspection stations can provide convenient facilities for reassembling and checking of all medical equipment following processing of components. The unit should have compressed air and electrical outlets and drawers for handy storage of small tools and supplies. It should also have the means to test the reprocessed equipment for the possibility of sparking and/or electrical-shock hazards.

Large equipment items such as beds, Stryker frames, and wheel chairs, as well as housekeeping items such as buckets and carts can be sanitized using a steam-gun set, consisting of a siphon gun, detergent tank, gloves, and brushes that attach to the siphon gun. Typically, such units operate on the central house-steam-supply system (60-80 psig) and cold water (30-40 psig). Items may be cleaned with detergent then rinsed and sanitized with flowing steam.

## *Distribution Carts*

Distribution carts should be processed after each trip to a using unit. Cart-washer systems, providing proper and effective processing necessary to combat cross-contamination within the hospital, are commercially available. Carts are manually attached to an undertow device. They automatically advance from the entrance (load) position to the wash-rinse position, then to the dry position, and finally to the exit (unload) position. At this position the carts are manually detached from the undertow device.

The dual chambers of the unit (wash-rinse and dry) may be in use simultaneously, allowing two carts to be processed at the same time. This could be a double-door unit, with the entry door in the decontamination area, and the exit door in the "clean" area.

## Terminal Process

This is the "clean" area where the processed supplies are prepared for terminal sterilization or for temporary storage (in the processed-stores area) until needed by using units.

The terminal process and packaging area is typically divided according to the types of reprocessables prepared, such as:

Instruments

Utensils and treatment trays

Linen packs

Solutions

Preparation for sterilization includes inspection, selection, assembly, and wrapping.

All clean supplies enter the preparation and packaging area from:

1. Decontamination area
   a. Washer-sterilizer.
   b. Pass-through window.
   c. Ethylene-oxide-gas sterilizer.
   d. General-purpose sterilizer.
2. General stores: New or disposable items for prepartion or trays and other using-unit commodities.
3. Laundry
   a. Wrappers for items that are to be sterilized.
   b. Linen packs.

Heat- and moisture-stable items in washer-sterilizer racks are unloaded from the racks and placed on mobile storage shelving for easy maneuverability within the area, and for transportation to work stations.

The mobile storage shelving generally consists of four chromate-finished steel-rod shelves on an aluminum dolly with casters. These units allow the processed items to be conveniently stored (temporarily) and, when desired, to be brought directly to the work stations, thus invoking labor-saving principles.

Empty racks from the "clean" terminal preparation and packaging area (TPPA) can be transported to the racking station in the decontamination area via one-way conveyors (overhead rack-return units) in such a way that no part of the device in the "dirty" area ever enters the "clean" area.

Heat- and/or moisture-sensitive items that have been manually processed in the decontamination area can enter via a pass-through window or, in some cases, through the gas sterilizer.

Surgical and obstetrical instruments and instrument sets must be prepared for terminal sterilization. Individual instruments need be inspected and wrapped. Mobile storage-shelving units with hinged, glazed, lockable doors can provide temporary yet orderly storage of certain instruments until needed.

A linen "pack" room is used for preparing packs for terminal sterilization. Linens, consisting of drapes, gowns, towels, and dressing materials, as well as all other fabrics requiring sterilization, can be delivered to and temporarily stored in such a room until they are needed for pack preparation.

**Terminal Sterilization**

When the activities of the various divisions of the TPPA have been performed, the prepared items should be finally terminally sterilized.

An equipment-storage area is needed to hold medical equipment that has been cleaned and sanitized until needed by using units.

Processed materials are stored in a designated area until required by using units. When the items from the preparation and packaging area enter such a process-stores area, they are removed from the sterilizer loading carts and placed onto storage units.

Finally, a staging and dispatch area is needed for loading and distribution carts and for dispatching of the carts to using units, as well as for any administrative functions such as inventory records, requisitioning, purchasing, and billing.

# Index

ABC analysis, 269, 270, 339, 373, 389
ABC inventory control, 389
ABC usage analysis, 374; work measurement, 373
Absorption, 389; costing, 389
Abstract symbol, 389
Accelerated depreciation, 389
Acceptable quality level (AQL), 389
Acceptance, 389
Access time, 389
Accounting, 31, 63
Accounting department, 83
Accumulation bin, 390
Acquisition cost ratio, 73, 74
Acquisitions, 6, 368
Active inventory, 390
Activities, 390
Activity ratio, 390
Activity reports, 157
Add-in memory, 390
Address, 390
Ad hoc reports, 157
Administration, 6
Administrative: costs, 4; council, 66; employees, 49
Administrator perspective, 12
Administrators, 1
Adoption notice, 390
ADP (automatic data-processing system), 390
Advertising, 390
Advice notice, 390
Agent wholesaler, 390
Aggregate inventory, 391
Aggregate-inventory management, 391
Aging schedule, 391
Air kems, 472
Alexander, M., 387
Algorithm, 229, 371
Aljian, G., 381
Allocation, 391; of CSR costs, 161
Alphanumeric, 391
Alteration, 67
Alternative sources, 163
Ambulance service, 55
American Association for Industrial Management, 345
Ammer, D.S., 331, 336
Amortize, 391
Amount to reorder, 391
Analog, 391; plotter, 391
Analogy, 6, 209
Analysis, 57, 361
Analytical model, 391

Anesthesia, 54, 55; supplies, 15
Annual budget, 1; cost, 222; usage, 373
Annual-usage value, 391
Annuity, 391
Anthony, M.F., 302, 303
Anticipation, 391; inventories, 392
Apfelbach, C., XXI
Application (computers), 392
Appropriation, 392
Approved supplier, 71
Arbitrage, 392
Architecture (computers), 392
Arrow, K.J., 238, 307
Artificial-kidney machines, 470
Asepsis, 44, 392
Assembly, 392
Assembly, 392; parts list, 392; production, 44
Assignment problem, 392
Assignments, 306
Attributes: of information, 393; of organizational structures, 35
Audio-response unit, 393
Audit procedures: applications and use of value analysis, 121; for central stores, 147; for charging procedures, 151; for purchasing-department account functions, 119; purchasing ethics, 140; purchasing functions, 131; receiving functions, 146; reporting functions, 131; receiving functions, 146; reporting functions, 205; supplier performance evaluation, 124; vendor competition, 115
Audit steps, 140
Audit trail, 393
Audits, 53; of management, 58
Authority, XIX, 10
Authorization, 140
Automated: data processing, 60; systems, 165
Automatic stocking, 393
Auxiliary storage, 393
Available: time, 393; stock, 393; work, 393
Availabilities, 64, 393
Average: costing, 393; demand rate, 217; inventory, 217, 278, 393; number in storage, 221

Backhaul allowance/pickup allowance, 393
Backlog of orders, 393
Backorders, 45, 46, 161, 163, 393
Backup, 393
Backward scheduling, 394

Balanced loading, 394
Balance-of-stores records, 394
Banasik, R.C., 387
Band, 394
Banister, R., 384
Bank, 394
Barnes, R.M., 59, 71, 91, 376, 379
Base: index, 394; inventory level, 394;
    pipeline stock, 394; series, 374; statistic
    parameters, 54; stock, 394; stock
    system, 394
Basic: producer, 395; stock, 395
Basin racks, 468
Batch, 395; processing, 395; production,
    395; systems, 165
Batty, G.R., 384
Baud (communications), 395
Bayha, F.H., 363
Begole, C., 387
Bellettini, J., 381
Benchmark, 395
Benge, E.J., 363
Bennett respirator, 472
Bid, 395
Bill: of lading, 395; of landing, 395; for IV
    solutions, 351; of materials, 350, 395; of
    sale, 395
Billing, 89
Bin cards, 395
Bin tag, 396
Bin trips, 396
Bin-location file, 396
Binary, 395
Bit, 396
Blaes, S.M., 381
Blessing, J.A., 387
Block, 396; control, 396; diagram, 396;
    scheduling, 396
Blood: bank, 54, 55; pump, 472
Bloom, A., 368
Bocchino, W.A., 59, 91
Boehmer, N., 384
Boergadine, L.C., 381
Bolton, R.A., 91
Bolz, E., 381
Book: inventory, 396; value, 396
Boudreau, E.M., 387
Boundary, 396
Branch, G.R., 386, 396
Branch warehouse, 396
Break, 396
Break-even: analysis, 65, 263, 396; chart,
    265, 267; limitations, 268; point, 387
Bregande, B.J., 44, 90
Bremhorst, P.J., 381
Bridging run, 397
Brigham, E.F., 307

Brown, R.O., 386
Buchan, J., 386
Buchsbaum, P., XXI
Budget, 397; cycle, 51; variance, 397
Buffa, E.S., 6, 20, 272, 307, 336, 376, 379
Buffer, 397; inventories, 69; stock, 216,
    217, 397
Bug, 397
Build schedule, 397
Building-block approach, 155
Bulb, 15
Bulk breaking, 397
Bulk-order quantity, 397
Bunching, 397
Bunetta, J.M., 384
Burst, 397
Burton, G.D., 381
Business analysis, 397; cycle, 397; Equip-
    ment Manufacturers Association, 340;
    risk, 397
Buxbaum, R., XXI
Buying, 398; center, 398
Byte, 398

Calendar time, 398
Calculation of inventory unit costs, 272
Call-off quantity, 398
Call reports, 398
Campbell, C.R., 381
Cancellation, 67
Cantor, J., 91
Capacity, 398; planning, 398
Capital: asset, 398; budgeting, 398; costs,
    398; materiel, 31
Capitalization rate, 398
Card, 398; column, 399; hopper, 399; row,
    399; stacker, 399; system, 25
Carroll, S.J., Jr., 47, 90
Carry-back, carry-forward, 399
Carrying cost, 212, 213, 273, 399
Cart-exchange system, 37
Cash: budget, 399; cycle, 399; discount,
    227; 379; flow, 6, 64, 178, 369, 399
Cash-receipt journal, 399
Cast cutter, 472; room, 56
Caster, J., XXI
Catalog number, 166, 399
Catheters, 15, 470
Cathode-ray tube (CRT), 165, 399, 406
CAT Scanner, 56
Cautery sets, 470
Ceiling price, 77
Census, 368
Central: control unit, 399; processing, 65;
    processing department, 299, 300; proc-
    essing unit (CPU), 400; processor, 400;
    Stockroom, 14, 31; storeroom, 158, 215;

Central: (cont.)
   stores, 84; stores activities, 83; stores
   audit procedures, 147
Centralization, 25, 26; advantages, 43;
   disadvantages, 43
Centralized: dispatching, 400; information
   systems, 163; materials-management
   systems, 163; organization, 33; system,
   400
Cerny, J., XXI
Certificate of compliance, 400
Chain of distribution, 400
Chambers, J.C., 216, 307
Chandrasekaran, R. 216, 307
Changed-Rush, 72
Channel: information, 400; physical goods,
   400
Chapin, N., 341, 363
Character, 400; data, 400
Charging, 89; and billing, 89; system, 50
Checklist, 19, 21, 52, 68, 73, 75, 81, 83, 89,
   93, 181, 307, 315, 319, 365
Chip, 400
Clark, J.D., 178, 192
Clarke, G., 306, 308
Classification-of-goods theory, 400
Clerical and administrative costs, 277
Clerical system, 400
Clinic, 54; services, 55
Closed-loop system, 401
Closed shop, 401
Cluster sampling, 371
COBOL (Common Business Oriented
   Language), 401
Code, 401; of ethics, 67, 82
Codec, 401
Cognitive dissonance, 401
Collate, 401
Collateral, 401
Collection, 153
Commissary, 401
Commitment fee, 401
Commodity records, 401
Common carrier, 401; goals, 49; parts, 402;
   system, 402
Communication, 57; 153; Access Method
   (CAM), 402
Compensating balance, 402
Competitive bidding, 66
Compile, 402
Complementary product, 402
Component, 65, 402; parts, 402
Composite cost of capital, 402
Computational aids, 228
Computer, 155, 166, 402; activity, 166;
   -controlled exchange (CBS), 402; mem-
   ory, 45, 46; programs, 45, 46, 236, 260,
   261, 262, 403; programmers, 403; run-
   ning time, 46; selection, 178; -selection
   considerations, 178; systems, 154

Concurrent processing, 403
Configuration, 359
Consignment goods, 403
Console (computer), 403
Consolidation, 279
Constant: demand 212; demand rate, 403;
   supply rate, 403
Consumables, 1, 13, 31, 64
Consumer, 1; information-retrieval system,
   403; product-safety commission, 403
Containerized freight, 403
Continuous budget, 403; production, 403
Contract, 67; carrier, 403; market, 404;
   types, 75
Contractual vertical-marketing systems, 404
Contracyclical buying, 404
Contribution, 404
Control, 40, 44, 63; board, 404; indexes,
   52; of forms, 58; procedures, 270
Converter, 404
Conveying equipment, 404
Coordinated orders, 404
Core storage, 404
Corporate vertical marketing, 404
Corrective action, 404
Correlation coefficient, 404
Cosmo cautery unit, 472
Cost, 295; accounting, 272, 405; -benefit
   analysis, 405; of capital, 2, 277, 405;
   center, 405; center code, 405; contain-
   ment, 1; effective management, 153; ef-
   fectiveness, 279, 405; factors, 405; of
   goods sold, 405; of holding, 12; of
   holding inventories, 405; of money, 2;
   plus, 76, 405; plus fixed fee, 78; plus in-
   centive fee, 78; sharing, 76, 78; -type
   contract, 77; without fee, 76, 78
Costs: 178; administrative, 4; of deprecia-
   tion, 277; developmental, 153; holding, 1,
   4, 12, 405; obsolescence, 4; operational,
   153; paper-work, 4; pilferage and loss, 4
Counterproductive, 53
Coupler, 405
Coupon system, 405
Covenant, 405
CPM (Critical-path method), 354, 405
CPU, 405
Crashing, 406
Crisis intervention, 12
Critical-path: method, 354; scheduling, 406
Critical rate, 406
Croupette, 472
Crutches, 472
CSR, 14, 42-47, 54, 56, 79, 158, 166
Cumulative scheduling, 406
Current purchase-unit price, 406
Current system, 181
Customer, 61; order, 406
Cycle, 406; stock, 406; time, 406
Cyclical-inventory count, 406

Dalleck, W.C., 386
Damages, 405
Darukhanavala, P., 216, 307
Data, 8, 48, 57, 63, 153, 156, 180, 367, 368, 375, 377, 407
Data-base management system (DBMS), 407
Data-retrieval-oriented systems, 164
Date: of arrival, 157; or order, 157; of withdrawal, 157
Deacon, A.R.L., 360, 364
Dead load, 407
Dean, B.V., 273, 279, 307, 309, 345, 363 368
Debug, 407
Decentralization, 25; advantages, 43, 44; disadvantages, 43, 44
Decentralized: dispatching, 407; information systems, 163; MMS, 35
Decision guidelines, 212
Decision rules, 8, 10, 11, 65, 209
Decision table, 344, 347, 407
Deck, 408
Decode, 408
Decontaminations, 305, 469; area, 300, 467, 474
Decontaminating, 299
Decoupling inventory, 408
Decrement, 408
Delay report, 408
Delivery: cost ratio, 74; date, 403; lead times, 8, 408; over time, 230, 231; period, 408; to, 408; time data, 46
Delphi method, 368
Demand, 40, 241, 408; dependent, 409; distribution, 408; during a lead time, 408; filter, 403
Demarketing, 408
Demodulation, 408
Departmental receipts, 373; report 159; stock, 409
Depreciation, 409
Descriptive text, 409
Design, 361; of forms, 58; modification, 409
Destructive testing, 369
Detailed scheduling, 409
Deterioration, 12, 52, 409
Deterministic model, 409
Developmental costs, 153
Diagnostic routine, 409
Dichloro-difluoromethane, 469
Dictionary, 409
Dietary, 15, 55, 65, 305; department, 232, 256
Digital computer, 409
Director of purchasing, 66; job description, 32
Direct access, 410; channel, 410; competition, 410; cost, 410; index, 410; labor, 410; materials, 410; ordering, 410; pickup, 410

Disbursement, 410
Disc, 410
Discount, 73, 75, 411; order quantity, 411
Discounted cash-flow analysis, 65
Discounted cash-flow techniques, 410
Discounting, 411; of accounts receivable, 411
Disk-drive storage device, 411
Dispatch, 305; area, 300
Dispatching, 411
Display, 411
Disposables, 1, 13, 31
Distribution, 6, 12, 40, 162, 411; carts, 473; channel, 411; checklist and audit procedures, 149; data processing (DDP), 411; -oriented information systems, 164; structures, 37; system, 411; vehicles, 300, 467
Distributor, 411
Diversion, 411
Document, 411
Document-retrieval-oriented systems, 164
Documentation, 181, 411; of systems and procedures, 181
Doll, C.L. 306, 308
DOLRIPECTOMS, 242
Double-bin system, 411
Downtime, 412
Dowst, S., 381
Drayage, 412
Due dates, 64, 412
Dumb terminals, 412
Dump, 412
Dunnage, 412
Duplication of inventory, 45, 46
Dynamic memory, 412
Dynamics, 361

Early deliveries, 163
Earmarked material, 412
ECG, 54
Echelon, 412
Economic stabilization program, 2, 3, 4
Economic lot-size, 65, 219, 232; lot-size equation, 220, 228; lot-size modifications, 228; ordering quantity, 65, 219, 338, 412; run length, 412; time cycle, 412
Economy, 362; of scale, 44
Edit, 412
EEG, 54, 56
Effectivity date, 413
Efficiency, 413
Effort, 376
Eighty/twenty (80/20) rule, 269, 413
Eilon, S., 386
EKG, 56
Elasticity, 413
Electromyography, 56
Electrotomes, 470
Electronic data processing, 413; system, 181

Elemental: parts, 413; times, 375
Ellis, B., 297, 308
Emergency, 279; room, 54, 55; orders, 413
Emerzian, A.D., 384
Empirical distribution, 413
Encode, 413
End item, 413
Engelman, R.M., 381, 384
Engineering: change, 413; drawing, 413
EOG, 65, 217, 222, 225; modification, 228
Equipment, 65; committee, 68; layout, 60; storage area, 300
Equivalent annual cost, 65
Escueta, E., XXI
Esophagoscopes, 470
Esta, D., 381
Esteem value, 70, 413
Ethylene oxide, 469
Ethylene-oxide-gas, 474; sterilizers, 471
Evaluation, 53, 361, 368; of supplier performance, 73
Exception reports, 157, 413
Excess: demand, 241; material requisition, 413
Exchange-cart system, 40, 41
Exclusive distribution, 414
Expansion potential, 178
Expected demand, 217, 414
Expediting, 279, 414
Expenditures, hospital, 4
Expense materials, 31
Explosion, 414; chart, 350, 352
Exponential: decay, 414; smoothing, 414
External: funds, 414; storage, 414

Facilities layout, 60, 215
Factory-owned retail outlet, 414
Failure rate, 414
Fairfield, F.R., 307
Feasible economic order quantity, 224
Feedback, 414
Feeder ships, 415
Feeding, 305
Fetch-and-carry system, 37
Fetter, R.B., 386
Field, 415; warehousing, 415; work, 370
FIFO (First-in, first-out), 415
File, 166, 415; maintenance, 415; management, 415; organization, 415
Final: assembly, 415; market, 415
Financial: considerations, 31; lease, 415; risks, 77; solvency, 74; statements, 5; structure, 415
Finished goods, 61, 415; inventory, 415; product, 415
Firm: fixed price, 76; program procedure, 415
First-off inspection, 416
Fisherman, A., 386

Fixed price, 76; contract, 75, 76; incentive, 76, 77; with escalation, 76; with redetermination, 76
Fixed: charges, 416; cost, 263, 416
Fixed-interval-reorder system, 416
Fixed-length record, 416
Fixed-order cycle, 416; quantity method, 213; system, 416
Fixed-period control system, 416
Fixed-reorder quantity, 209
Fixed-review-time method, 212
Fixed-time method, 209
Flasked solution, 472
Flexible: budget, 416; price, 76, 77
Flip-flop, 416
Floating-order point, 416
Floppy disc, 416
Flow: chart, 340, 345, 417; chart symbols, 340; process chart, 417; production, 417; racks, 417; shop, 417
Fluids and solutions, 300
FOB (Free on board), 417; destination, 417; point, 417
Follow-up, 417
Forcing orders, 417
Forecast, 417; error, 417; interval, 417; usage, 8
Forecasting, 40, 417
Form: control, 58; design, 58
FORTRAN (FORmula TRANslating system), 417
Forward load, 417
Fox, M.S., 384
Free stock, 418
Freeze period, 418
Freight, 75; cost, 73
Frequency, 306, 375
Friedman, W.R., Jr., 382
Frozen order, 418
Functional responsibility, 35
Future needs, 155

Gallagher, J.D., 155, 192
Gantt chart, 354, 355, 356
Gantt, H.L., 354
Garrett, R.D., 59, 91
Garrity, J.T., 154, 192
General: accounting, 57; ledger, 161; purpose racks, 468; purpose sterilizer, 472; stores, 305; supplies, 300
Generalized systems flow chart, 358
Generator, 418
GFE, 418
Gilbreth, D.L., 59, 91
Giroux, F., 386
Glassware racks, 468
Glossary, 389
Goal-setting, 51
Goals, 51, 155
Goods receiving, 418

Goods-in-process inventory, 418
Goods-received note, 418
Grant, E.L., 363
Gravity feed, 418
Great-leap-forward approach, 155
Greene, E.A., 384
Gross requirements, 419
Grouping orders, 419
Gudapati, D., 307
Gudapati, K., 216
Gunn, T.W., 384

Hadley, G., 240, 307, 386
Handling, 12, 419; or labor costs, 277; and
    storage costs, 419
Hanssmann, F., 386
Hard copy, 165, 419
Hard data, 367
Hardware, 419; characteristics, 178
Harris, J.L., 387
Harris, Ford W., 238, 307
Harris, T., 238, 307
Hayes, E.H., 370, 379
Head, 419
Health maintenance organization, 31, 42,
    45, 156, 158, 183, 218, 225, 290, 368, 369
Heat-sensitive items, 467, 469
Heat-stable items 467
Hedging, 419
Heinritz, S.F., 382
Helmer, O., 368
Hemostat sterilization, 338
Henning, W.K., 1, 2, 20, 384
Henry, J.B., 382
Henry, M.D., 192
Heuristic, 419
High-level language, 420
Historical data, 375
History of inventory control, 238
H.H. Franklin Manufacturing Company,
    238
Hodgins, B., 382
Hoel, P.O., 370, 379
Hold: order, 420; points, 420
Holding: costs, 1, 4, 220, 221; or carrying
    cost, 420
Home health service, 55
Hospital expenditures, 4
Hospitals, 2, 20, 38
Hospital statistics, 2
Hossner, L., XXI
House accounts, 420
Housekeeping, 56, 65; supplies, 15
Housley, C.E., 37, 38, 41, 42, 43, 90, 279,
    308, 332, 336, 384, 387

Ice: bag, 472; collar, 472
Idea generation, 420
Ideal capacity, 420
Iglehart, J.K., 385

Illegal character, 420
Immediate access, 420
Impact, 420; printer, 420
Implementation, 46, 60
Impulse goods, 420
Inactive inventory, 420
Incidence-type diagram, 181
Incidence: matrix, 348; table, 349
Increment, 420
Incremental cost of capital, 421
Independent demand, 421
Independent-demand items, 421
Index, 421
Indexed sequential, 421
Indirect channel, 421; cost, 421; materials,
    421
Individual purchase orders, 72
Infectious items, 467, 471
Information, 6, 153, 421; disclosures, 142;
    flow, 6, 215, 218, 421; processes, 343;
    processing, 340; retrieval, 59, 421;
    system, 10, 153, 421; systems
    characteristics, 163
Infrastructure, management, 1
In-process inventory, 421
Input, 421; validation, 422
Input-output: devices, 422; matrix, 353;
    table, 353
Inservice education, 57
Insistance, 422
Inspection, 6; order, 422
Institutional objectives, 306
Instruction, 422
Instrument recovery, 302
Instruments, 474; and equipment, 470, 471;
    and instrument sets, 300
Integrated data processing, 422
Integrated system, 422
Intelligent terminal, 422
Intensive distribution, 422
Interactive computing, 422
Interactive: computer program, 236; mode,
    236, 422
Interface, 422
Intermediaries, 422
Intermediate: clause, 423; market, 423;
    nursing care, 55
Internal: auditor, 68; storage, 423
Interval time, 423
Intravenous solution prescription, 340
Intrinsic forecast, 423
Inventory, 5, 38, 423; analysis, 423; carry-
    ing costs, 277, 278, 423; control, 6, 64,
    65, 273, 423; -control setup/change
    form, 166; cost of capital, 423; cost
    method, 423; database, 6, 423; efficiency,
    242; file, 423, formal, 5; on hand, 17,
    18, 157; informal, 5, 209; investment,
    423; -item file, 166; level, 45, 46, 212,
    217; models, 423; perpetual, 179;

Inventory (cont'd)
     policy, 424; record, 218; shorts list, 424;
     shrinkage, 424; simulation, 424; stan-
     dard, 424; team, 424; turnover, 424;
     turns ratio, 52; usage, 424; value, 424
Invoice, 424
I/O, 424
Ireson, W.C., 363
Isolation cart, 472
Issue-unit designation, 178
Item, characterization, 241; substitution,
     292, 293, 294
IV: sets, 470; supplies, 15

Jaffee, M., 368
Jankowski, T.E., 54, 58, 90
Javad, S., XXI, 2, 20, 43, 44, 90, 241, 307
JCL (Job-control language), 424
Jessen, R.J., 370, 379
Job: descriptions, 31, 32; evaluation, 376;
     scheduling, 424; status, 425
Job-order costing, 424
Job-shop operation, 425
Jones, R.M., 385
Joslen, R.A., 382
Judgment items, 425; sampling, 369

Kardex system, 153
Karger, D.W., 363
Key, 425
Keypunch, 425; machine, 425
Keypunching, 277
King, J.G., 382
Knocked down, 425
Koenigsberg, E., 386
Kohn, J., 382, 387
Koleski, R.A., 368
Kotha, S., XXI
Kowalski, J., 385
Kress, A.L., 363
Krumrey, N.A., 387
Kutilek, R.J., 385
K words, 179

Lab: clinical, 55; pathology, 55
Labor, 76; claim, 425; costs, 2; and
     delivery, 55; relations, 74; supplies, 15;
     ticket, 425
Lammers, L., 43, 44, 90
Lamps, 470
Laufman, H., 387
Laundry, 65, 305, 474; and linen, 56
Lauzon, C., 382
Layout, 60, 425
LCL, 425
LeGwin, L.C., Jr., 385
Lead time, 1, 44, 45, 46, 64, 69, 162, 214,
     215, 241, 425; demand, 426; demand
     distribution, 426; offset, 426; replenish-
     ment, 1

Leading indicators, 426
Learning curve, 426
Lease-versus-buy, 64
Lee, L., Jr., 382
Leenders, M.R., 91
Legal department, 67
Length: of operation procedure, 54; of
     treatment, 54
Letter contracts, 76, 78
Level, 426; of effort, 76
Level-by-level planning, 426
Leventhal, E., 385
Levinson, P., 382
Library routine, 426
Lien, 426
Life-cycle status, 426
LIFO (Last-in, first-out), 427
Limiting operation, 427
Line: balancing, 427; of credit, 427;
     management, 427; printer, 427; respon-
     sibility, 35
Linear programming, 427
Linen: changing, 305; pack room, 300;
     packs, 300, 474
Link trainer, 360
List price, 73, 427
Live load, 427
Livy, B., 363
Lloyd, R.S., 387
Lo, J.S., 385
Load, 427; leveling, 428
Loading, 428; racks, 467, 468; time, 428
Locator file, 428
Logic diagram, 339
Logistical component, 299
Logistics management, 428
Lot size, 217, 221, 428
Lott, M.R., 363
LTL, 428
Lucia, S.R., 8, 20
Lytle, C.W., 363

Machine: address, 428; center, 428;
     language, 428; sensible, 428; utilization,
     428
Macroinstruction, 428
MAD (mean absolute deviation), 428
Maddison, L.W., 382
Magar, V.D., 360, 364
Magnetic-ink-character reader, 428
Magnetic tape, 429
Main frame, 429
Main memory, 429
Maintenance, 65; supplies, 61
Make or buy, 271; decisions, 271
Make to order, 429
Make to stock, 429
Make-versus-buy, 64
Makespan, 429
Makridakis, S., 216, 307

Management infrastructure, 1, 8, 10, 25
Management: audits, 58; engineering, 57; by exception, 429; information system (MIS), 429, 430
Managerial infrastructure, 25
Mantel, S.J., Jr., 368, 379
Mantell, J., 155, 156, 192
Manual systems, 165
Manufacturing, 65, 429; forecast, 429; order, 429; process, 429
Margin, 429
Marginal: cost, 429; revenue, 429
Markdown pricing, 429
Market, 429; classification, 430; segmentation, 430; share, 430; stability, 430; testing, 430
Marketing, 430; concept, 430; cycle, 430; mix, 430; plan, 430; research, 430
Marschak, J., 238, 307
Marshaling, 430; list, 430
Master: file, 430; procurement plan, 431; production schedule, 431; record, 180; tariff, 431; warehouse, 431
Materials, 76, 431; availability, 64; -charging functions checklist, 151; control, xix, 431; distribution, 302, 303; distribution structures, 37; distribution subsystem, 301; flow, 6, 215, 300; flow-process chart, 431; hold tag, 431; management, XIX, 432; management components, 8; management department checklist, 21; management documentation, 14; management environment, 1; management infrastructure checklist, 95; management information system, 8, 84, 153, 154, 155, 156, 160, 161, 166, 182, 432; management manual, 82; management organization, 27; management system checklist, 109; management system, XIX, 6; management system components, 10; obsolescense report, 431; ordering system, 432; pickup, 303; planning, 432; processing equipment, 467; processing procedures, 467; purchasing functions, 125; requirement plan, 431; requisition, 431; schedule, 432; storage, 86; transfer, 431; usage report, 161
Materiel, 2
Mathematical model, 45
Matrix: 432; bill of material, 432
Matrix-type organization, 34, 35
Matrix organization: advantages, 36; disadvantages, 36
Max-min, 432
Maximum: level, 432; revenue, 264
Maynard, H.B., 59, 91, 273, 303, 363, 376, 379
MBO (management by objectives), 47, 48, 50, 51, 52; audit procedures, 107; checklist, 52, 95; processes, 103

Measurement, 48, 370; of work, 59
Measures of materials service performance, 242
Medical-surgical supplies, 15, 55
Medical: care review, 57; equipment, 300, 467; library, 57; records, 55; staff administration, 57; treatment, 305; photography and illustration, 57
Memory, 432
Merchandise inventory, 432
Meyer, E.M. 385
MICR (magnetic in-character recognition), 433
Microinstruction, 433
Microprogramming, 433
Middle-management report, 159
Middleman, 433
Miller, J.G., 20
Miller-Abbott tubes, 471
Min max, 65; method, 214; replenishment policy, 216; system, 433
Minicomputer, 433
Minimal inventory, 180
Minimum stock, 433
Minimum cost solution, 224
Mitchell, R.C., 53, 90
Mix control, 433
MMIS (materials management information system), 84, 153, 154, 155, 156, 160, 161, 166, 182; characteristics, 163; checklist, 163, 181; checklists and audit procedures, 193; reports requested, 160; specifications, 160
MMS (materials management system), 45, 47, 50, 51, 58
Mnemonic, 433
Mode, 433
Model, 433
Modeling, 241
Modular bill of materials, 433
Modularity, 434
Modulation, 434
Module, 14, 47, 158, 215
Moisture-sensitive items, 467, 469; -stable items, 467
Moore, G.C., 385
Morrison, D., 216, 307
Motivation, 180; research, 434
Mottice, H.J., 59
Move: order, 434; ticket, 434; time, 434
Movement inventory, 434
Moving annual total, 434
Moving weighted average, 434
Moy, J., XXI
MRP (materials-requirements planning), 434
Mullick, S.K., 216, 307
Multiechelon materials management, 182
Multiechelon inventory systems, 20
Multifacility health center, 14, 215
Multilevel bill of materials, 434

Multiplexing, 434
Multiprocessing, 435
Multiprogramming, 435
Multiproduct, EOQ, 234

Nanosecond, 435
Nebulizers, 470
Need date, 435
Needs, 435
Net change, 435
Net: delivery price, 73, 75; requirement, 435; requirements schedule, 435; revenue, 263; value cost, 74, 75
Network, 435; analysis techniques, 435; description table (NDT), 435; planning, 435
Neuman, P., 79
Nevers, M.R., 382
Nichols, R., 388
NMS organization, 31
Node, 435
Nominal interest rate, 436
Noncurrency, 52
Nonlinear programming, 436
Nonsignificant part numbers, 436
Nonstandard stock, 33, 57, 184, 185, 186, 187, 188, 189, 190, 191
Normal probablity distribution, 436
Normalize, 436
Norris, F.S., 385
Nuclear medicine, 54, 56
Number: of items, 241; of patients, 54; of stockouts, 163; of supply echelons, 241
Numeric data, 436
Numerical analysis, 436
Numerical solution, 267
Nurses, 46
Nursing administration, 57

O'Connell, J.A., 382
Objectives, 44, 155, 241, 368, 370
Objective probability distribution, 436
Object program 436
Obsolescence, 4, 279, 436; costs, 4
Off line, 436
Office equipment ordering, 339
On hand, 436; inventory, 17, 18
On line, 436; inquiry, 153
Open: account purchase, 437; insurance policy, 437; item, 437; purchase-order report, 437; shop, 437; to buy, 437
Operating level, 437
Operation: card, 437; research, 437; process chart, 340; scheduling, 437
Operational costs, 153
Operations, 65; function flow, 359; research, 437; sequence, 437
Opthalmoscopes, 470
Optical scan, 438
Optimal, 438

Optimization, 438
Optimum, 222
Oral, M., 273, 279, 303, 307
Order, 438; backlog, 438; control, 438; cost, 273, 438; entry, 277; frequency, 212; intake control, 438; number, 438; point, 217, 438; procedures, 270; quantity, 219, 438
Ordering, 438; cost, 438; cycle, 210, 241; procedures, 103; rules, 45, 46
Organ acquisitions, 56
Organizational: chart, 27, 28, 342; levels, 47; performance, 51; structure, 25, 26, 33
Osborne, R., XXI
Out-of-stock, 163
Outgoing materials systems, 439
Output, 439; control, 439; data, 439
Overhead, 439; account, 439
Overrun, 439
Overstock, 180
Overstocking, 46
Oversupply, 163
Ownership of materials, 439
Oxygen: gauge, 472; tents, 471, 472

Packaging area, 300
Paper work, 45, 46; costs, 4
PAR-level system, 37, 39, 41
Parking, 56
Pass, 439
Pass-through window, 474
Patient: accounting, 57; care, 15; charge, 40; charge item, 439; kits, 300
Payback period, 65, 439
Payment, 73; flow, 440
Penetration pricing, 440
Percent: defective, 256; of fill, 440; short, 242
Percentage of cost, 77
Performance, 376
Periodic: inventory, 440; inventory system, 440; reports, 157
Peripheral function, 440
Perkins, J.H., 385
Perpetual inventory, 179, 216, 440; -inventory record, 440; -inventory system, 440; stockchecking, 440
Personnel, 57
Perspective: administrator, 12; manager, 13; user, 11
PERT (program evaluation and review technique), 354, 440; chart, 355; cost chart, 357; diagram, 356; network, 356
Pharmaceuticals, 15, 230, 232
Pharmacy, 55, 65, 256, 305
Physical distribution, 440
Physical file, 440
Physical inventory, 16, 45, 46, 368, 441
Picking: list, 441; sheet, 441
Piece parts, 441
Pilferage: 44; and loss costs, 4

Pill, J., 368, 379
Placement of orders, 72
Planning, 57, 441; horizon, 441; period, 220, 221
Plant, 65; maintenance, 56; operation, 56
Plotter, 441
Plowden, M.D., 382
Plug-compatible unit, 441
Plugged level, 441
Pollard, T., 383
Portable sonic cleaners, 469
Posting time, 179
Postinventory review, 441
Pottery, 471
Powell, P.B., 383
Precedence: diagram, 349; matrix, 349, 350
Prepaid: expenses, 441; plans, 225
Preproduction planning, 441
Prescheduling, 442
Present: value (PV), 442; worth, 65
Price, 442; breaks, 1, 64, 442; break point, 224; hike, 279; information, 64; lining, 442; maintenance, 442; prevailing at the date of shipment, 442; protection, 442; quote, 75; redetermination, 77; variance, 442
Priest, J.L., 385
Primary file, 442
Prime cost, 442; operations, 442; rate, 442; vendor, 218
Principals and standards of purchasing practice, 67
Priority list, 442; rules, 442
Probability sampling, 370, 372
Probabilistic demand, 210, 240, 443; distribution, 443; model, 443
Procedural guidelines, 66
Procedure-oriented language, 443
Process: average, 443; component, 299; control, 443; costing, 443; industry, 443; planning, 443; time, 215, 443
Processed-stores area, 300
Processed stores, 305
Processing, 6, 30, 65, 153, 443, 444; department 26; times 45, 46, 218
Processor, 444
Procurement, 162; procedures, 184, 185, 186; time, 444
Product, 74, 279, 444, 445
Production, 232, 234, 256, 273, 445, 446
Product-flow process diagram, 338
Product service, 444, 445
Professionalism, 26
Program, 446; evaluation and review technique, 354
Programmed decision, 446
Programming, 446
Progress, 447
Promises-kept penalty, 74
Promotional mix, 447

Protection time, 447
Provisioning, 447
Pull strategy, 447
Pulse-code modulation (PCM) and delta modulation, 447
Pump motors, 471
Punch card, 447
Purchases, 56
Purchase value, 15
Purchasing, 6, 61, 65
Purchasing, 28, 33, 61, 65, 66, 67, 68, 69, 81, 82, 117, 131, 134, 140, 142, 179, 216, 273, 277, 447, 448
Push strategy, 448

Quality, 64; control, 448; cost ratio, 73
Qualitative standards, 448
Quantitative standards, 448
Quantity: desired, 256; discount, 163, 223, 448; on hand, 69, 162; received, 157; started, 257; ordered, 157, 162; withdrawn, 157
Quarterly-ordering system, 448
Queueing time, 448
Quick-deck explosion, 448
Quota sampling, 371
Quotas, 370

Racks, 468
Radiology, 15, 54, 55
Random, 448, 449
Randomness, 377
Range of items stocked, 449
Rate-of-return, 65, 449
Raw materials, 61, 65, 449
Raymond, F.E., 238
Reaction time, 449
Real time, 449; processing, 449; systems, 165, 166
Recall, 279
Receipt of requisitions, 69
Receiving, 6, 46, 63, 83, 84, 85, 145, 146, 162, 305, 449
Reconciling inventory, 449
Reconsignment, 450
Record, 450
Records, 59
Recreation therapy, 54, 56
Regional warehouse, 215
Regression analysis, 450
Regulatory power, 450
Reich, R., 368
Reiger, H., 368
Reinvestment rate, 450
Relative value units, 54
Release, 450
Reliability, 377, 450
Remittance advice, 450
Remote access, 450
Remote batch processing, 450

Renal dialysis, 56
Reorder: costs, 1, 12, 64, 220; point, 65,
    218, 450; quantity, 450; report, 450
Replacement: cost accounting, 451; order,
    451
Replenishment: lead time 1, 211, 218, 451;
    order, 219, 373; quantity, 210
Report, 157, 158, 163; analysis, 58; depart-
    mental, 159; middle-management, 159;
    top management, 158
Reporting functions, audit procedures, 205
Reprocessing, 305
Reproductibility, 362
Requirements, 451; planning, 65; schedul-
    ing, 451
Requisitioner, 69
Requisitioning, 162
Research projects, 56
Research and development, 451
Reserve material, 216, 451
Residential care, 55
Responsibility, XIX, 10, 49; area, 30; func-
    tional, 35; line, 35
Restraint of competition-collusion, 143
Restraints, 472
Retailers, 451
Retrieval, 153
Retrieve, 451
Retrieval and recovery of reusables, 301
Return to vendors, 163
Returns, 451
Reusables, 1, 13, 31, 297, 298, 300
Review, 213; cost, 213; interval, 451; period,
    451; of requisitions, 69
Rework order, 451
Riggs, J.L., 71, 91, 385
Risk premium, 451
Risk-taking, 49
Roenfeldt, R.L., 382
Rolling forecast, 451
Romig, H.C., 370, 379
Ronis, R., 368
Rose, G.W., 44, 90
Routine, 452
Rubin, R., 383
Rubinstein, J., 368
Ruchlin, H.S., 54, 90
Running: parallel, 452; time, 452
Rush order, 452
RVU, 54, 55

Safety: reserve, 216; reserve quantity, 217,
    218; stock, 452; time, 452
Sale and leaseback, 452
Sales, 452
Salmonowitz, P., XXI
Salvador, M., 273, 279, 307, 308
Salvage, 452; and supplies disposal, 452;
    value, 452
Sample, 368, 453

Sampling, 270, 271, 367, 369, 375, 453
Sand bag, 472
Sawtooth diagram, 453
Schabracq, A., 385
Scharf, T.G., 180, 192
Schedule, 46, 306, 453
Scheduling, 453
Schema, 453
Schlag, D.W., 386
Schmitz, H.H., 59, 90
Schrock, R.D., 386
Schropp, M.L., 388
Schultz, R.L., 156, 192
Schwab, J.L., 376
Schwartz, B.L., 279, 308
Scientific inventory control, 453
Scrap, 453; loss, 256, 257
Sealed-bid pricing, 453
Secured account, 454
Security, 45, 46, 56
Selection, 71
Selective distribution, 454
Semiconventional system, 454
Semifinished goods, 454
Sensitivity, 361
Sequence number, 454
Sequencing, 454
Sequential: access, 454; control, 454
Service, 454; cost ratio, 74; level, 1, 53, 163,
    255, 455; parts-transfer order, 455; per-
    formance measures, 242; time, 455
Service, A., 368
Setback time, 455
Setup, 12, 220, 273, 455
Setup or ordering costs, 273
Setup/change form, 166
Shaughnessy, S., 383
Shelf life, 455
Shipment, 63
Shipping, 162, 455; authorization, 455;
    costs, 64; order, 455
Shop, 455, 456
Shopping goods, 456
Short: date, 456; sale, 456
Shortage, 1, 235, 456; allowed, 230, 231,
    232, 236; control, 456; costs, 1, 273,
    278, 279, 456; note, 456
Shrinkage, 12, 44, 52, 456
Shrode, W.A., 59
SHUR statistics, 55, 90
Silva, J., 155, 156, 192
Silver, 302
Simple random sampling, 370
Simplification of work, 59
Simulation, 359, 361, 362, 456
Single-source-supplier, 79
Slevin, D.P., 156, 192
Sluga, J., XXI
Smith, M.A., 388
Smith, D.D., 216, 307

Smoothing constant, 457
Social services, 54, 56
Soft data, 367
Software, 457; rating, 179
Solution method, 241
Solutions, 474
Sort file, 457
Source: document, 457; program, 457
Space: relationship, 305; requirements, 45; usage, 12
Spare parts, 457
Specifications, 62, 64, 83, 160, 457
Specific identification, 457
Speech: pathology, 56; therapy, 54
Split: lots, 457; solutions, 457
Square root table, 226, 256
Stadnik, J.K., 385
Staff functions, 458
Stafford, D., 387
Standard, 458; cost, 458; data, 375; definitions, 343; deviation, 458; forms, 63; hour, 459; industrial classification, 76; purchase order, 458; purchase unit price, 458; stock, 31; system, 66; times, 458
Standardization, 26, 296
Standardization committees, 296
Standard-stock: items, 14, 16; sutures, 17; syringes, 18
Starr, M.K., 386
Statistical data, 375; theory, 371
Status reports, 157
Stegmerten, D.J., 376, 379
Step, 458
Sterilizing equipment, 469
Sterilizer, 474
Stewart, C.E., 387
Stochastic demand, 240; process, 458
Stock, 249, 458, 459
Stocking, 40; cost, 266; location, 459
Stockouts, 1, 45, 46, 52, 161, 255, 279, 459
Stockpiling, 52
Stockyard, 459
Storage, 6, 64, 86, 87, 88, 153, 162, 164, 220, 221, 277, 459
Storeroom, 459
Storing, 6, 459
Strategy, 459
Stratification, 370
Stratified random sampling, 370, 372
Subassembly, 65, 459
Subjective: data, 368; evaluation, 376; probability distributions, 459
Suboptimization, 459
Subordinate management, 51
Subroutine, 460
Substitutions, 47, 279
Substitutable items, 163
Substitute products, 460
Substituteability, 257, 279, 287, 290, 295
Supervisor reliability, 377

Supplies, 65, 460
Supplier: ability, 74; competence, 74; performance evaluation, 73, 122, 124; rating, 74; selection, 71
Suppliers, 62
Supply: distribution, 29; quotes, 39; tradeoffs, 64
Survey, 370; sampling, 368
Svestka, J.A., 345, 363
Synthesis, 361
System, 460; engineers, 460; test, 460
Systematic storage procedures, 86
Systematic sampling, 371
Systems: analysis, 58, 60, 367, 374; automated, 165; batch, 165; description, 14, 58; design, 58; manual, 165; and procedures, 52, 53, 60, 156; real-time, 165, 166; study, 368

Tape drive, 460
Target price, 77
Target-inventory level, 460
Task: delegation, 346; force, 156
Taylor, F.W., 59, 91, 363
Technical: ability, 74; development, 460
Teletype terminal, 236
Term: discount, 461; loan, 461
Terminal, 461; process, 473; sterilization, 475
Test: marketing, 461; tubes, 470
Testing: destructive, 369; nondestructive, 369
Theft, 12
Therapy, 54
Thueson, J., 386
Time: clerk, 461; compression, 362; division multiplex, 461; period, 241; series planning, 461; sharing, 461; standard, 461; ticket, 461
Tisdale, T., XXI
Tosi, H.L., Jr., 47
Total: cost, 263, 264; cover, 462; inventory report, 462; revenue, 264; supply-cart-exchange system, 39; system, 462
Toughness/fragility, 462
Toys, 471
TPOP (time-phase order point), 462
TPPA, 474, 475
Traction: accessories, 472; cart, 472
Trafas, C.J., 383
Traffic, 462; control, 462
Training, 361
Transactions, 157, 462; control block (TCB), 462; file, 462
Transfer price, 462
Transit time, 462, 215, 218
Translator, 463
Transportation: costs, 463; distribution issues; 306; inventories, 463; problem, 463
Traska, M.R., 302, 308
Turnaround time, 463
Turnover, 161, 463

Turns ratio, 52, 278
Two-bin: method, 210, 214; system, 463
Two-level reorder system, 463

Uniform delivered price, 463
Unit: of capability, 53; costs, 8, 209, 272; of issue, 464; load, 463; prices, 163; of purchase, 464; of service provided, 53
Units: demanded, 255; supplied, 255
Unplanned-production orders, 464
Unreliability, 52
Usage, 1, 40, 45, 46, 52, 162, 214, 218, 373, 374, 461, 464
Use, 153; value, 70, 464
User: locations, 1; perspective, 11
Utilization factor, 464

Value: analysis, 26, 69, 70, 279, 296; engineering, 70; of information, 153, 165
Variable, 464; costs, 263, 464; length record, 464; profit, 77
Vehicle routing, 306
Vendors, 64, 67, 69, 111, 115, 162, 179, 215, 464
Vertical distribution (marketing), 464
Virtual access, 464
Visual-review system, 465
Vital-capacity apparatus, 472
Voich, D. Jr., 59, 91
Volatile storage, 465
Volatility/stability, 465

Volume discounts, 223, 229
Voucher, 465

Wage and increase series, 76
Wallgren, L.R., 388
Wangensteen, 472
Warehousing, 6
Warehouse, 46, 158, 373, 465
Warranty, 74
Washer-sterilizer, 467, 468, 469, 474
Waybill, 465
Weighted cost of capital, 465
Weston, J.F., 307
Westwick, C.A., 257, 307
Wheeler, D.L., 383
Wheelwright, S.C., 216, 307
White, A.F., 386
Whitin, T.M., 238, 240, 307, 386
Whybark, D.C., 216, 307
Widman, P., XXI, 66
Wilson, R.H., 238
Wilson, G., 302, 303
Wire cutter, 472
Won (impact printer), 465
Wooldridge, M.C., 383
Word, 466
Work-in-process inventory, 466
Working capital, 466; days, 255; stock, 466
Wright, J.W., 306, 308

Yield, 466; factor, 466
Yu, C.S., 279, 308
Yuen, J.Y.S., 383

# About the Author

**Arnold Reisman** is professor of operations research at the Case Western Reserve University in Cleveland, Ohio. He also holds joint appointments in the Schools of Library Science, Medicine, and Engineering. He received the B.S., M.S., and Ph.D. degrees in engineering from the University of California, Los Angeles. Professor Reisman is author of eight books, including one on inventory control and another on health-care-delivery planning. His book *Managerial and Engineering Economics* won the Lanchester Prize (Honorable Mention) in 1971. In addition he has authored more than ninety papers, articles, and chapters in books.

In 1971 Professor Reisman was voted for inclusion in *Outstanding Educators in America* and in 1973 he was named Engineer of the Year by the Cleveland chapters of eleven engineering societies. He is listed in many biographies, including *Who's Who in America, Who's Who in the World,* and *American Men and Women of Science.* He is a member of many professional, scientific, and honor societies and is a Fellow of the Society for Advanced Medical Systems and of the American Association for the Advancement of Science and has served on its council. He has been retained as a consultant by many organizations and has performed systems studies for more than twenty hospitals, including the Kaiser-Permanente System, the Cleveland Clinic Foundation, and the University Hospitals of Cleveland. He is the founder of and serves on the board of the Greater Cleveland Coalition on Health Care Cost Effectiveness and is a principal in Case Western Reserve's Center for Health Systems Management. As consultant to the Pan American Health Organization he has traveled widely in the Americas.